Inhibition of Tumor Induction and Development

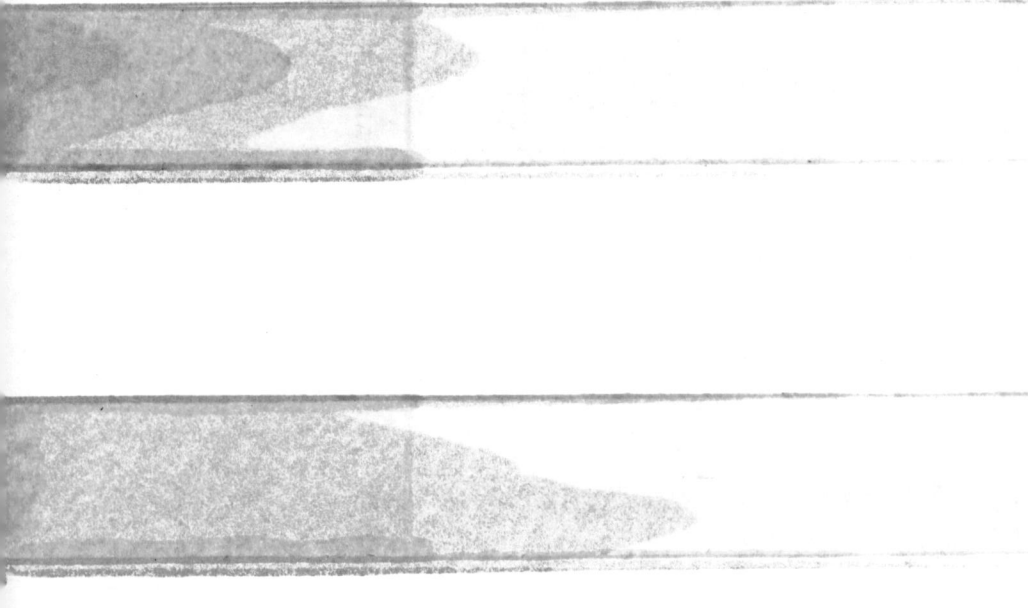

Inhibition of Tumor Induction and Development

Edited by **Morris S. Zedeck**
and **Martin Lipkin**

Memorial Sloan–Kettering Cancer Center
New York, New York

SPRINGER SCIENCE+BUSINESS MEDIA, LLC

Library of Congress Cataloging in Publication Data

Main entry under title:

Inhibition of tumor induction and development.

Includes bibliographical references and index.
Contents: Inhibition of chemical carcinogenesis by phenols, coumarins, aromatic isothiocyanates, flavones, and indoles/Lee W. Wattenberg and Luke K. T. Lam – Inhibition of carcinogen metabolism and action by disulfiram, pyrazole and related compounds/Emerich S. Fiala – Retinoids and chemoprevention of cancer/Michael B. Sporn and Dianne L. Newton – [etc.]

1. Tumors—Prevention. 2. Antineoplastic agents—Physiological effect. 3. Carcinogens—Metabolism. I. Zedeck, Morris S. II. Lipkin, Martin. [DNLM: 1. Carcinogens, Environmental—Antagonists and inhibitors. 2. Neoplasms—Prevention and control. 3. Neoplasms—Immunology. QZ 202 I54]

RC268.I53	616.99'205	81-7324
ISBN 978-1-4615-9220-4 ISBN 978-1-4615-9218-1 (eBook)		AACR2
DOI 10.1007/978-1-4615-9218-1		

© 1981 Springer Science+Business Media New York
Originally published by Plenum Press in 1981
Softcover reprint of the hardcover 1st edition 1981

All rights reserved

No part of this book may be reproduced, stored in a retrieval system, or transmitted, in any form or by any means, electronic, mechanical, photocopying, microfilming, recording, or otherwise, without written permission from the Publisher

Contributors

Bertram Ira Cohen, Veterans Administration Medical Center, New York, New York 10010; and Department of Medicine, New York University School of Medicine, New York, New York 10016

Emerich S. Fiala, Naylor Dana Institute for Disease Prevention, American Health Foundation, Valhalla, New York 10595

A. Clark Griffin, Department of Biochemistry, The University of Texas System Cancer Center, M.D. Anderson Hospital and Tumor Institute, Houston, Texas 77030

Maryce M. Jacobs, Eppley Institute for Research in Cancer, University of Nebraska Medical Center, Omaha, Nebraska 68105

Luke K. T. Lam, Department of Laboratory Medicine and Pathology, University of Minnesota, Minneapolis, Minnesota 55455

Martin Lipkin, Memorial Sloan-Kettering Cancer Center, New York, New York 10021

William J. Mergens, Hoffmann-LaRoche, Hoffmann-LaRoche, Inc., Nutley, New Jersey 07110

Sidney S. Mirvish, Eppley Institute for Research in Cancer, University of Nebraska Medical Center, Omaha, Nebraska 68105

Harold L. Newmark, Hoffmann-LaRoche, Hoffmann-LaRoche, Inc., Nutley, New Jersey 07110

Dianne L. Newton, Laboratory of Chemoprevention, National Cancer Institute, Bethesda, Maryland 20205

Robert Franklin Raicht, Veterans Administration Medical Center, New York, New York 10010; and Department of Medicine, New York University School of Medicine; New York, New York 10016

Rulon W. Rawson, Bonneville Center for Research on Cancer Cause and Prevention, University of Utah Research Institute, Salt Lake City, Utah 84108

Hans Olov Sjögren, The Wallenberg Laboratory, University of Lund, Lund, Sweden

Michael B. Sporn, Laboratory of Chemoprevention, National Cancer Institute, Bethesda, Maryland 20205

Lee W. Wattenberg, Department of Laboratory Medicine and Pathology, University of Minnesota, Minneapolis, Minnesota 55455

Morris S. Zedeck, Memorial Sloan-Kettering Cancer Center, New York, New York 10021

Preface

The primary purpose of this book is to bring to the attention of members of the medical and scientific communities, as well as to other interested persons, a new and expanding area of investigation that features the use of chemicals for the prevention of tumor induction and development. This novel use of chemical compounds has succeeded in producing a remarkable series of discoveries in recent years. Some of these are beginning to be evaluated in the field of clinical oncology in a manner that has potentially enormous public health implications. It is anticipated, therefore, that increasing amounts of time, energy, and financial resources will be devoted to the further development and expansion of this work. The major contribution of this book at the present time is that it summarizes and brings up to date the pioneering efforts of the various scientists who originated this new and exciting field of scientific activity.

The thoughts expressed by Louis Pasteur in 1884 may soon be applicable in the fight against cancer: "When meditating over a disease, I never think of finding a remedy for it, but instead a means of preventing it." The emphasis on cancer prevention currently underway is the result, in part, of an increased awareness that the environment—geographical, cultural, and occupational—has a role in development of the disease. Accordingly, it is now technically feasible to detect many of the known carcinogens in the environment, and the search for means to minimize exposure to such environmental factors or to prevent the effects of these agents is a rational approach. Knowledge of the biology of cancer is being amassed rapidly; understanding the mechanisms of carcinogen formation, carcinogen absorption, and metabolic activation of carcinogen interaction with cell macromolecules, of cellular changes leading to the state of transformation, of cell differentiation, and of metastasis allow for many avenues of approach toward inhibiting neoplasia. In fact, although there are relatively few compounds available to date that have proven to be effective in preventing tumorigenesis experimentally, their mechanisms of action involve several of these approaches. It is also of interest that the active substances are chemically very diverse in nature and include vitamins and vitamin analogues, food preservatives, trace elements, and plant products. It may be anticipated that, because of the complexity of the neoplastic process, many substances, both natural and synthetic, differing markedly in their chemical structure, will be needed to influence the many steps leading to tumor growth.

Thus, much new information has recently been gathered in the field of cancer prevention, and several of the findings have progressed to the stage of clinical investigations that are currently under way. This book serves not only as a reference for the work accomplished to date but also, by focusing on the problems that exist, as a stimulus for future endeavors.

Morris S. Zedeck
Martin Lipkin

Contents

Chapter 1
Inhibition of Chemical Carcinogenesis by Phenols, Coumarins, Aromatic Isothiocyanates, Flavones, and Indoles
Lee W. Wattenberg and Luke K. T. Lam

I. Introduction	1
II. Inhibitors of Chemical Carcinogens	4
A. Phenols	4
B. Coumarins and Other Simple Lactones	9
C. Aromatic Isothiocyanates	10
D. Flavones	12
E. Indoles	13
F. Possible Hazards from Inducers of Increased Microsomal Mixed-Function Oxidase Activity	15
III. Discussion	16
References	19

Chapter 2
Inhibition of Carcinogen Metabolism and Action by Disulfiram, Pyrazole, and Related Compounds
Emerich S. Fiala

I. Introduction	23
II. Disulfiram	24
A. Commercial and Medicinal Use	24
B. Toxicity	25
C. Effects on Enzyme Systems	25
D. Metabolism	27

III. Sodium Diethyldithiocarbamate and Dithiocarbamate
    Pesticides 28
    A. Commercial and Medicinal Use 28
    B. Toxicity 29
    C. Effects on Enzyme Systems 30
IV. Carbon Disulfide 30
    A. Commercial Use 30
    B. Effects on Enzyme Systems 31
V. Pyrazole 31
    A. Metabolism, Toxicity, and Enzyme Inhibition 31
VI. Polycyclic Aromatic Hydrocarbons: Benzo[a]pyrene and
    7,12-Dimethylbenz[a]anthracene 32
    A. Metabolism 32
    B. Effects of Thiono Sulfur Compounds on Carcinogenicity .. 33
VII. Hydrazo and Azoxy Carcinogens 35
    A. 1,2-Dimethylhydrazine 35
    B. Procarbazine 45
VIII. N-Nitrosamines 47
    A. Dimethylnitrosamine and Diethylnitrosamine 47
    B. N-Nitrosopyrrolidine 50
    C. N-n-Butyl-N-(4-hydroxybutyl) nitrosamine 51
IX. Arylamines 52
    A. 2-Acetylaminofluorene 52
    B. 3,2'-Dimethyl-4-aminobiphenyl 54
X. Azo Dyes: 3'-Methyl-4-dimethylaminoazobenzene 55
XI. Ultraviolet Light 57
XII. Spontaneous Tumors 57
XIII. Other Effects of Thiono Sulfur Compounds 59
    References 60

Chapter 3
Retinoids and Chemoprevention of Cancer

Michael B. Sporn and Dianne L. Newton

I. Introduction 71
II. Retinoids and Epithelial Cell Differentiation 72
III. Suppression of Malignant Transformation and Tumor
    Promotion by Retinoids 73
IV. Retinoid Deficiency and Carcinogenesis 76

V. Natural Retinoids and Prevention of Carcinogenesis 77
VI. Structure–Activity Relationships of New Synthetic Retinoids .. 81
VII. Prevention of Cancer in Experimental Animals with New Synthetic Retinoids 90
VIII. Mechanism of Action of Retinoids in Chemoprevention of Cancer 92
IX. Mechanism of Toxicity of Retinoids 94
X. Combination Chemoprevention with Retinoids 95
References 96

Chapter 4
Ascorbic Acid Inhibition of N-Nitroso Compound Formation in Chemical, Food, and Biological Systems
Sidney S. Mirvish

I. Introduction 101
II. *In Vitro* Studies 101
   A. Studies in Acidic Aqueous Solutions 101
   B. Use of Ascorbate in the Meat Industry 108
   C. Nitrosation in Lipids and by Nitrogen Oxides 110
III. *In Vivo* Studies 111
   A. Acute Toxicity Experiments 111
   B. Carcinogenicity Experiments 112
   C. Chemical Analysis of Biological Materials 115
IV. Tests on Carcinogenicity and Mutagenicity of Ascorbic Acid .. 116
V. Effects of Ascorbic Acid on Carcinogenicity and Mutagenicity of N-Nitroso Compounds 117
VI. Ascorbic Acid and Carcinogenesis in Man 119
VII. Summary and Conclusions 120
References 122

Chapter 5
α-Tocopherol (Vitamin E) and Its Relationship to Tumor Induction and Development
Harold L. Newmark and William J. Mergens

I. Introduction 127
   A. Mechanisms of Tumor Induction/Inhibition 128

II. Vitamin E as an Antitumor Agent 129
   A. Ultraviolet Light-Induced Carcinogenesis 129
   B. Polynuclear Aromatic Hydrocarbons 130
III. Nitroso Compounds 132
   A. Carcinogenicity 133
   B. Mutagenicity 134
   C. Mechanism of Activation 134
   D. Implications for Carcinogenesis 135
IV. Formation of N-Nitroso Compounds 136
   A. General Principles 136
   B. Aqueous Systems 138
   C. Nonaqueous Systems 139
   D. Transnitrosation 140
V. Blocking N-Nitroso Compound Formation 141
   A. Principles 141
   B. Blocking Agents 145
   C. Integration of Blocking Systems........................ 150
VI. α-Tocopherol Applications 152
   A. Bacon 152
   B. Other Foods 153
   C. Rectal and Colonic Carcinogenesis 154
   D. Lung Cancer 155
   E. Bladder Cancer 156
   F. N-Nitroso Compounds in Blood 157
   G. Gastric Cancer 157
VII. Ascorbic Acid and Tocopherol Effect on Preformed
     Nitrosamines 158
VIII. Summary 159
     References 160

Chapter 6
Trace Elements and Metals as Anticarcinogens
Maryce M. Jacobs and A. Clark Griffin

I. Introduction 169
II. Selenium 170
   A. Clinical 170
   B. Animal 172
   C. Bacterial 174
   D. Other *in Vitro* Systems 176

Contents

III. Zinc	177
IV. Copper	179
V. Other Trace Elements and Metals	180
A. Metal–Metal Anticarcinogenicity	180
B. Nutritional Factors	182
C. Other Trace Element Effects	182
VI. Closing Remarks	184
References	184

Chapter 7

Plant Sterols: Protective Role in Chemical Carcinogenesis

Bertram Ira Cohen and Robert Franklin Raicht

I. Background	189
II. Plant Sterols: Structure and Function	190
III. Animal Test Systems	192
IV. Results	195
A. Effect of N-Methyl-N-nitrosourea on Tumor Formation in Animals Given Plant Sterol and/or Bile Acid	195
V. Discussion	196
References	199

Chapter 8

Immunoprevention

Hans Olov Sjögren

I. Introduction	203
II. Detection of Tumor-Associated Antigens in Experimental Rat Bowel Carcinomas	203
III. Evidence that Embryonic Antigens are Associated with Bowel Carcinomas	204
IV. Enhanced 1,2-Dimethylhydrazine-Induced Tumorigenesis in Immunosuppressed Rats	206
V. Inhibitory Effect on Bowel Carcinogenesis by Immunization with Transplantable Syngeneic Colon Carcinoma	206
VI. Inhibitory Effect on Bowel Carcinogenesis by Immunization with Fetal Tissue	208

VII. Inhibition of 1,2-Dimethylhydrazine-Induced
   Carcinogenesis in Multiparous Rats 210
VIII. Effect of Tumor Resection on the Development
   of Additional Primary Tumors 210
IX. Regression of Early Primary Bowel Carcinomas
   by Multimodal Immunological Treatment 211
X. Conclusions 213
   References 215

Chapter 9
Summation and Future Challenges
Rulon W. Rawson, Martin Lipkin, and Morris S. Zedeck

I. Introduction 219
II. Challenges to Chemists and Molecular and Cell Biologists 220
III. Challenges to Epidemiologists and Oncologists 222

Index 225

1

Inhibition of Chemical Carcinogenesis by Phenols, Coumarins, Aromatic Isothiocyanates, Flavones, and Indoles

LEE W. WATTENBERG and
LUKE K. T. LAM

I. Introduction

An increasing number and diversity of compounds have been found to inhibit the neoplastic effects of chemical carcinogens when administered prior to and/or simultaneously with the carcinogen. These inhibitors include naturally occurring constituents of foods, particularly vegetables and fruit, and also synthetic compounds, some of which are food additives (Wattenberg, 1979a,b). The inhibitors encompass a wide range of chemical structures (Fig. 1). The time relationship between administration of the inhibitors and carcinogens as well as direct studies of mechanisms of inhibition indicate that these inhibitors can act by preventing carcinogenic species from reaching or reacting with critical cellular targets. In essence, they exert a barrier function.

LEE W. WATTENBERG and LUKE K. T. LAM • Department of Laboratory Medicine and Pathology, University of Minnesota, Minneapolis, Minnesota 55455.

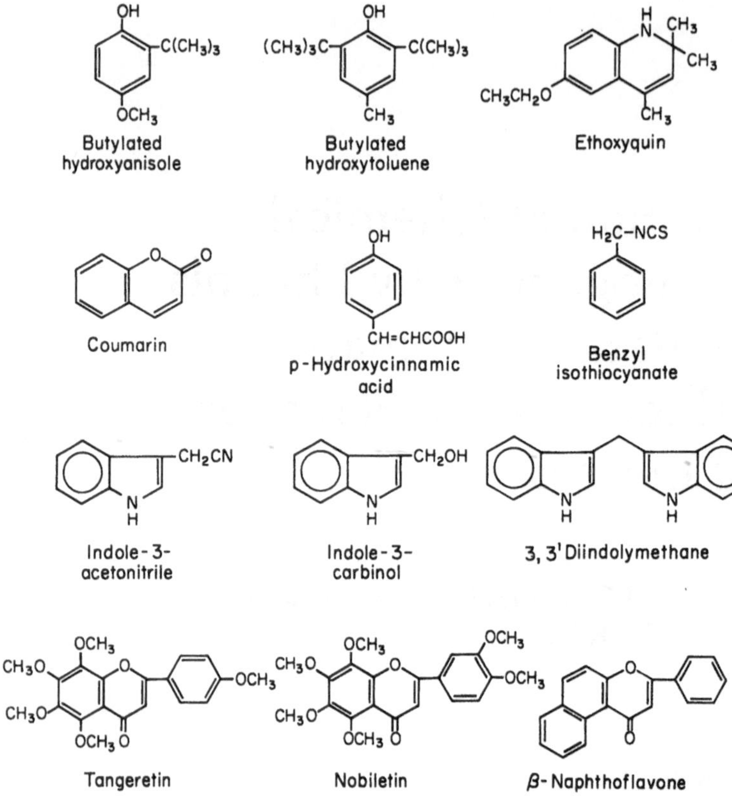

FIGURE 1. Some inhibitors of chemical carcinogens.

Most inhibitors appear to act by enhancing host detoxification systems. Some produce a selective effect by preventing enzymatic activation of specific carcinogens to their ultimate carcinogenic forms (Fiala *et al.*, 1977). Other inhibitors enhance detoxification systems that have the capacity to inhibit a wide range of carcinogens. Inhibition can also occur by interaction of carcinogenic electrophiles with compounds having the capacity to scavenge reactive species of this type (Marquardt *et al.*, 1974). Five groups of inhibitors will be discussed: phenols, coumarins and other simple lactones, aromatic isothiocyanates, flavones, and indoles. Members of all of these groups occur in food consumed by man. In addition to the compounds that are found in food, related chemicals will also be discussed where these chemicals provide information as to structure–activity relationships or mechanism of inhibitor action.

TABLE 1. Inhibition of Carcinogen-Induced Neoplasia by Phenols

Carcinogen	Antioxidant	Species	Site of neoplasm inhibited	Reference
Benzo(a)pyrene	BHA	Mouse	Lung	Wattenberg (1973)
Benzo(a)pyrene	BHA, BHT	Mouse	Forestomach	Wattenberg (1972a)
7,12-Dimethylbenz(a)anthracene	BHA	Mouse	Lung	Wattenberg (1973)
7,12-Dimethylbenz(a)anthracene	BHA	Mouse	Forestomach	Wattenberg (1972a)
7,12-Dimethylbenz(a)anthracene	BHA, BHT	Mouse	Skin	Slaga and Bracken (1977)
7,12-Dimethylbenz(a)anthracene	BHA, BHT	Rat	Breast	Wattenberg (1972a)
7-Hydroxymethyl-12-methyl-benz(a)anthracene	BHA	Mouse	Lung	Wattenberg (1973)
Dibenz(a,h)anthracene	BHA	Mouse	Lung	Wattenberg (1973)
Diethylnitrosamine	BHA	Mouse	Lung	Wattenberg (1972b)
4-Nitroquinoline-N-oxide	BHA	Mouse	Lung	Wattenberg (1972b)
Uracil mustard	BHA	Mouse	Lung	Wattenberg (1973)
Urethane	BHA	Mouse	Lung	Wattenberg (1973)
Methylazoxymethanol acetate	BHA	Mouse	Large intestine	Wattenberg and Sparnins (1979)
trans-5-Amino-3[2-(5-nitro-2-furyl)-vinyl]-1,2,4-oxadiazole	BHA	Mouse	Forestomach, lung	E. Bueding, H. Dunsford, and P. Dolan (personal communication)
β-Propiolactone	BHA	Mouse	Forestomach	L. W. Wattenberg (unpublished data)
N-2-Fluorenylacetamide	BHT	Rat	Liver	Ulland et al. (1973)
N-Hydroxy-N-2-fluorenylacetamide	BHT	Rat	Liver, breast	Ulland et al. (1973)
4-Dimethylaminoazobenzene	BHT	Rat	Liver	Frankfurt et al. (1967)
Azoxymethane	BHT	Rat	Large intestine	Weisburger et al. (1977)

II. Inhibitors of Chemical Carcinogens

A. Phenols

1. Carcinogens Inhibited

Investigations of the inhibitory effects of two phenolic antioxidants, butylated hydroxyanisole (BHA) and butylated hydroxytoluene (BHT), have been carried out with a number of chemical carcinogens. These two antioxidants are of interest in that they are widely employed as food additives. Inhibition occurs under a variety of experimental conditions and with a broad range of carcinogens as shown in Table 1.

A diversity of experimental models and administration schedules have been used in the experiments listed in Table 1. In a typical case, the inhibitor is fed in the diet for about a week prior to an initial administration of the carcinogen, and the feeding is continued until all doses of the carcinogen have been given. One variation of this procedure is for the inhibitor to be administered either by oral intubation or parenterally prior to each administration of the carcinogen. A second variation is to include both the inhibitor and carcinogen in the diet. All of these time relationships between inhibitor and carcinogen administrations are those to be expected from inhibitors that enhance carcinogen detoxification or in some other manner prevent the active form of the carcinogen from reaching or reacting with critical cellular target sites.

In addition to inhibition of carcinogenesis, BHA has been found to inhibit mutagenesis resulting from administration of known carcinogens and some additional mutagenic compounds in which the capacity to produce neoplasms has not yet been established. Two procedures have been employed, both of which entail use of *Salmonella typhimurium* tester strains TA-100 and TA-98. The first is a host-mediated procedure in which the organisms are introduced into the peritoneal cavity. The test compound is administered either i.m. or p.o., and BHA is added to the diet. An alternate method entails determination of the effect of dietary BHA on excretion of mutagenic metabolites of test compounds. Butylated hydroxyanisole was found to inhibit host-mediated mutagenesis of benzo(*a*)pyrene (BP), hycanthone, metronidazole, metrifonate, praziquantel, and mebenzadole. Butylated hydroxyanisole also reduced the excretion of mutagenic metabolities of these six compounds as well as diazepam (Batzinger *et al.*, 1978).

2. Studies of the Mechanisms by which BHA Inhibits Carcinogen-Induced Neoplasia

The phenol most extensively studied for its mechanism of inhibition of chemical carcinogenesis has been BHA. This compound is quite remarkable in terms of the range of carcinogens as well as mutagens it inhibits. Studies carried out thus far indicate that an important mechanism of this inhibition resides in the capacity of BHA to cause enhanced detoxification. Mice that have been fed BHA for a period of 1–2 weeks at dose levels used for carcinogen inhibition experiments have been employed for studies of this nature. The microsomal monooxygenase system is the initial enzyme system shown to be altered. This alteration can be demonstrated by incubating BP with liver microsomes, cofactors required for mixed function oxidase activity, and added DNA. Under these conditions, reactive metabolites of BP bind to DNA. If liver microsomes from mice fed BHA are employed, approximately one-half as much binding of BP metabolites to DNA occurs as compared to incubation with control microsomes (Speier and Wattenberg, 1975). High-pressure liquid chromatography (HPLC) studies of metabolites of BP produced by incubation of this carcinogen with microsomes from mice fed BHA as compared to controls also show changes. Two metabolic alterations are found that could result in inhibition of carcinogenesis. The first is a decrease in epoxidation of BP, which is an activation process, and the second is an increase in formation of 3-hydroxybenzo(a)pyrene, a metabolite of detoxification (Lam and Wattenberg, 1977).

Subsequent work has focused on the effects of BHA on the activities of conjugating enzymes. The initial work of this nature showed that addition of BHA to diets results in large increases in glutathione-S-transferase activity. Four substrates were employed, i.e., 1,2-dichloro-4-nitrobenzene, 1-chloro-2,4-dinitrobenzene, p-nitrobenzylchloride, and Δ^5-androstene-3,17-dione. After 12 days of feeding BHA, the glutathione-S-transferase activity, as determined with the first three of these substrates, was increased over ten times that of control animals; a fivefold increase was found with the fourth substrate. Ethoxyquin also induced and increased glutathione-S-transferase activity but was about half as effective as BHA (Benson et al., 1978). In related investigations, it was found that the administration of BHA produced an increase in the levels of reduced thiols in liver, kidney, lung, and duodenum (Benson et al., 1978).

A second conjugating enzyme investigated is UDP-glucuronyl transferase. Studies carried out under similar conditions to those for glutathione-S-

transferase have showed that feeding a diet containing BHA results in slightly greater than a fourfold increase in liver UDP-glucuronyl transferase activity using p-aminophenol as the substrate (Cha and Bueding, 1979). BHT also has been shown to induce an increase in activity of this enzyme (Grantham et al., 1973). In addition to its effects on the two conjugating enzymes, the feeding of a diet containing BHA causes an increase in epoxide hydratase and glucose-6-phosphate dehydrogenase activities (Cha and Bueding, 1979).

The increases in enzyme activities described above have been observed in animals fed a diet containing BHA for at least 3 days. Little data are available for shorter time intervals. These are inducible enzymes, and it would be anticipated that a substantial period of time would be required for the activity to increase. No increase in liver glutathione-S-transferase activity occurs for at least 6 hr subsequent to BHA administration (L. W. Wattenberg and V. L. Sparnins, unpublished data). However, in the case of liver microsomal metabolism of BP, changes of another type can be found as early as 2 hr after a single oral administration of BHA. At that time, the microsomal metabolism of BP to metabolites binding to DNA has been reduced to one-half that found with microsomes from control animals (Speier et al., 1978). The reduction is of the same order of magnitude as that in mice fed BHA for a week or more. Changes in the BP metabolite pattern similar to those found after prolonged feeding occur 4 hr after a single administration of BHA, the earliest time interval studied thus far (Speier et al., 1978). A point of considerable importance is that no increase in the overall metabolism of BP, as determined by HPLC, occurs at any time interval after administration of BHA either by oral intubation or in the diet. Similarly, studies of BP metabolism using the determination of aryl hydrocarbon hydroxylase (AHH) activity do not show an increase (Lam and Wattenberg, 1977; Speier et al., 1978).

A perusal of the enzyme activities increased by BHA reveals that they include both microsomal enzymes (UDP-glucuronyl transferase and epoxide hydratase) and enzymes located in the cytosol of the cell (glutathione-S-transferase and glucose-6-phosphate dehydrogenase). This diversity of enzyme inductions suggests a relationship to observations made by Poland et al., on the inducing effects of some xenobiotic compounds chemically different from BHA. These include 2,3,7,8-tetrachlorodibenzo-p-dioxin (TCDD) and polycyclic aromatic hydrocarbons. Their mechanism of induction has been extensively studied using the extremely potent compound TCDD (Poland and Kende, 1977). Work carried out by these investigators has demonstrated that TCDD binds a cytoplasmic receptor. This complex enters the nucleus

Inhibition of Chemical Carcinogenesis

and causes the induction of increased activity of major detoxification systems including UDP-glucuronyl transferase, epoxide hydratase and glutathione-S-transferase (Poland *et al.*, 1979). Induction of increased AHH activity also occurs, as does the activity of a number of other enzymes (Poland and Kende, 1977; Fig. 2). The sequence of events has similarities to that existing with steroids in which a steroid binds to a cytoplasmic receptor, the complex enters the nucleus, and a coordinated series of biochemical changes ensues.

Methylcholanthrene (MC) and BP have been found to be competitive inhibitors for the binding of TCDD to the cytoplasmic receptor. Many of the

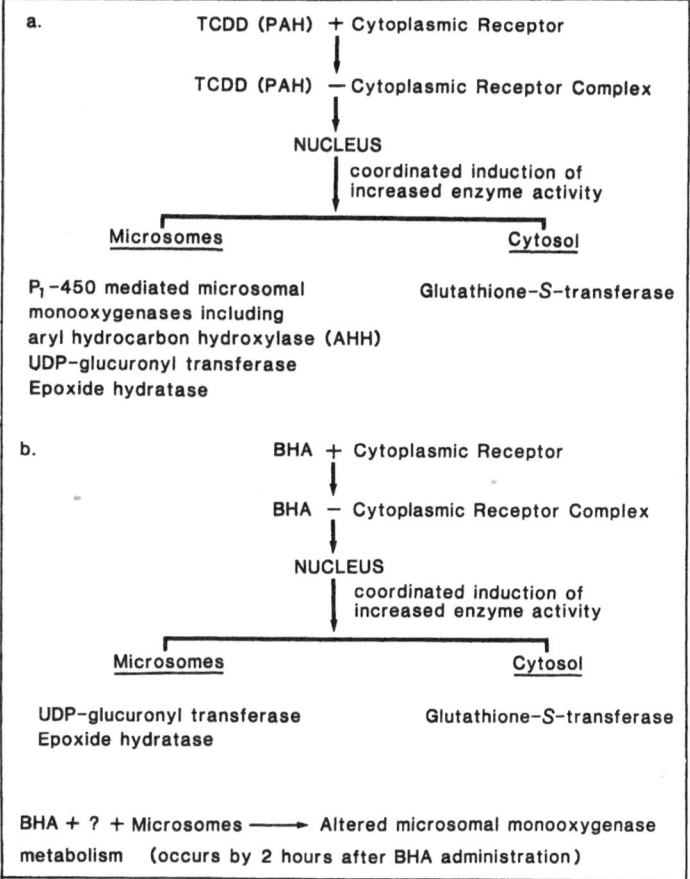

FIGURE 2. (a) Coordinated induction by 2,3,7,8-tetrachlorodibenzo-p-dioxin (TCDD) and polycyclic aromatic hydrocarbons (PAH) of some enzymes important for the detoxification and excretion of polycyclic aromatic hydrocarbons and related compounds. (b) Coordinated response to BHA administration.

same enzyme inductions are produced by these compounds as are produced by TCDD, suggesting that the three compounds act through the same receptor. This is not the case for phenobarbital, diphenylhydantoin, phenylbutazone, and pregnenolone-16-α-carbonitrile, all of which also induce increased activity of hepatic microsomal enzymes (Poland and Kende, 1977).

Butylated hydroxyanisole evokes a coordinated group of reactions involving some of the same enzymes that are induced by TCDD. These enzymes have the overall effect of enhancing detoxification. We would postulate that this coordinated response to BHA is likely to be the result of a similar series of events to that found with TCDD, although differences in magnitude and diversities of enzymes induced clearly exist (Fig. 2). Identification of a putative cytoplasmic receptor for BHA has not been accomplished. It is probable that it would differ from that for TCDD and related compounds. If one assumes that at least some potentially toxic xenobiotic chemicals induce a coordinated enzyme response that enhances their own detoxification and that of chemically related compounds, then the differences between the coordinated responses to a phenol such as BHA and those to compounds such as polycyclic aromatic hydrocarbons and TCDD are understandable. Thus, phenols contain a hydroxy group that is available for conjugation. Increased activity of conjugating systems would be the main requirement for detoxification and excretion of these compounds. An increase in AHH activity is not necessary for this purpose. In contrast, a compound such as MC or other polycyclic aromatic hydrocarbons requires the presence of one or more polar groups in order for conjugation to occur. Thus, an increase in AHH activity as well as increased activity of conjugating enzymes are necessary for detoxification and excretion. In Fig. 2, differences in the coordinated enzyme responses are depicted.

The alteration of the microsomal monooxygenase system that is observed 2 hr after BHA administration is an interesting finding in terms of its temporal occurrence. It is possible that a totally coordinated detoxification system would have an early component to protect the organism until enhanced activity of inducible enzymes has occurred. The rapid alteration in the microsomal monooxygenase system following BHA administration may represent such an event. If this is in fact the case, then there may be some relationship among BHA, its putative cytoplasmic receptor, and the microsomal monooxygenase system that, overall, results in alteration of the monooxygenase system. Alternatively, it is possible that a direct interaction of BHA or one of its metabolites with the monooxygenase system occurs. At present, these are theoretical considerations that require experimental exploration.

B. Coumarins and Other Simple Lactones

The coumarins comprise an important group of natural products and are present in a variety of vegetables and fruits consumed by man (Späth, 1937; Robinson, 1963; Dean, 1963). An initial report by Feuer *et al.,* (1976) showed that DMBA-induced mammary tumor formation is inhibited by coumarin. Subsequently, this result was confirmed, and further studies of the effects of three naturally occurring simple derivatives of coumarin have been carried out (Wattenberg *et al.,* 1979). Additional compounds have also been investigated in an attempt to obtain information about the relationships of chemical structure and inhibitory potency. In these studies, two animal test systems have been used. The first is DMBA-induced mammary tumor formation in female Sprague–Dawley rats, and the second is BP-induced neoplasia of the forestomach in ICR/Ha mice. In the experiments with DMBA-mammary tumor formation, the effects of administration of coumarin and three of its derivatives, i.e., umbelliferone (7-hydroxycoumarin), scopoletin (7-hydroxy-6-methoxycoumarin), and limettin (5,7-dimethoxycoumarin) were investigated. Coumarin was found to be a moderately potent inhibitor as demonstrated by a decrease in the number of animals bearing mammary neoplasms and the number of tumors per animal. Limettin was less effective, and scopoletin had only a marginal inhibitory effect. Umbelliferone did not inhibit DMBA-induced neoplasia under the conditions employed (Wattenberg *et al.,* 1979).

The same coumarins have also been studied to determine their capacities to inhibit BP-induced neoplasia of the mouse forestomach. Overall, the coumarins were less effective in this experimental model than in the rat mammary tumor experiments. Coumarin inhibited BP-induced neoplasia of the forestomach. Limettin, umbelliferone, and scopoletin were inactive. Several additional compounds have been studied for their effects on BP-induced neoplasia of the forestomach. Two five-membered benzolactones, 2-coumaranone and phthalide, were investigated. Neither compound was effective. Of four alicyclic lactones studied, only α-angelicalactone inhibited BP-induced neoplasia and was considerably more potent than coumarin. The other three, i.e., γ-valerolactone, L-ascorbic acid, and isocitric lactone, were without inhibitory effects (Wattenberg *et al.,* 1979). Several structure–activity relationships are evident from data currently available. With the coumarins, increased polarity of substituents results in decreasing activity as inhibitors. For both the coumarins and the five-membered ring lactones studied, protic groups, such as hydroxy and carboxy groups, abolish the capacity to inhibit. Although unsaturation in the lactone ring does not always lead to inhibitory activity, the presence of at least one double bond is essential. Thus, the property of inhibiting BP and DMBA is not a general characteristic of all coumarins and alicyclic lactones but is restricted to those with specific structural features.

The mechanism or mechanisms by which the coumarins and α-angelicalactone cause inhibition of DMBA- or BP-induced neoplasia has not been established. Feuer *et al.* observed that coumarin administration decreased the activity of the coumarin-3-hydroxylase system. A reduction in coumarin-3-hydroxylase activity was also observed by these investigators in pregnant rats in which DMBA-induced neoplasia of the mammary gland was suppressed (Feuer and Kellen, 1974a,b; Feuer *et al.*, 1976). On the basis of these two sets of observations, they postulated that a reduction in microsomal enzyme activity might be responsible for the protective effect of coumarin. However, no direct investigations of DMBA metabolism were carried out. The assumption that parallel changes occur in the activity of coumarin-3-hydroxylase and the activity of the microsomal enzyme system metabolizing DMBA to an ultimate carcinogenic form has not been demonstrated experimentally.

Although the inhibitory effect of coumarin on DMBA- and BP-induced carcinogenesis may be explained by an alteration of the microsomal metabolism of the carcinogens, other mechanisms exist including a direct reaction between active forms of the carcinogen and the inhibitor (Georgieff, 1971). Alternatively, the ring-opened products of these lactones may serve as nucleophiles to scavenge the reactive ultimate carcinogenic metabolites. Studies in solution chemistry have shown that the ring opening of coumarins to substituted phenols occurs only at $pH > 7$ (Bowden *et al.*, 1968; Hershfield and Schmir, 1973). This reaction would not appear to be favorable in the gastric contents. However, under the complex conditions existing *in vivo*, it is conceivable that ring opening might occur. This would have potential importance since several phenols have been shown to inhibit chemical carcinogens (Wattenberg, 1978a,b). The above considerations indicate that there are several possible mechanisms that singly or in combination could account for the inhibitory effects of coumarins and α-angelicalactone.

C. Aromatic Isothiocyanates

Benzyl isothiocyanate and phenethyl isothiocyanate occur in cruciferous plants. Some of these plants, such as brussels sprouts, cabbage, cauliflower, and broccoli, are consumed by man. The two isothiocyanates have been studied for their inhibitory effects against BP and DMBA in animal models in which neoplasia was produced in three organs, i.e., forestomach, lung, and mammary gland. In addition to the naturally occurring isothiocyanates, several synthetic compounds also have been investigated: phenyl isothiocyanate, diphenylmethyl isothiocyanate, and allyl isothiocyanate.

Benzyl isothiocyanate, phenethyl isothiocyanate, and phenyl isothiocyanate inhibit DMBA-induced neoplasia of the mammary gland in female Sprague–Dawley rats. Inhibition occurs when the isothiocyanates are administered by oral intubation 4 hr prior to DMBA. Further work on the effects on inhibition of altering the time of administration of the isothiocyanate relative to that of the carcinogen have been carried out using benzyl isothiocyanate. Inhibition is obtained when this test compound is given 2 hr prior to DMBA. Inhibition is markedly diminished when the time interval is increased to 24 hr prior to DMBA. No inhibition occurs if the isothiocyanate is given 4 hr after the DMBA (Wattenberg, 1977).

Addition of benzyl isothiocyanate or phenethyl isothiocyanate to a diet containing DMBA inhibits neoplasia of the forestomach in ICR/Ha mice. Benzyl isothiocyanate also inhibits BP-induced neoplasia of the forestomach under comparable conditions. Other experiments have been carried out with isothiocyanates added to the diet but in which BP was given by oral intubation rather than added to the diet. By employing this method, it was again found that benzyl isothiocyanate inhibited BP-induced neoplasia of the forestomach. Phenyl isothiocyanate also inhibited BP-induced neoplasia, but sodium thiocyanate was inactive.

Studies of inhibition of pulmonary neoplasia have been carried out using two experimental systems. The first entailed addition of carcinogen and test substance to the diet of ICR/Ha mice. Benzyl isothiocyanate inhibits DMBA-induced neoplasia of the lung under these conditions (Wattenberg, 1977). A second experimental model employed female A/HeJ mice. The test substance was fed in the diet through the entire period of carcinogen administrations. Nine days after the start of the diets, the first dose of carcinogen was administered by oral intubation. Two weeks later, a second administration of carcinogen was given. Twenty-four weeks after the first dose of carcinogen, mice were sacrificed and pulmonary adenomas counted. Using DMBA as the carcinogen, the inhibitory capacities of the following compounds were studied: benzyl isothiocyanate, phenethyl isothiocyanate, benzyl thiocyanate, diphenylmethyl thiocyanate, phenyl thiocyanate, and allyl isothiocyanate. Results, in parentheses, are expressed as the ratio of tumor counts in the animals receiving the test substance divided by the counts in the controls. Inhibition was produced by benzyl isothiocyanate (0.52*), phenethyl isothiocyanate (0.64*), phenyl thiocyanate (0.56*), and diphenylmethyl thiocyanate (0.32*). In contrast, benzyl thiocyanate (0.82) and allyl isothiocyanate (1.2) were inactive as inhibitors.

The work described above has demonstrated that the two naturally occurring isothiocyanates, benzyl isothiocyanate and phenethyl isothiocyanate, inhibit polycyclic aromatic hydrocarbon-induced neoplasia at three target sites: breast, lung, and forestomach. Two of these target sites are remote from the portal of entry of the isothiocyanates. In the case of the forestomach, there is direct contact of inhibitor and target site. Of importance is the fact that protection has been observed under conditions in which the inhibitor was given prior to or prior to and simultaneously with the carcinogen but does not occur when the isothiocyanate is given subsequent to the carcinogen. However, the mechanism of inhibition by this class of inhibitors is unknown.

D. Flavones

The study of flavones as possible inhibitors of chemical carcinogens was undertaken as a result of data that showed that a number of inducers of increased microsomal mixed-function oxidase activity inhibit chemical carcinogens (Wattenberg, 1978a,b). In initial work, several flavones were found to induce increased AHH activity using BP as the substrate (Wattenberg et al., 1968). Flavone itself is a moderately potent inducer. In the compounds studied, hydroxylation reduced inducing activity, but corresponding methoxy compounds were active. The vast majority of naturally occurring flavones are polyhydroxy derivatives. A small number contain only methoxy groups. Two of these, tangeretin (5,6,7,8,4'-pentamethoxyflavone) and nobiletin (5,6,7,8,-3',4'-hexamethoxyflavone) were active inducers of increased AHH activity (Fig. 1).

An investigation of inhibition of BP-induced carcinogenesis was carried out with three flavones. The compounds chosen for study were β-naphthoflavone (5,6-benzoflavone), quercetin pentamethyl ether, and rutin (3,3',4',5,7-pentahydroxyflavone-3-rutinoside). β-Naphthoflavone, a synthetic compound, is the most potent flavone found thus far in terms of its capacity to induce increased AHH activity. Quercetin pentamethyl ether is a

*$p < 0.05$.

moderately potent inducer of increased AHH activity. This compound is synthetic and was used as a substitute for tangeretin which could not be obtained in sufficient quantity for carcinogen-inhibition studies. Both compounds are pentamethoxy flavones with similar inducing capacities. Rutin is a naturally occurring compound with very weak AHH-inducing activity. The three flavones were added to the diet of A/HeJ mice that subsequently were challenged with BP given by oral intubation. β-Naphthoflavone caused almost total inhibition of pulmonary adenoma formation; quercetin pentamethyl ether reduced the number of these neoplasms by half. The number of adenomas in animals fed rutin and the control diet was the same. Thus, the inhibitory effects on BP-induced neoplasia paralleled the potency of the three flavones in inducing increased AHH activity (Wattenberg and Leong, 1970). In other experiments in which the only flavone employed was β-naphthoflavone, this compound inhibited DMBA-induced mammary tumor formation in the rat and BP-initiated epidermal neoplasia in the mouse (Wattenberg and Leong, 1968, 1970).

E. Indoles

Indole-3-carbinol, 3,3'-diindolylmethane, and indole-3-acetonitrile occur in edible cruciferous vegetables such as brussels sprouts, cabbage, cauliflower, and broccoli which are consumed by large numbers of individuals. These three indoles have been studied for their effects on BP- and DMBA-induced neoplasia in rodents. When added to the diet, all three indoles inhibited BP-induced neoplasia of the forestomach. Addition to the diet was also found to inhibit BP-induced pulmonary adenoma formation. In other experiments, indole-3-carbinol and diindolylmethane inhibited DMBA-induced mammary tumor formation in female Sprague–Dawley rats, but indole-3-acetonitrile was inactive in this experimental model (Wattenberg and Loub, 1978).

The original rationale for the use of the three indoles is based on their ability to alter microsomal mixed-function oxidase activity. All three compounds induce increased activity of this system towards BP (designated AHH activity) and other substrates (Loub *et al.*, 1975; Pantuck *et al.*, 1976, 1979). The most potent inducer is indole-3-carbinol, and the least active is indole-3-acetonitrile. Since a number of compounds inducing increased microsomal mixed-function oxidase activity protect against carcinogen-induced neoplasia (Wattenberg, 1978a,b), the three indoles were selected for study of their capacities to act as inhibitors in the investigations summarized above. In experiments in which neoplasms occur at a site distant from that of administration of the carcinogen, as with mammary tumor formation resulting from oral administration of DMBA or pulmonary adenoma formation from oral administration of BP, indole-3-carbinol is effective as an inhibitor. In contrast, indole-3-acetonitrile, a weak inducer of microsomal mixed-function oxidase activity does not inhibit DMBA-induced mammary tumor formation and is considerably less active than indole-3-carbinol in inhibiting BP-induced pulmonary adenoma formation. These findings are in accord with previously found relationships between potency of induction of increased AHH activity and effectiveness as inhibitors of BP- or DMBA-induced neoplasia (Wattenberg, 1978a,b).

In the case of the BP-induced neoplasia of the forestomach, a different situation exists. Although indole-3-carbinol is a more potent inducer of increased AHH activity than indole-3-acetonitrile in this tissue, the two compounds inhibit tumor formation to the same degree. The effect of administration of indoles on the metabolite pattern of carcinogens has not yet been determined. It is possible that in the forestomach, in contrast to other tissues, indole-3-acetonitrile is particularly favorable in terms of deviating metabolism of BP towards detoxification. The AHH determination gives data on the overall enzyme activity but not on metabolite pattern. The precise nature of the metabolites is of obvious importance. If these are detoxification products, then protection will occur. Even a weak inducer or a compound such as BHA, which alters the metabolite pattern without enhancing overall microsomal mixed-function oxidase activity, can be an effective inhibitor by reducing the relative amount of carcinogen converted to a reactive electrophilic species. Other possible mechanisms of inhibition exist. The fact that in inhibition of forestomach tumor formation indole-3-acetonitrile comes into direct contact with the target tissue must be considered. Thus, there may be different tissue responses depending on direct contact of this indole with the target tissue as contrasted to target sites remote from that of the indole administration.

Studies comparable to those employing indole-3-acetonitrile have been carried out with phenyl acetonitrile and octanenitrile in order to determine whether inhibition of BP-induced forestomach neoplasia was a general property of nitriles. This is not the case. These two nitriles did not exert an inhibitory effect. Since indole-3-acetonitrile is the most abundant of the indoles found in many edible cruciferous vegetables, elucidation of its mechanism of inhibition is of particular importance.

F. Possible Hazards from Inducers of Increased Microsomal Mixed-Function Oxidase Activity

Having presented information that shows a protective effect from administration of inducers of increased microsomal monooxygenase activity, i.e., flavones and indoles, we must now consider possible hazards from compounds having this type of biological effect. It has been demonstrated for many chemical carcinogens that the microsomal monooxygenase system converts these compounds to a proximate carcinogenic form. However, there is frequently a competing detoxification pathway or pathways. The classic example of this is the aromatic amines. With these compounds, ring hydroxylation results in detoxification whereas hydroxylation of the nitrogen is an activation reaction (Miller and Miller, 1969). Thus, administration of inducers of increased monooxygenase activity in these instances may result in a relatively greater proportion of the carcinogen being detoxified rather than activated to a carcinogenic metabolite.

An additional consideration is that, quite independent of competing detoxification reactions, increased rates of carcinogen activation may not increase the carcinogenic response. Rapid activation is of importance in situations involving a reversible effect in which there is a substantial threshold. Rapid activation may result in achieving such a threshold. However, in the case of chemical carcinogenesis, different conditions exist. In this instance, there appears to be either no threshold or a very low threshold. Thus, one might anticipate that for a given amount of carcinogen, slow activation would result in as great or even a greater carcinogenic effect than rapid activation. With slow activation there would be less likelihood of wastage of activated species of carcinogen from cells through production of an amount in excess of that most effective for the number of critical binding sites. An additional consideration is that some inducers of increased AHH activity also induce increased activity of conjugating enzymes. This could enhance detoxification as has been discussed in the section on phenolic antioxidants and ethoxyquin (Section II.A).

In spite of the above considerations, the complexity of the microsomal monooxygenase system is sufficiently great so as to make it possible that under some circumstances an induction of increased activity of one or more of its cytochrome P-450 species would enhance carcinogenesis. This may be the case with safrole. Administration of phenobarbital in the drinking water of rats concurrently fed safrole in the diet results in a greater number of tumors of the liver than in animals not receiving the phenobarbital (Wislocki et al., 1977). However, phenobarbital is a compound with multiple biological actions, and this lends an element of uncertainty as to the mechanism by which it enhances the carcinogenic response to safrole. One of these biological actions is its capacity to act as a tumor promoting agent. When phenobarbital is administered subsequent to the hepatocarcinogens 2-acetylaminofluorene, diethylnitrosamine, and 2-methyl-N,N-dimethyl-4-aminoazobenzene, it increases the neoplastic response (Peraino et al., 1973, 1977; Kitagawa et al., 1979). A somewhat similar situation exists for BHT. This compound, like phenobarbital, can induce increased microsomal monooxygenase activity. In addition, when BHT is given subsequent to carcinogens, it, like phenobarbital, can enhance a neoplastic response. Administration of BHT subsequent to urethane increases the number of pulmonary adenomas formed (Witschi et al., 1977). If administered after 2-acetylaminofluorene, an increase in hepatic tumors is observed (Peraino et al., 1977). The neoplasia-enhancing effects of phenobarbital and BHT represent a hazard that requires evaluation with respect to other compounds having the capacity to induce increased microsomal monooxygenase activity. It remains to be determined whether tumor promotion is a related or an unrelated characteristic of a particular class or classes of inducers.

III. Discussion

The identification of a substantial number of compounds having the capacity to inhibit the neoplastic effects of chemical carcinogens gives rise to two questions. The first is, "What is the current role that these compounds play in reducing the impact of chemical carcinogens on man?" and the second, "What is the optimal role that they could have?" The first question can be rephrased in two additional ways that may have some conceptual value, i.e., "Is there a significant balance between carcinogens and anticarcinogenic agents that determines whether an individual will develop cancer?" and "To what extent do variations in cancer incidence among groups of individuals reflect differences in magnitude of exposure to carcinogens, and to what extent to protective agents?" Evidence suggesting that inhibitors do play a role in man is of three types: the nature of the inhibitory compounds themselves, the mechanisms of inhibition, and epidemiological data.

The inhibitors found thus far are very diverse in chemical structure and are widely distributed in the environment. Indeed, their chemical diversity makes it likely that other inhibitors exist that have not yet been identified.

Diversity and wide distribution are factors enhancing the probability that inhibitors have an impact on man. The second type of supporting evidence is the nature of the mechanisms of inhibition. A considerable amount of data indicates that many inhibitors are effective by virtue of enhancing host detoxification systems. These systems have been discussed previously in Section II.A. An important characteristic of these detoxification pathways is that their activities can be changed by xenobiotic compounds occurring in the environment. The microsomal mixed-function oxidase system has the capacity to inhibit chemical carcinogens. This system is particularly notable for its response to xenobiotic compounds. The activity for the microsomal mixed-function oxidase system in metabolizing at least some carcinogens in tissues of the major portals of entry of carcinogens (intestinal tract and lungs) appears to be almost totally determined by exogenous environmental factors (Wattenberg, 1970). Thus, animals fed purified diets and kept in animal quarters with filtered air show almost no mixed-function oxidase activity with polycyclic aromatic hydrocarbons and azo dyes as substrates. The implication of these findings is that the nature of the diet as well as other environmental exposures will determine the activity and characteristics of this important carcinogen-metabolizing system in tissues that come into initial contact with chemical carcinogens.

Some epidemiological data support the possibility that inhibitors in the environment protect against the occurrence of neoplasia. An apparent protective effect of consumption of vegetables against several common cancers, particularly those of the alimentary tract, has been found. Vegetables are a source of many inhibitors of chemical carcinogens since they contain phenols, coumarins, aromatic isothiocyanates, and indoles. Cruciferous vegetables such as cabbage, brussels sprouts, and cauliflower are a particularly rich source of known inhibitors (Wattenberg, 1972c). One of the most dramatic epidemiological investigations is a case-control study by Graham et al., 1978) that shows an inverse correlation between the magnitude of consumption of cabbage and the occurrence of cancer of the colon. The relative risk in individuals with the highest consumption of cabbage as compared to those with little or no intake of this vegetable is about one-third. In a second study, an analysis of risk factors for lung cancer in Singapore Chinese has shown that the relative risk was less in those consuming mustard greens and kale regularly than in individuals with infrequent intake of these vegetables (MacLennan et al., 1977). Several investigations have been published in which an inverse relationship has been found between magnitude of consumption of other vegetables including lettuce, celery, and tomatoes and cancer of the stomach or precursor lesions in that organ (Haenszel *et al.,* 1972, 1976). The reduced incidence of cancer in Seventh Day Adventists, a group that has a vegetarian diet, is well documented and is in accord with the other data discussed above (Phillips, 1975).

The group of epidemiological studies cited is of interest because of the occurrence of inhibitors of chemical carcinogenesis in vegetables. However, these studies cannot be considered as conclusive. At least two major areas of uncertainty exist. The first is a lack of evidence that the relatively high consumption of vegetables has actually enhanced the effectiveness of protective systems against chemical carcinogens in the individuals at risk. Obtaining quantitative data of this nature is critical for establishing firmly a relationship between dietary factors and risk. The second uncertainty is whether there might be important undefined correlates between magnitude of consumption of vegetables and aspects of life style or diet that are the true variables altering the responses of the individual to carcinogens. These obviously are difficult problems and require solutions.

Considerations of the optimal role that compounds that prevent cancer-producing agents from reaching or reacting with critical target sites might play entail evaluations of their deliberate use. At present, it clearly would be premature to undertake such measures. We simply do not have an adequate base of information. However, at a future time when more data are available on mechanisms of inhibition, diversity of inhibitors, and their toxicity, such an investigation might be undertaken. Accordingly, there would be some value in considering factors entailed in making decisions concerning the deliberate use of inhibitors of chemical carcinogenesis. For any normal group of individuals, a critical restraint is the possibility of toxicity. Inhibitors would have to be taken by individuals for many years in order to be effective. Even a low toxicity could outweigh any benefits. However, there are selected situations in which this formidable obstacle might be overcome. One specific instance is carcinogens within the gastrointestinal tract. In this case, it is conceivable that an inhibitor could be designed that would not be absorbed. Under these conditions, a compound with little or no toxicity might be available. The importance of considerations of this type is made more compelling by recent findings of mutagenic substances in the feces (Varghese *et al.,* 1977). If these mutagens are in fact carcinogens, efforts at finding effective inhibitors active within the large bowel might be warranted. In other sites, specific situations amenable to selective approaches could exist as well.

A conceivable basis for introduction of an inhibitor into the environment would be the acquisition of favorable data from epidemiological investigations. Such data should include firm evidence that a population group with a significant intake of a particular inhibitor has a diminished incidence of one or more neoplasms. Mechanistic data relating the intake of the inhibitor to carcinogen inhibition such as tissues from the particular population group showing an increased capacity to detoxify carcinogens would be important. In addition, there should be clear evidence of lack of toxicity from the inhibitor. Under these conditions, consideration of the use of the material bringing about the inhibition might be warranted. This, in essence, is a natural or unplanned type of experiment. Depending on the magnitude of the inhibition and reliability of estimates of lack of adverse side effects, convincing data could be provided for deliberate use of the substance.

There do exist individuals who because of genetic or acquired characteristics are at increased risk from chemical carcinogens. Under these conditions, less rigid requirements for lack of toxicity of inhibitors might be justified. With regard to this possibility, an exceedingly important prohibition is that inhibitors not be used as a mechanism for allowing increased exposures to carcinogens or increasing tolerance levels to cancer-producing substances.

ACKNOWLEDGMENTS. Investigations included in this presentation were supported by Public Health Service Grants CA-09599, CA-15638, and CA-14146 from the National Cancer Institute.

References

Batzinger, R. P., Ou, S. L., and Bueding, E., 1978, Antimutagenic effects of 2(3)-tert-butyl-4-hydroxyanisole and of antimicrobial agents, *Cancer Res.* **12**:4478–4485.

Benson, A. M., Batzinger, R. P., Ou, S. L., Bueding, E., Cha, Y. N., and Talalay, P., 1978, Elevation of hepatic glutathione-S-transferase activities and protection against mutagenic metabolites by dietary antioxidants, *Cancer Res.* **12**:4486–4495.

Bowden, K., Hanson, M. J., and Taylor, G. R., 1968, Reactions of carbonyl compounds in basic solutions. Part I. The alkaline ring fission of coumarins, *J. Chem. Soc. (B)* 174–177.

Cha, Y. N., and Bueding, E., 1979, Effects of 2(3)-tert-butyl-4-hydroxyanisole administration on the activities of several hepatic microsomal and cytoplasmic enzymes in mice, *Biochem. Pharmacol.* **28**:1917–1921.

Dean, F. M., 1963, *Naturally Occurring Oxygen Ring Compounds,* pp. 176–219, Butterworths, London.

Feuer, G., and Kellen, J. A., 1974a, Inhibition of enhancement of mammary tumorigenesis by 7,12-dimethylbenz(*a*)anthracene in the female Sprague–Dawley rats, *Int. J. Clin. Pharmacol.* **9**:62–69.

Feuer, G., and Kellen, J. A., 1974b, Link between carcinogenicity and hepatic metabolism of 7,12-dimethylbenz(*a*)anthracene, *Oncology* **30**:499–508.

Feuer, G., Kellen, J. A., and Kovacs, K., 1976, Suppression of 7,12-dimethylbenz(*a*)anthracene-induced breast carcinoma by coumarin in the rat, *Oncology* **33**: 35–39.

Fiala, E. S., Bobotas, G., Kulakis, C., Wattenberg, L. W., and Weisburger, J. H., 1977, The effects of disulfiram and related compounds on the in vivo metabolism of the colon carcinogen 1,2-dimethylhydrazine, *Biochem. Pharmacol.* 26: 1763–1768.

Frankfurt, O. S., Lipchina, L. P., Bunto, T. V., and Emanuel, N. M., 1967, The influence of 4-methyl-2,6-di-tertbutylphenol (Ionol) on the development of hepatic tumors in rats, *Bull. Exp. Biol. Med.* 8:86–88.

Georgieff, K. K., 1971, Free radical inhibitory effect of some anticancer compounds, *Science* 173: 537–539.

Graham, S., Dayai, H., Swanson, M., Mittelman, A., and Wilkinson, G., 1978, Diet in the epidemiology of cancer of the colon and rectum, *J. Natl. Cancer Inst.* 61:709–714.

Grantham, P. H., Weisburger, J. H., and Weisburger, E. K., 1973, Effects of the antioxidant butylated hydroxytoulene on the metabolism of the carcinogens N-2-fluorenylacetamide and N-hydroxy-N-2-fluorenylacetamide, *Food Cosmet. Toxicol.* 11:209–217.

Haenszel, W., Kurihara, M., Segi, M., and Lee, R. K. C., 1972, Stomach cancer among Japanese in Hawaii, *J. Natl. Cancer Inst.* 49:969–988.

Haenszel, W., Correa, P., Cuello, C., Guzman, N., Burbano, L., Lores, H., and Munoz, J., 1976, Gastric cancer in Colombia: Case-control epidemiological study of precursor lesions, *J. Natl. Cancer Inst.* 57:1021–1026.

Hershfield, R., and Schmir, G. L., 1973, The lactonization of ring-substituted coumarenic acids. Structural effects on the partitioning of tetrahedral intermediate in esterification, *J. Am. Chem. Soc.* 95:7359–7369.

Kitagawa, T., Pitot, H. C., Miller, E. C., and Miller, J. A., 1979, Promotion by dietary phenobarbital of hepatocarcinogenesis by 2-methyl-N,N-dimethyl-4-aminoazobenzene in the rat, *Cancer Res.* 39:112–115.

Lam, L. K. T., and Wattenberg, L. W., 1977, Effects of butylated hydroxyanisole on the metabolism of benzo(*a*)pyrene by mouse liver microsomes, *J. Natl. Cancer Inst.* 58:413–417.

Loub, W. D., Wattenberg, L. W., and Davis, D. W., 1975, Aryl hydrocarbon hydroxylase induction in rat tissues by naturally occurring indoles of cruciferous plants, *J. Natl. Cancer Inst.* 54:985–988.

MacLennan, R., Da Costa, J., Day, N. E., Law, C. H., Ng, Y. N., and Shanmugaratnam, K., 1977, Risk-factors for lung cancer in Singapore Chinese, a population with high female incidence rates, *Int. J. Cancer* 20:854–860.

Marquadt, H., Sapozink, M., and Zedeck, M., 1974, Inhibition by cysteamine-HCl of oncogenesis induced by 7,12-dimethylbenz(*a*)anthracene without affecting toxicity, *Cancer Res.* 34:3387–3390.

Miller, J. A., and Miller, E. C., 1969, The metabolic activation of carcinogenic aromatic amines and amides, *Prog. Exp. Tumor Res.* 11:273–301.

Pantuck, E. J., Hsiao, K. C., Loub, W. D., Wattenberg, L. W., Kuntzman, R., and Conney, A. H., 1976, Stimulatory effect of vegetables on intestinal drug metabolism in the rat, *J. Pharmacol. Exp. Ther.* 198:277–283.

Pantuck, E. J., Pantuck, C. B., Garland, W. A., Mins, B., Wattenberg, L. W., Anderson, K. E., Kappas, A., and Conney, A. Y., 1979, Effects of dietary brussels sprouts and cabbage on human drug metabolism, *Clin. Pharmacol. Ther.* 25:88–95.

Peraino, C., Fry, R. J., Staffeldt, E., and Kisieleski, W. D., 1973, Effects of varying exposure to phenobarbital on its enhancement of 2-acetylaminofluorene-induced hepatic tumorigenesis in the rat, *J. Natl. Cancer Inst.* 33:2701–2705.

Peraino, C., Fry, R. J., Staffeldt, E., and Christopher, J. P., 1977, Enhancing effects of phenobarbitone and butylated hydroxytoluene on 2-acetylaminofluorene-induced hepatic tumorigenesis in the rat, *Food Cosmet. Toxicol.* 15:93–6.

Phillips, R. L., 1975, Role of life-style and dietary habits in risk of cancer among Seventh-Day Adventists, *Cancer Res.* 35:3513–3522.

Poland, A., and Kende, A., 1977, The genetic expression of aryl hydrocarbon hydroxylase activity: Evidence for a receptor mutation in nonresponsive mice, in: *Origins of Human Cancer* (H. H. Hiatt, J. D. Watson, and J. A. Winstein, eds.), pp. 847–867, Cold Spring Harbor Laboratory, New York.

Poland, A., Greenlee, W. F., and Kende, A. S., 1979, Studies on the mechanism of action of the chlorinated dibenzo-*p*-dioxins and related compounds, in: *The Scientific Basis for the Public Control of Environmental Health Hazards*, Vol. 320, pp. 214–230, New York Academy of Sciences, New York.

Robinson, T., 1963, *The Organic Constituents of Higher Plants*, pp. 45–69, Burgess Publishing Co., Minneapolis.

Slaga, T. J., and Bracken, W. M., 1977, The effects of antioxidants on skin tumor initiation and aryl hydrocarbon hydroxylase, *Cancer Res.* **37**:1631–1635.

Spath, E., 1937, Die naturlichen Cumarine, *Ber. Dtsch. Chem. Ges.* **70**:83–117.

Speir, J. L., and Wattenberg, L. W., 1975, Alterations in microsomal metabolism of benzo-(*a*)pyrene in mice fed butylated hydroxyanisole, *J. Natl. Cancer Inst.* **55**:469–472.

Speier, J. L., Lam, L. K. T., and Wattenberg, L. W., 1978, Effects of administration to mice of butylated hydroxyanisole by oral intubation on benzo(*a*)pyrene-induced pulmonary adenoma formation and metabolism of benzo(*a*)pyrene, *J. Natl. Cancer Inst.* **60**:605–609.

Ulland, B. M., Weisburger, J. H., Yammamoto, R. S., and Weisburger, E. K., 1973, Antioxidants and carcinogenesis: Butylated hydroxytoluene, but not diphenyl-*p*-phenylene-diamine, inhibits cancer induction by *N*-2-fluorencylacetamide and by *N*-hydroxy-*N*-2-fluorenylacetamide in rats, *Food Cosmet. Toxicol.* **11**:199–207.

Varghese, A. J., Land, P., Furrer, R., and Bruce, W. R., 1977, Evidence for the formation of mutagenic *N*-nitroso compounds in the human body, *Proc. Am. Assoc. Cancer Res.* **18**:80.

Wattenberg, L. W., 1970, The role of the portal of entry in inhibition of tumorigenesis, *Prog. Exp. Tumor Res.* **14**:89–104.

Wattenberg, L. W., 1972a, Inhibition of carcinogenic and toxic effects of polycyclic hydrocarbons by phenolic antioxidants and ethoxyquin, *J. Natl. Cancer Inst.* **48**:1425–1430.

Wattenberg, L. W., 1972b, Inhibition of carcinogenic effects of diethylnitrosamine and 4-nitroquinoline-*N*-oxide by antioxidants, *Fed. Proc.* **31**:633.

Wattenberg, L. W., 1972c, Enzymatic reactions and carcinogenesis, in: *Environment and Cancer* (R. D. Cumley, ed.), pp. 241–255, William & Wilkins, Baltimore.

Wattenberg, L. W., 1973, Inhibition of chemical carcinogen-induced pulmonary neoplasia by butylated hydroxyanisole, *J. Natl. Cancer Inst.* **50**:1541–1544.

Wattenberg, L. W., 1977, Inhibition of carcinogenic effects of polycyclic hydrocarbons by benzyl isothiocyanate and related compounds, *J. Natl. Cancer Inst.* **58**:395–398.

Wattenberg, L. W., 1978a, Inhibition of chemical carcinogenesis, *J. Natl. Cancer Inst.* **60**:11–18.

Wattenberg, L. W., 1978b, Inhibitors of chemical carcinogens, *Adv. Cancer Res.* **26**:197–226.

Wattenberg, L. W., 1979a, Inhibitors of carcinogenesis, in: *Carcinogens: Identification and Mechanism of Action* (A. C. Griffin and C. R. Shaw, eds.), pp. 299–316, Raven Press, New York.

Wattenberg, L. W., 1979b, Naturally-occurring inhibitors of chemical carcinogenesis, in: *Naturally-Occurring Carcinogens—Mutagens and Modulators of Carcinogenesis. Proceedings of the Sixth International Symposium of the Princess Takamatsu Cancer Research Fund*, pp. 315–329, University of Tokyo Press, Tokyo.

Wattenberg, L. W., and Leong, J. L., 1968, Inhibition of the carcinogenic action of 7,12-dimethylbenz(*a*)anthracene by beta-napthoflavone, *Proc. Soc. Exp. Biol. Med.* **128**:940–943.

Wattenberg, L. W., and Leong, J. L., 1970, Inhibition of the carcinogenic action of benzo(*a*)pyrene by flavones, *Cancer Res.* **30**:1922–1925.

Wattenberg, L. W., and Loub, W. D., 1978, Inhibition of polycyclic hydrocarbon-induced neoplasia by naturally occurring indoles, *Cancer Res.* **38**:1410–1413.

Wattenberg, L. W., and Sparnins, V. L., 1979, Inhibitory effects of butylated hydroxyanisole and methylazoxymethanol acetate-induced neoplasia of the large intestine and on nicotinamide adenine dinucleotide-dependent alcohol dehydrogenase activity in mice, *J. Natl. Cancer Inst.* **63**:219–222.

Wattenberg, L. W., Page, M. A., and Leong, J. L., 1968, Induction of increased benzopyrene hydroxylase activity by flavones and related compounds, *Cancer Res.* **28**:934–937.

Wattenberg, L. W., Lam, L. K. T., and Fladmoe, A. V., 1979, Inhibition of carcinogen-induced neoplasia by coumarins and α-angelicalactone, *Cancer Res.* **39**:1651–1654.

Wislocki, P. G., Miller, E. C., Miller, J. A., McCoy, E. C., and Rosenkranz, H. S., 1977, Carcinogenic and mutagenic activities of safrole, 1'-hydroxysafrole, and some known or possible metabolites, *Cancer Res.* **37**:1883–1891.

Weisburger, E. K., Evarts, R. P., and Wenk, M. L., 1977, Inhibitory effect of butylated hydroxytoluene (BHT) on intestinal carcinogenesis in rats by azoxymethane, *Food Cosmet. Toxicol.* **15**:139–121.

Witschi, H., Williamson, D., and Lock, S., 1977, Enhancement of urethan tumorigenesis in mouse lung by butylated hydroxytoluene, *J. Natl. Cancer Inst.* **58**:301–305.

2

Inhibition of Carcinogen Metabolism and Action by Disulfiram, Pyrazole, and Related Compounds

EMERICH S. FIALA

I. Introduction

In order to manifest their carcinogenic activity, procarcinogens of widely diverse chemical classes such as the polycyclic aromatic hydrocarbons, the N-nitrosamines, the aromatic amines and azo dyes, the aliphatic hydrazo and azoxy compounds, and others (Miller, 1970) must undergo metabolic transformations to their ultimate reactive species. For all of the above procarcinogens, strong evidence has accumulated that these ultimate species have in common the feature of a high degree of electron deficiency, or electrophilicity, and the ability to react with macromolecules such as DNA, RNA, and proteins to produce genetic and epigenetic cellular alterations. Since metabolism is a prerequisite for their carcinogenicity, it is clear that inhibitors and inducers of enzymes involved in the activation or detoxication reactions of these compounds can also profoundly modify their carcinogenic potency.

Although chemical carcinogenesis involves several discrete, progressive stages, any one of which can be subject to modification by chemical or other factors as discussed by the other authors in this volume, for reasons of

---

EMERICH S. FIALA • Naylor Dana Institute for Disease Prevention, American Health Foundation, Valhalla, New York 10595.

personal research interests, I have limited my contribution to the examination of current literature on the effects of the thiono sulfur and pyrazole inhibitors on carcinogen metabolism and action. Thiono sulfur compounds such as the aromatic isothiocyanates, which occur in cruciferous plants consumed by man, and the thiocarbamates and xanthates, which are used in vast quantities as agricultural pesticides, have been shown to be powerful inhibitors of chemical carcinogenesis in animal models (Wattenberg, 1978a,b). Thus, it may not be unreasonable to expect that human exposure to these agents could also, to an as yet undefinable degree, modify the incidence of chemically induced human cancer. The thiono sulfur compounds as well as the pyrazoles, in addition, may prove to be useful tools in the clarification of the metabolic routes of various carcinogens (Grab and Zedeck, 1977; Fiala *et al.*, 1977a,b, 1978a,b). Finally considerations of the mode of action of these inhibitors may be of use in the design of more effective and less toxic agents which could find application in the event that deliberate exposure of human populations to inhibitors of chemical carcinogenesis is seriously considered (Wattenberg, 1978a).

As will become apparent, except in one or two cases, our knowledge of the mechanism of action of these inhibitors is even at best scanty and incomplete. I hope that the present contribution will serve to point out these gaps in our knowledge and stimulate further research in this area which is both intensely interesting and of potential human benefit.

II. Disulfiram

A. Commercial and Medicinal Use

Disulfiram (tetraethylthiuram disulfide, Antabuse®) finds its major commercial use in the processing of natural and synthetic rubbers, with an estimated world production for this purpose of approximately half a million kilograms annually (International Agency for Research on Cancer, 1976). A closely related analogue, tetramethylthiuram disulfide (Thiram®) is an extensively used agricultural fungicide and an accelerator in the compounding of rubber, with an estimated U.S. production, during the 1970s, in the millions of kilograms (International Agency for Research on Cancer, 1976). Medicinally, disulfiram has been in use for the past 30 years in the aversion therapy of chronic alcoholism. The intake of alcohol following the administration of disulfiram (typically 500 mg p.o. daily for 2–3 weeks or 1000–1600 mg/kg by subcutaneous implantation) produces a variety of unpleasant effects including flushing, pounding of the heart and head, dyspnea, and nausea, all of which tend to discourage further drinking. This reaction and other side effects of disulfiram therapy can be quite severe and may even be fatal (Hald and Jacobsen, 1948a; Haley, 1979). The pharmacological and psychological aspects of disulfiram therapy have been described in detail in a recent review (Kwentus and Major, 1979).

The exact mechanism of the disulfiram–alcohol reaction is still controversial (de Saint-Blanquat and Derache, 1976; Faiman, 1979), but a major factor appears to be the inhibition of alcohol metabolism at the level of aldehyde dehydrogenase, thus resulting in the accumulation of toxic acetaldehyde (Hald and Jacobsen, 1948b; Truitt and Walsh, 1971; Deitrich and Erwin, 1971; Kitson, 1976). Disulfiram is also a strong inhibitor of dopamine-β-hydroxylase (Goldstein *et al.*, 1964; McKenna and Di Stefano, 1977), and a mechanism to explain the antialcohol response by depletion of tissue norepinephrine has also been proposed (Truitt and Walsh, 1971). It is of interest that a disulfiramlike reaction to the ingestion of alcohol can also be evoked by a number of compounds structurally unrelated to disulfiram, such as monomethylhydrazine (Abelin *et al.*, 1958), calcium carbimide (Ferguson, 1956), N-(1-hydroxycyclopropyl)-L-glutamine (coprine) (Carlsson *et al.*, 1978; Wiseman and Abeles, 1979), and others (Kitson, 1977; Faiman *et al.*, 1978).

B. Toxicity

The LD_{50} for disulfiram administered p.o. to Wistar rats ranged from 8.6 g/kg when water was the vehicle to 1.3 g/kg when cottonseed oil was used. The Webster mouse is apparently more resistant to the toxic effects of disulfiram; as much as 10 g/kg could be administered p.o. in water with minimal toxic effects (Child and Crump, 1952). Chronic feeding of 0.5 and 1 g of disulfiram per kilogram of diet resulted in significant growth retardation and decrease in longevity of Wistar-derived rats, but concentrations in the diet of 0.125 and 0.25 g/kg were without significant effect (Holck *et al.*, 1970).

C. Effects on Enzyme Systems

Although *in vivo*, the biological effects of disulfiram are not easily separated from those of its pharmacologically active metabolites diethyldithiocarbamate and CS_2, in model systems *in vitro*, disulfiram has been found to inhibit enzymes such as D-amino acid oxidase by reacting with protein sulfhydryl groups (Neims *et al.*, 1966a,b). During this reaction, one-half of the disulfiram molecule binds to a protein–SH group while the other half is liberated as diethyldithiocarbamate:

$$\text{Protein—SH} + (CH_3CH_2)_2N-\underset{\underset{\text{disulfiram}}{}}{\overset{\overset{S}{\|}}{C}}-S-S-\overset{\overset{S}{\|}}{C}-N(CH_2CH_3)_2 \longrightarrow$$

$$\text{Protein—S—S—}\overset{\overset{S}{\|}}{C}-N(CH_2CH_3)_2 + (CH_3CH_2)_2N-\underset{\text{diethyldithiocarbamate}}{\overset{\overset{S}{\|}}{C}}-S^-$$

This thiol–disulfide exchange mechanism is also believed to play a role in the inhibition by disulfiram of aldehyde dehydrogenase (Deitrich and Erwin, 1971), probably of esterases (Zemaitis and Greene, 1976), of hexokinase (Strömme, 1963), and of monoamine oxidase (Schurr *et al.*, 1978).

A second mechanism whereby disulfiram may affect the metabolism of various substrates for the mixed-function oxidase system is by direct binding to cytochrome P-450, producing a type I difference spectrum (Zemaitis and Greene, 1976, 1979; Malejka-Giganti *et al.*, 1980). Chronic treatment (Zemaitis and Greene, 1976; Lang *et al.*, 1976) (300–400 mg/kg daily, 4–12 days) or a single large dose (Hunter and Neal, 1976) (741 mg/kg) of disulfiram produces a depression of rat liver microsome P-450 content with a concomitant decrease in the metabolism of various mixed-function oxidase substrates. At lower levels of chronic feeding (100 mg/kg daily), disulfiram produces only a transient decrease in cytochrome P-450 which eventually returns to normal levels during the feeding, as does enzyme activity toward certain substrates, e.g., ethylmorphine demethylase, although inhibition of other enzyme activities, e.g., hydroxylation of aniline, persists (Zemaitis and Greene, 1976).

Besides its inhibitory effects on enzyme systems *in vitro* and *in vivo*, disulfiram has also been found to increase the levels of certain rat liver enzymes, in particular those involved in the glucuronic acid pathway. Thus, the activities of UDP glucose dehydrogenase, UDP glucuronyltransferase, UDP glucuronate pyrophosphatase, and L-gulonate dehydrogenase were found to be significantly increased after the intragastric administration of the drug (300 mg/kg daily, 4 times) (Marselos *et al.*, 1976). In addition, the levels of liver microsomal cytochrome b_5 and NADPH-cytochrome c reductase were also observed to be significantly increased (Zemaitis and Greene, 1976) after similar treatment.

D. Metabolism

In rats, disulfiram (*1* in Fig. 1) is rapidly absorbed after either oral or i.p. administration. Using ^{35}S-labeled disulfiram, Faiman *et al.* (1978) observed that after 1/2 hr, ^{35}S was found in the thyroid, brain, liver, testis,

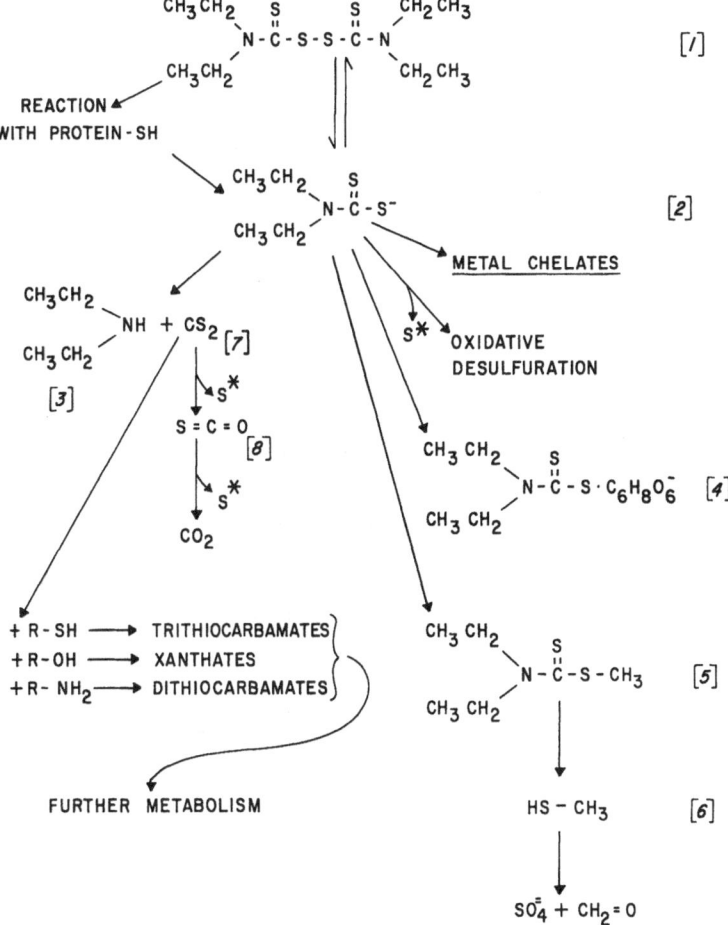

FIGURE 1. Metabolism of disulfiram [*1*]. Diethyldithiocarbamate [*2*]; diethylamine [*3*]; glucuronide of diethyldithiocarbamate [*4*]; methyl ester of diethyldithiocarbamate [*5*]; methyl mercaptan [*6*]; carbon disulfide [*7*]; carbonyl sulfide [*8*].

kidneys, lung, spleen, and plasma. The main excretory route for disulfiram metabolites is the urine (65% of the dose); approximately 20% is excreted in the feces (Strömme, 1966). As much as 12% of the dose may appear in the exhaled air in the form of CS_2 (Faiman et al., 1978; Strömme, 1965a).

The proximate metabolite of disulfiram is diethyldithiocarbamate (2 in Fig. 1) which is formed as a result of a reversible reduction (Strömme, 1963; Zemaitis and Greene, 1976) and also as a result of binding to –SH-containing proteins by a reaction resulting in mixed disulfide formation (Strömme, 1965a,b). The dithiocarbamate is conjugated with glucuronic acid to diethyldithiocarbamate-S-glucuronide (4 in Fig. 1) (Kaslander, 1963). An alternate conjugation reaction involves the formation of the methyl ester (5 in Fig. 1), with S-adenosylmethionine as the methyl donor (Gessner and Jakubowski, 1972). The methyl ester is metabolized further to SO_4^{-2} and formaldehyde, probably via the methyl mercaptan (6 in Fig. 1) intermediate (Gessner and Jakubowski, 1972; Mazel et al., 1964). Alternately, diethyldithiocarbamate is reversibly cleaved to diethylamine (3 in Fig. 1) and CS_2 (Faiman et al., 1978; Linderholm and Berg, 1951). Carbon disulfide is metabolized in vivo as well as in vitro by rat liver microsomes through two successive desulfuration steps to CO_2, with carbonyl sulfide (8 in Fig. 1) as an intermediate (Bond and De Matteis, 1969; Dalvi et al., 1975; Dalvi and Neal, 1978). Additional metabolic reactions of CS_2 may include condensations with thiols, including —SH groups of proteins, alcohols, and amines to form trithiocarbamates, xanthates, and dithiocarbamates, respectively (Kromer and Freundt, 1976; Souček and Mádlo, 1953; McKenna and Di Stefano, 1977). These products presumably could be metabolically recycled in addition to undergoing desulfuration reactions directly. Such recycling, as well as the fact that both the reduction of disulfiram to diethyldithiocarbamate and the cleavage of the latter to CS_2 and diethylamine are reversible in vivo, presents a rather complex situation. Since several of the intermediates in the metabolism of disulfiram possess significant biological activity dependent on quite differing mechanisms, it is clear that attempts to ascribe the in vivo effects of disulfiram to any one metabolite or mechanism may represent at best an oversimplification.

III. Sodium Diethyldithiocarbamate and Dithiocarbamate Pesticides

A. Commercial and Medicinal Use

Sodium diethyldithiocarbamate is produced commercially for use in the rubber industry and in the manufacture of fungicides (International

Agency for Research on Cancer, 1976). The compound is a powerful chelating agent and has been used in the treatment of nickel carbonyl poisoning (Sunderman, 1967). Diethyldithiocarbamate is fairly stable in slightly alkaline (pH 8–9) aqueous solution but rapidly decomposes at pH 4.0, with a half-life of 30 sec to diethylamine and CS_2 (Neims *et al.*, 1966b). Several related dithiocarbamates such as zinc dimethyldithiocarbamate (Ziram®), ferric dimethyldithiocarbamate (Ferbam®), manganese ethylene bis-(dithiocarbamate) (Maneb®), zinc ethylene bis-(dithiocarbamate) (Zineb®), disodium ethylene bis-(dithiocarbamate) (Nabam®), and tetramethyl thiuram disulfide (Thiram®) are extensively used in agriculture as pesticides. The structures of these compounds are shown in Fig. 2.

B. Toxicity

The toxicity, possible carcinogenicity, and environmental health aspects of the dithiocarbamates have been discussed in several reviews (In-

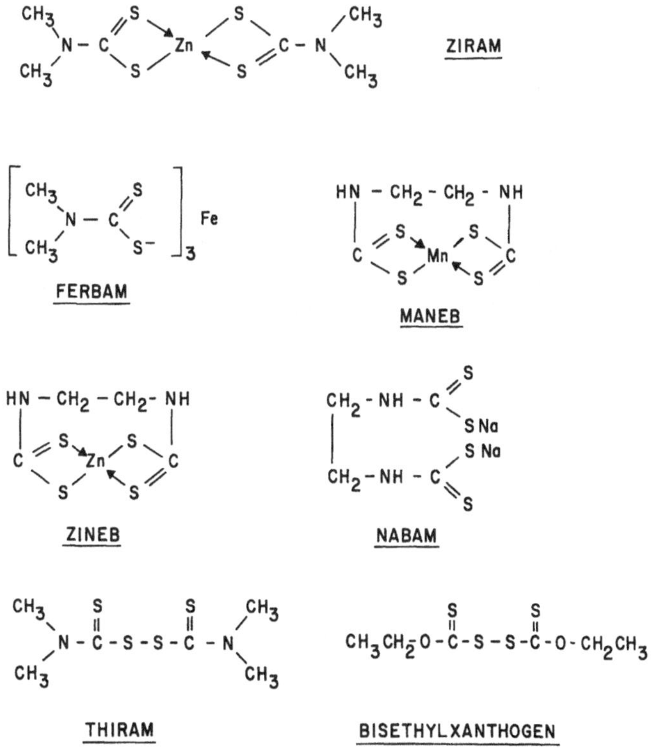

FIGURE 2. Structures of some thiocarbamate pesticides.

ternational Agency for Research on Cancer, 1976; Fishbein, 1976; Lee *et al.*, 1978). The LD_{50} of sodium diethyldithiocarbamate, i.p., in rats is reported as 1.5 g/kg (West and Sunderman, 1958). When fed at levels of 1250 or 2500 ppm in the diets of male and female F344 rats for 104 weeks and at levels of 500 or 4000 ppm in the diets of male and female B6C3F1 mice for 108–109 weeks, sodium diethyldithiocarbamate did not significantly affect longevity in rats but significantly ($p = 0.025$) increased the longevity of female mice (National Cancer Institute, 1979a).

C. Effects on Enzyme Systems

Because of its potent chelating ability, diethyldithiocarbamate can directly inhibit the activity of some metalloenzymes. Thus, the compound has been found to inhibit the copper-containing enzyme superoxide dismutase (Heikkila *et al.*, 1976) which plays a major role in the detoxication of the highly reactive and cytotoxic superoxide radical produced during the biological reduction of molecular oxygen. The inhibition of dopamine-β-carboxylase (Goldstein *et al.*, 1964; McKenna and Di Stefano, 1977) has been suggested to involve a similar mechanism.

The administration of a single large dose (5 mmol/kg) of diethyldithiocarbamate to control or to phenobarbital- or 3-methylcholanthrene-pretreated rats results in a significant decrease of liver microsomal cytochrome P-450 and in inhibition of benzphetamine metabolism. A decrease in cytochrome P-450 is also observed when diethyldithiocarbamate is incubated with rat liver microsomes in the presence of NADPH. Since the decrease does not occur in the absence of NADPH, active metabolism of diethyldithiocarbamate, probably involving oxidative desulfuration, is required for the effect (Hunter and Neal, 1975). Oxidative desulfuration and interactions with sulfhydryl compounds also play major roles in the metabolism and biological activities of the dithiocarbamate fungicides (Fishbein, 1976).

In contrast to disulfiram, neither diethyldithiocarbamate nor the related dimethyl analogue produces measurable binding spectra when added to microsomes, nor do they inhibit the microsomal metabolism of ethylmorphine, a type I compound (Zemaitis and Greene, 1979).

IV. Carbon Disulfide

A. Commercial Use

Carbon disulfide is widely used industrially as a solvent and in the manufacture of viscose rayon, a process involving the formation of polymeric cellulose xanthates. The estimated U.S. production of CS_2 in 1978 was approximately 210,000 metric tons (Stanford Research Institute, 1978). Excessive exposure to CS_2 vapor by viscose rayon workers has been associated with an increased risk for coronary heart disease (Hernberg *et al.*, 1976) as well as other toxic manifestations.

B. Effects on Enzyme Systems

In rats, exposure to CS_2 causes inhibition of various metabolic reactions associated with the microsomal mixed-function oxidase system such as aliphatic C-hydroxylations, aromatic hydroxylations, and oxidative dealkylations (Freundt *et al.*, 1976; Kromer and Freundt, 1976). High doses of CS_2 cause a decrease in the levels of liver microsomal cytochrome P-450, and the decrease is dependent on the metabolism of CS_2 to CO_2. The decrease in cytochrome P-450 caused by CS_2 is stimulated by phenobarbital pretreatment and is reduced by mixed-function oxidase inhibitors such as SKF-525A (De Matteis, 1973; Dalvi *et al.*, 1975; De Matteis and Seawright, 1973). Although evidence exists for a direct, reversible binding of CS_2 at two different sites to microsomal enzymes (Kromer and Freundt, 1976) which may account for the observed loss of enzymatic activity, a second mechanism involving the binding of an active form of sulfur to enzyme protein during the metabolic desulfuration of CS_2 to COS and of COS to CO_2 also plays a role (Dalvi and Neal, 1978; Dalvi *et al.*, 1975). Such binding of sulfur with consequent decrease of enzymatic activity also occurs during the oxidative desulfuration of parathion, phenylthiourea, 1-naphthylisothiocyanate (De Matteis, 1974), and probably of other thiono sulfur compounds such as diethyldithiocarbamate, methimazole, and propylthiouracil (Hunter and Neal, 1975).

V. Pyrazole

A. Metabolism, Toxicity, and Enzyme Inhibition

Pyrazole

and some of its derivatives, in particular 4-methylpyrazole, are known to be potent inhibitors of alcohol dehydrogenase. Pyrazole forms a ternary complex with the enzyme and NAD and acts as a competitive inhibitor with respect to alcohol (Theorell and Yonetani, 1963). Pyrazole is metabolized by the rat to the 3- and 4-hydroxy and to the 3,4-dihydroxy and 1,3,4-trihydroxy derivatives which are excreted as conjugates of pentoses and of glucuronic acid (Clay et al., 1977).

In addition to inhibiting alcohol dehydrogenase both *in vivo* and *in vitro*, pyrazole also inhibits tryptophan pyrrolase (Rouach et al., 1976) and catalase (Feytmans et al., 1973) *in vivo* but not *in vitro*, indicating that metabolism of the drug is necessary for these effects. Pyrazole also inhibits the microsomal metabolism of aniline and pentobarbital as well as benzo[a]pyrene *in vitro* (Lieber et al., 1970) and produces a type II binding spectrum with hepatic microsomes (Rubin et al., 1971). Thus, it is apparent that pyrazole is not only an inhibitor of alcohol dehydrogenase *in vivo* but affects other enzyme systems as well.

The acute LD_{50} of pyrazole in mice or rats has been reported as ranging from 878 to 1360 mg/kg (references in Deis and Lester, 1979), although a single dose of 140 mg/kg p.o. was reported to produce a 50% mortality in female Sprague–Dawley rats as well as a 90–100% incidence of necrosis of the thyroid follicular epithelium 5 days after administration (Szabo et al., 1978). A review of the biochemical pharmacology of the pyrazoles has been published recently (Deis and Lester, 1979).

VI. Polycyclic Aromatic Hydrocarbons: Benzo[a]pyrene and 7,12-Dimethylbenz[a]anthracene

A. Metabolism

A summary of the metabolic steps leading to the production of reactive electrophiles from benzo[a]pyrene (BP) and 7,12-dimethylbenz[a]anthracene (DMBA) is shown in Fig. 3.

For BP (*1* in Fig. 3), the first activation step is epoxidation by the mixed-function oxidase (MFO) cytochrome P-450 system. The epoxide (*2* in Fig. 3) is then hydrated by epoxide hydrase to yield the 7,8-dihydrodiol (*3* in Fig. 3) which is further oxidized at the 9,10 double bond to yield the 7,8-diol-9,10-epoxide (*4* in Fig. 3) believed to be the ultimate carcinogen (Levin et al., 1977, and references therein).

A similar multiple-step sequence plays a role in the biological activation of DMBA (*5* in Fig. 3) in which the 3,4-dihydroxy-1,2-epoxy-1,2,3,4-

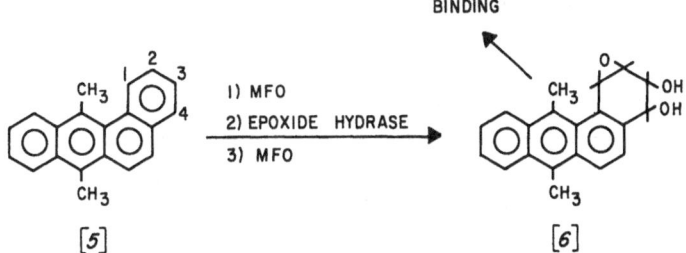

FIGURE 3. Summarized metabolic activation pathways of benzo[a]pyrene [1] and dimethylbenz[a]anthracene [5].

tetrahydro-7,12-dimethylbenz[a]anthracene (6 in Fig. 3) is believed to be the ultimate carcinogen (Bigger et al., 1980, and references therein).

For a complete discussion of the chemistry, metabolism, and carcinogenicity of these and other polycyclic aromatic compounds, the interested reader is referred to a review by Dipple (1976) and to a comprehensive series of reviews edited by Gelboin and Ts'O (1978).

B. Effects of Thiono Sulfur Compounds on Carcinogenicity

Using female ICR/Ha mice fed a diet containing 0.3 mg/g BP, Wattenberg (1974) demonstrated a complete inhibition of tumorigenicity for the forestomach when disulfiram at 0.03 mmol/g (8.9 mg/g) was also included in the diet. In the same report, the effects of disulfiram, dimethyldithiocarbamate, benzyl thiocyanate ($\phi-CH_2-S-C\equiv N$), and other sulfur-containing compounds such as cystine, L-methionine, N-acetyl-L-methionine, and N-acetyl-L-methionine methyl ester were studied with respect to their ability to influence DMBA-induced mammary tumors and adrenal necrosis in female Sprague–Dawley rats. With a single 12-mg dose of DMBA (olive oil; oral intubation), disulfiram at 0.03 mmol/g of diet, dimethyldithiocarbamate at 0.06 mmol/g, and benzyl thiocyanate at 0.03 mmol/g produced significant reduction in both the incidence and multiplicity of mammary tumors. Cystine (0.03 mmol/g), L-methionine, N-acetyl-L-methionine, and N-acetyl-L-methionine methyl ester (all at 0.06 mmol/g diet) had no effect in this respect. It is of interest that disulfiram, dimethyldithiocarbamate, and benzyl isocyanate also prevented the adrenal necrosis induced by a single large (30 mg) intragastric dose of DMBA. As in the case of mammary carcinogenesis, the other sulfur compounds listed above were without protective effect. Using the DMBA-induced adrenal necrosis model, Wattenberg determined a dose–response relationship with disulfiram. Thus, 1 week of feeding of disulfiram at levels of 0.0003, 0.001, and 0.003 mmol/g diet prior to administration of DMBA had no protective effect; 0.01 mmol/g disulfiram had a significant effect, and 0.03 mmol/g afforded complete protection.

These studies were extended by Borchert and Wattenberg (1976) who confirmed the previously observed complete inhibition of the carcinogenicity of BP for the forestomach of ICR/Ha mice and also found a partial inhibition of BP-induced pulmonary tumors by disulfiram. Moreover, using ^{14}C- as well as ^{3}H-labeled BP, Borchert and Wattenberg found significant inhibition of the binding of label to protein, RNA, and DNA isolated from the stomachs of mice on disulfiram-containing diets compared to mice on control diet. Interestingly, no differences caused by disulfiram were detected in the binding of label to macromolecules isolated from the livers of these mice. Binding to lung macromolecules was not determined in these experiments.

In contrast to the inhibition of BP-induced forestomach tumors in mice and of both DMBA-induced mammary carcinogenesis and adrenal necrosis by benzyl thiocyanate in rats, this compound was found to have no protective effect on the induction of forestomach tumors by dietary DMBA (0.05 mg/g) in female ICR/Ha mice (Wattenberg, 1977). However the isomer, benzyl isothiocyanate ($\phi-CH_2-N=C=S$) as well as phenethylisothiocyanate significantly inhibited forestomach tumors induced by DMBA. Although the incidence of pulmonary tumors was unaffected, the number of tumors per mouse decreased significantly. Benzyl isothiocyanate also completely inhibited BP-induced forestomach tumors. When given as a single large dose of 50 mg prior to the administration of 12 mg DMBA p.o. to female Sprague–Dawley rats, benzyl isothiocyanate was found to inhibit the carcinogenicity of the latter for the mammary gland. However, the effect was dependent on the time of administration of the inhibitor: if given 2 or 4 hr prior to the carcinogen, significant inhibition was seen. If given 24 hr before or 4 hr after the carcinogen, much less inhibition was observed (Wattenberg, 1978a).

The exact mechanisms whereby disulfiram, dimethyldithiocarbamate, and the isothiocyanate derivatives exert their inhibitory effects on BP and DMBA carcinogenicity are unknown. It is tempting to suggest that inhibition of the mixed-function oxidase, probably during the oxidative desulfuration of these compounds, with consequent decrease in epoxide formation plays a major role. It would be of interest, in this connection, to examine the effects of CS_2 on the carcinogenicity of BP and DMBA since an inhibitory effect would also be expected if this indeed were the mechanism. Additionally, it would seem desirable to determine the effects of these compounds on the nature of the BP and DMBA metabolites produced *in vitro* by microsomal systems, since such experiments could provide information as to which specific metabolic steps are affected.

VII. Hydrazo and Azoxy Carcinogens

A. 1,2-Dimethylhydrazine

1,2-Dimethylhydrazine is a potent carcinogen which induces tumors of the small and large intestines of mice, rats, and hamsters with a high degree of selectivity (Druckrey *et al.*, 1967b; Oswald and Krüger, 1969; Thurnherr *et al.*, 1973). The organ specificity of the carcinogen is associated with the methyl groups; in contrast to 1,2-dimethylhydrazine, the 1,2-diethyl analogue produces brain, olfactory, and mammary gland tumors (Druckrey *et al.*, 1966). Hydrazine, monomethylhydrazine, and 1,1-dimethylhydrazine are much less carcinogenic, and, depending on the species, strain, and route of administration, produce tumors variously in the liver, kidney, and lung (Toth,

1969, 1973; Biancifiori et al., 1966; Toth and Shimizu, 1973). 1,2-Dimethylhydrazine is effective in producing intestinal tumors when administered repeatedly in small doses, e.g., 7-21 mg/kg, s.c., weekly, 10-20 weeks, and also when given as a single large dose, e.g., 40-200 mg/kg (Martin et al., 1974; Druckrey, 1970).

1,2-Dimethylhydrazine is easily oxidized to azomethane gas either by oxygen in the presence of catalytic amounts of heavy metals (Aebi et al., 1965) or by chemical oxidants such as mercuric oxide (Horisberger and Matsumoto, 1968). The carcinogenic properties of this poisonous and explosive gas have not been studied. Further oxidation, carried out with perbenzoic acid or m-chloroperbenzoic acid (Horisberger and Matsumoto, 1968), converts azomethane to azoxymethane in high yield. Interestingly, azoxymethane is also produced during the treatment of methylamine with various oxidizing agents (Fiala, 1980). Azoxymethane is much more powerful a carcinogen than 1,2-dimethylhydrazine, yet its organospecificity is essentially identical (Druckrey, 1970; Ward, 1975). Bromination of azoxymethane and subsequent reaction with silver acetate produces methylazoxymethyl acetate (Horisberger and Matsumoto, 1968), again a powerful carcinogen with much the same organospecificity as its chemical precursors (Laqueur et al., 1967; Zedeck and Sternberg, 1974). Methylazoxymethyl acetate, a stable liquid, is easily hydrolyzed by various esterases (Poynter et al., 1971/72; Fiala et al., 1976a; Grab and Zedeck, 1977) to the unstable methylazoxymethanol. The latter may also be obtained by β-glucosidase hydrolysis of the naturally occurring carcinogen, cycasin (Matsumoto and Strong, 1963). Various aspects of the use of these carcinogens in experimental intestinal cancer research have been described in several excellent reviews (Weisburger, 1971; Laqueur and Spatz, 1975; Pozharisski et al., 1979).

1. Metabolism

The chemical precursor-product relationship among these carcinogens is also reflected in their metabolism, as shown in Fig. 4. Originally proposed by Druckrey (1969, 1970), the metabolic pathway for the activation of 1,2-dimethylhydrazine has been shown to indeed operate *in vivo*. Thus, after the administration of 1,2-dimethylhydrazine (*1* in Fig. 4) to rats, azomethane (*2* in Fig. 4) was detected in the exhaled air (Fiala et al., 1976b; Rogers and Pegg, 1977), and azoxymethane (*3* in Fig. 4) and methylazoxymethanol (*4* in Fig. 4) were detected in the urine (Fiala, 1977). In addition, the hydroxylation of

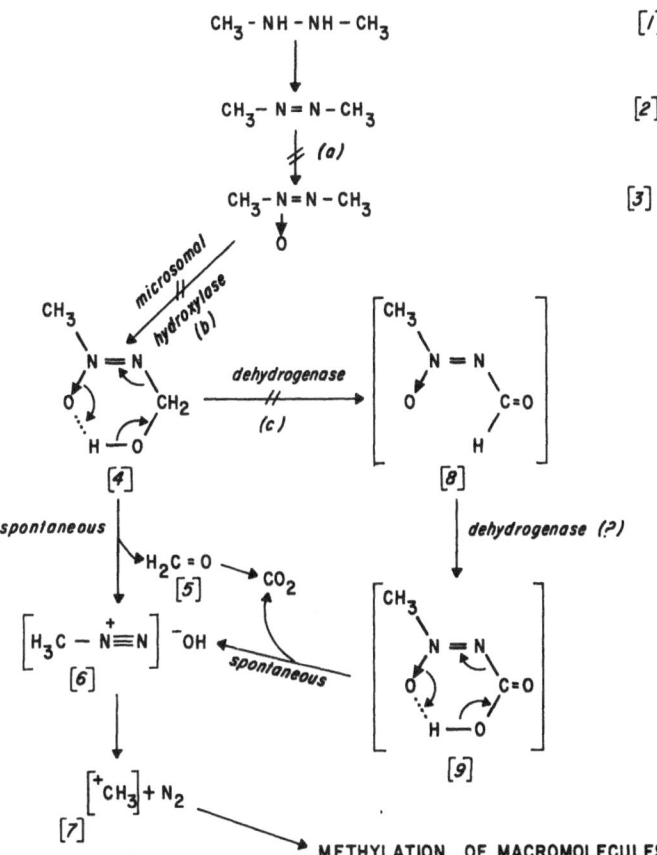

FIGURE 4. Known and postulated steps in the metabolic activation of 1,2-dimethylhydrazine [1]. Azomethane [2]; azoxymethane [3]; methylazoxymethanol [4]; formaldehyde [5]; methyl diazonium ion [6]; methyl carbonium ion [7]; methylazoxyformaldehyde [8]; methylazoxy formic acid [9]. Steps (a) and (b) are blocked by thiono sulfur compounds. Steps (b) and (c) are blocked by pyrazole.

azoxymethane to methylazoxymethanol by rat liver microsomes *in vitro* and also *in vivo* has been demonstrated (Fiala *et al.*, 1977a,b, 1978a).

Methylazoxymethanol is unstable at temperatures above 0°C and, at 37°C, has a half-life in solutions of physiological pH of approximately 8.5 to 12 hr (Fiala *et al.*, 1976a; Grab and Zedeck, 1977). The products of the spontaneous decomposition include formaldehyde (5 in Fig. 4) and the unstable methyl diazonium ion (6 in Fig. 4) (Druckrey, 1970; Nagasawa *et al.*, 1976) which can methylate nucleic acids (Matsumoto and Higa, 1966) and other receptor molecules (Benn and Kazmaier, 1972) through the release of the highly electrophilic methyl carbonium ion (7 in Fig. 4) and N_2. This pathway of successive oxidations of 1,2-dimethylhydrazine leading to the production of the highly reactive electrophile (7 in Fig. 4) was believed to be responsible for the genotoxic (Druckrey, 1973) effects of the carcinogen through the alkylation of colon, liver, and kidney DNA as observed *in vivo* (Hawks and Magee, 1974; Likhachev *et al.*, 1977; Cooper *et al.*, 1978; Zedeck and Brown, 1977; Pegg, 1978; Rogers and Pegg, 1977). However, the breakdown of methylazoxymethanol to a methylating species by a spontaneous process could not, by itself, account for the narrow range of organospecificity of 1,2-dimethylhydrazine and its metabolic or chemical derivatives, since such an event could presumably take place in all tissues with equal facility.

To account for the selective production of intestinal tumors, an elegant mechanism was proposed by Weisburger (1971). In Weisburger's scheme, 1,2-dimethylhydrazine was metabolized in the liver to methylazoxymethanol and the latter conjugated with glucuronic acid. The stable glucuronide was postulated to be transported via the bile to the gut and to be cleaved there by bacterial β-glucuronidase to the unstable alcohol. It is of interest that the β-glucuronide of methylazoxymethanol has been synthesized (Matsumoto *et al.*, 1979) and shown to be mutagenic after hydrolysis with β-glucuronidase (Matsushima *et al.*, 1979). However, it has been shown in both Magee's laboratory (Hawks and Magee, 1974) and our own (Fiala and Weisburger, 1975) that biliary metabolites account for only a very small fraction (*ca.* 0.7–1%) of the 1,2-dimethylhydrazine dose administered. Moreover, several laboratories have demonstrated that 1,2-dimethylhydrazine, azoxymethane, and methylazoxymethyl acetate administered parenterally are active in producing tumors in portions of the colon that are surgically isolated from the fecal stream, indicating that the carcinogens and/or their metabolites reach the intestinal mucosa primarily by the bloodstream rather than the bile (Wittig *et al.*, 1971; Campbell *et al.*, 1975; Matsubara *et al.*, 1978; Rublo *et al.*, 1980).

An alternative explanation for the organospecificity of 1,2-dimethylhydrazine and its derived carcinogens was provided by the discovery by Zedeck and collaborators (Grab and Zedeck, 1977; Zedeck *et al.*, 1979) that cytosol fractions of various rat tissues as well as solutions of purified horse liver alcohol dehydrogenase were able to catalyze the reduction of NAD using methylazoxymethanol as substrate. Moreover, the activity of the various tissues could be directly correlated with their sensitivity to methylazoxymethyl acetate carcinogenesis. Using ammonium sulfate purification followed by column chromatography, Grab and Zedeck demonstrated a close association between rat liver alcohol dehydrogenase and the enzyme utilizing methylazoxymethanol as substrate ("methylazoxymethanol dehydrogenase"). Interestingly, the possibility of the involvement of alcohol dehydrogenase in the metabolism of both N-nitrosamines and methylazoxymethanol had been predicted in 1973 by Schoental. The product of this reaction, presumably methylazoxyformaldehyde (*8* in Fig. 4), has not yet been isolated or chemically synthesized, and thus its chemical and physical properties are unknown. It has been suggested that methylazoxyformaldehyde could be further metabolized by an aldehyde dehydrogenase to the carboxylic acid (*9* in Fig. 4) which by a concerted reaction mechanism might yield the methyl diazonium ion (*6* in Fig. 4) by a loss of CO_2 (Fiala *et al.*, 1978a). Alternately, since alcohol dehydrogenase has known dismutase activity (Abeles and Lee, 1960):

$$\begin{array}{c} R-CH{=}O + NAD \longrightarrow R-COOH + NADH \\ R-CH{=}O + NADH \longrightarrow R-CH_2OH + NAD \\ \hline 2\,R-CH{=}O \longrightarrow R-COOH + R-CH_2OH \end{array}$$

it is possible that this enzyme alone may suffice for the conversion of methylazoxymethanol to the hypothetical unstable acid (*9* in Fig. 4). It must be emphasized that these schemes are highly speculative, with no supporting evidence at this time, and are presented solely with the intent of stimulating further research in this interesting area.

2. Effects of Thiono Sulfur Compounds on Carcinogenicity, Metabolism, and Mutagenicity

The inhibition of the carcinogenicity of 1,2-dimethylhydrazine by disulfiram was first reported by Wattenberg (1975) in what has by now become a classic and widely emulated study. In these experiments, female CF1 mice on control diets or diets containing 5 mg/g disulfiram, 5 mg/g butylated hydroxyanisole, or 1.25 mg/g benzyl isothiocyanate were given 16 weekly injections of 0.7 mg of 1,2-dimethylhydrazine. Whereas all of the mice on the control and benzyl isothiocyanate diets were found to have colon tumors at 36 weeks, no tumors were found in the disulfiram group. In the group receiving

BHA, a 26% reduction of tumors of the colon was found. In similar studies, Wattenberg et al. (1977) found that sodium diethyldithiocarbamate, at levels of 1.5 or 7.5 mg/g diet, and bisethylxanthogen or Maneb® at levels of 5 mg g diet also completely inhibited 1,2-dimethylhydrazine carcinogenicity in mice.

Having developed the necessary methods for the study of 1,2-dimethylhydrazine metabolism (Fiala et al., 1976a, at about the same time that Wattenberg's studies came to our attention, our laboratory had an obvious interest in determining the effects of disulfiram on the metabolism of the carcinogen. Following the protocol of Schmähl and Krüger (1972), we pretreated male F344 rats with 1 g/kg disulfiram p.o. and gave s.c. injections of either 21 mg/kg or 200 mg/kg of [^{14}C]1,2-dimethylhydrazine 2 hr later (Fiala et al., 1977a). The rats pretreated with disulfiram and given 21 mg/kg [^{14}C]1,2-dimethylhydrazine exhaled 36% of the dose in the form of azomethane. This represented an increase of some 180% with respect to control rats pretreated p.o. with vehicle (4% starch) only. At the same time, the amount of $^{14}CO_2$, the ultimate metabolic product of the labeled carcinogen in the exhaled air, was decreased from approximately 10% of the dose in the controls to approximately 2% in the rats pretreated with disulfiram. Analysis of the urines of the disulfiram-pretreated rats by high-pressure liquid chromatography showed an almost complete absence of 1,2-dimethylhydrazine metabolites such as azoxymethane and methylazoxymethanol, in contrast to the controls. Although the increase in exhaled azomethane by disulfiram might conceivably have been caused by a stimulation of the oxidation of 1,2-dimethylhydrazine, the decreases in exhaled $^{14}CO_2$ and in urinary metabolites indicated, rather, that the oxidation of 1,2-dimethylhydrazine to azomethane proceeded normally in these animals but that the further metabolism of azomethane was blocked. Thus, azomethane accumulated and was excreted in higher amounts. A block at the stage of N-oxidation of azomethane to azoxymethane would also prevent the formation of methylazoxymethanol and the proximate carcinogen, the methyl diazonium ion. Thus, these experiments explained Wattenberg's observations on the inhibition of 1,2-dimethylhydrazine carcinogenicity by disulfiram in biochemical terms.

The conclusion that disulfiram would block the formation of an alkylating species from 1,2-dimethylhydrazine was directly confirmed by Swenberg et al. (1979). These workers found that the inclusion of 5 mg/g disulfiram in the diet of BP rats lowered the amount of DNA alkylation by 1,2-dimethylhydrazine, as reflected in 7-methyl- and O^6-methylguanine content, to less than 1% of the control (no disulfiram) levels. Similar results were obtained by Likhachev et al. (1978).

We obtained clear-cut evidence for the inhibition of azomethane N-oxidation only at the lower of the two doses of 1,2-dimethylhydrazine used. At the 200-mg/kg dose of the carcinogen, disulfiram increased the amount of azomethane exhaled by only 27%. Also, high-pressure liquid chromatography of the urines of the disulfiram-pretreated rats showed the presence of both methylazoxymethanol and azoxymethane, although in lower amounts than in the control rats. This indicates that the inhibitory effect of disulfiram on the carcinogenicity of 1,2-dimethylhydrazine would probably also be dependent on the dose of the carcinogen.

Having localized the action of disulfiram to the inhibition of the N-oxidation of azomethane, we further sought to determine what structural feature of the disulfiram molecule was required for this effect. For this purpose we compared the effects of disulfiram and its metabolites, diethyldithiocarbamate, diethylamine, and carbon disulfide on the ability to inhibit [^{14}C]1,2-dimethylhydrazine metabolism. Also included in this series of experiments were bisethylxanthogen (Fig. 2) which contains the —O—(C=S)—S— group rather than the >N—(C=S)—S— group of disulfiram, sec-butyldisulfide which contains the —S—S— group but not a thiono sulfur group, and triethylamine. The last, a tertiary amine, was used because it could not be completely excluded that possible N-oxidation of disulfiram was competing with the N-oxidation of azomethane.

The results obtained (Fiala *et al.*, 1977a) showed that disulfiram, diethyldithiocarbamate, carbon disulfide, and bisethylxanthogen had virtually identical effects: these compounds increased the amounts of azomethane and decreased the amounts of $^{14}CO_2$ in the exhaled air. They significantly decreased the urinary levels of azoxymethane, methylazoxymethanol, and other products of 1,2-dimethylhydrazine metabolism and also decreased the levels of ^{14}C in various organs such as the colon mucosa, liver, kidney, spleen, and lung. In contrast, treatments with equimolar amounts of diethylamine, triethylamine, or sec-butyldisulfide were completely ineffective in these respects.

These results showed that the presence of the thiono sulfur group >C=S, rather than the presence of a nitrogen or a disulfide bond, is necessary for the inhibition of 1,2-dimethylhydrazine metabolism. Furthermore, the results suggested that carbon disulfide itself should inhibit the carcinogenicity of 1,2-dimethylhydrazine. This prediction was tested in animal experiments by Wattenberg and Fiala (1978). While approximately 50% of female CF1 mice treated with 1,2-dimethylhydrazine (0.4 mg per week for 8 weeks, then 0.6 mg per week for 8 weeks) developed neoplasms of the large intestine and anus, no neoplasms developed when each injection of the carcinogen was preceded by the p.o. administration of 2.5 or 5.0 mg of carbon disulfide.

A second block in the metabolic activation of 1,2-dimethylhydrazine by disulfiram and carbon disulfide was demonstrated when we showed that these compounds inhibited the *in vivo* (Fiala, 1977) metabolism of ^{14}C-labeled azoxymethane. Both compounds given orally 2 hr prior to the s.c. administration of [^{14}C]azoxymethane completely inhibited the metabolism of the carcinogen to $^{14}CO_2$ for approximately 6 hr. After this time, metabolism resumed, probably because of the limited half-life of the inhibitors in the rat. High-pressure liquid chromatographic examination of the urines of the rats treated with the inhibitors showed a virtual absence of metabolites with nonmetabolized [^{14}C]azoxymethane as the major labeled urinary component, in contrast to the urines of control animals which contained significant amounts of [^{14}C]methylazoxymethanol, [^{14}C]urea, and other metabolites of the carcinogen. These results, which indicated that disulfiram and CS_2 inhibit the hydroxylation of azoxymethane to methylazoxymethanol, were confirmed by *in vitro* studies (Table 1). The addition of either disulfiram or CS_2 to a rat liver microsomal system resulted in an almost complete inhibition of the conversion of azoxymethane to methylazoxymethanol as detected by a high-pressure liquid chromatographic method (Fiala, 1977). Similar inhibition of azoxymethane hydroxylation was obtained with liver microsomes from rats pretreated with disulfiram (Table 1).

The inhibition of the *in vitro* metabolism of azoxymethane by disulfiram was also demonstrated by Campbell *et al.* (1978). The inclusion of disulfiram in the diet (0.25%, 2 days prior to sacrifice) was found to reduce by 70% the rate of rat liver microsome-mediated metabolism of azoxymethane to formaldehyde, although the cytochrome P-450 levels were not significantly altered. The demethylation of azoxymethane to formaldehyde by rat liver microsomes had been reported earlier by Preussman *et al.* (1969); this reaction may represent an initial hydroxylation to methylazoxymethanol followed by spontaneous breakdown to formaldehyde and the methyldiazonium ion (Fig. 4).

Disulfiram was found to inhibit the carcinogenicity of azoxymethane in mice by Wattenberg *et al.* (1977) and in rats by Nigro and Campbell (1978). However, in contrast to the results obtained with 1,2-dimethylhydrazine where complete inhibition of carcinogenicity was observed, disulfiram had only a partial protective effect in both cases. The difference is probably explained by the fact that in the case of 1,2-dimethylhydrazine, disulfiram inhibits two consecutive steps in the activation sequence, whereas in the case

TABLE 1. Inhibition of Hydroxylation of Azoxymethane to
Methylazoxymethanol by CS_2 and Disulfiram

System	Methylazoxymethanol formed (nmol/mg microsomal protein)
Complete[a]	15.3 ± 3.2 (8)[b]
Minus NADPH generating system	0 (2)
Minus NADPH generating system plus NADH	0 (2)
Complete minus O_2	0–3 (3)
Complete plus 3 μmol disulfiram	<1 (3)
Complete plus 3 μmol CS_2	<1 (3)
Complete; rats pretreated with disulfiram (1 g/kg, 3 hr prior to sacrifice)	<1 (3)

[a] 1.5 ml incubation mixtures contained 5 μmol azoxymethane, 15 μmol $MgCl_2$, 15 μmol glucose-6-phosphate, 30 μg glucose-6-phosphate dehydrogenase, 300 nmol NADP, 2.4 mg (protein) rat liver microsomes, and 1.2 ml 0.07 M sodium phosphate buffer, pH 7.8. Incubations were carried out at 37° for 15 min. Methylazoxymethanol was determined as described previously (Fiala, 1977).
[b] Values in parenthesis represent replicate determinations.

of azoxymethane, only one metabolic step is inhibited. Thus, even if the inhibitions of N-oxidation and the hydroxylation reactions by disulfiram were incomplete, a greater net effect in the case of 1,2-dimethylhydrazine would be expected.

The effects of disulfiram on the carcinogenicity of methylazoxymethyl acetate in mice were also studied by Wattenberg (personal communication) but, in this case, no protection was found. This suggests that if disulfiram or its metabolites act as scavengers for the ultimate reactive species in the 1,2-dimethylhydrazine activation pathway, such a role is very minor. Also the lack of effect of disulfiram, a potent inhibitor of certain forms of aldehyde dehydrogenase, may be an argument against the suggested role of this enzyme in the further activation of methylazoxyformaldehyde (8 in Fig. 4).

Using the *Salmonella* assay (Ames *et al.*, 1975), Rosin and Stich (1979) found no inhibition by disulfiram of the mutagenicities of the direct acting carcinogens N-methyl-N'-nitro-N-nitrosoguanidine or of N-acetoxy-2-acetyl-aminofluorene, although cysteamine, sodium bisulfite, selenite, and propyl gallate inhibited the mutagenicity of the former, and propyl gallate, selenite, and cysteamine inhibited the mutagenicity of the latter carcinogen. On the other hand, using 1,2-dimethylhydrazine and azoxymethane in the *Salmonella* host-mediated assay, Moriya *et al.* (1978, 1979) found inhibition of mutagenicity by disulfiram, diethyldithiocarbamate, CS_2, and Maneb® as well as by pyrazole and aminoacetonitrile. Sodium selenite in the same assay produced no inhibition of mutagenicity.

3. Effects of Pyrazole

As described above, Grab and Zedeck (1977) showed that methylazoxymethanol served as substrate for the reduction of NAD catalyzed by purified horse liver alcohol dehydrogenase and by cytosol preparations of rat liver, colon, and cecum. Such reactions were found to be inhibited by the addition of pyrazole to the incubation mixture, affording additional evidence that the enzyme responsible for the metabolism of the carcinogen was alcohol dehydrogenase.

In the same series of experiments, Grab and Zedeck (1977) were able to either partially or completely inhibit the lethality of large doses of methylazoxymethyl acetate in weanling male Sprague–Dawley rats by pyrazole. The lethal effects of dimethylnitrosamine, methyl(acetoxymethyl)nitrosamine, and N-methyl-N-nitrosourea were not significantly affected by the drug. Interestingly, disulfiram given 2 hr prior to methylazoxymethyl acetate considerably increased the lethality of the carcinogen (Zedeck *et al.*, 1979). Pyrazole also decreased the inhibition of colonic DNA synthesis induced by methylazoxymethyl acetate; in contrast, disulfiram potentiated this effect of the carcinogen. Whereas rats treated with the carcinogen only (single dose of 35 mg/kg) developed tumors of the colon and duodenum, rats pretreated with pyrazole developed no intestinal tumors but tumors of the kidney, of Zymbal's gland, and skin squamous papillomas (Zedeck and Tan, 1978). These results were interpreted by Zedeck to indicate that methylazoxyformaldehyde (*8* in Fig. 4) represents the ultimate active metabolite of methylazoxymethanol.

While treatment with pyrazole prevents the formation of methylazoxyformaldehyde *in vitro* and *in vivo*, treatment with disulfiram may prevent its further oxidation by aldehyde dehydrogenase and thus cause its accumulation with a concomitant increase in toxicity (Zedeck *et al.*, 1979). The inhibition of carcinogenicity in certain organs (colon), but not others (Zymbal's gland), that was obtained with pyrazole by Zedeck may be consistent with the fact that various alcohol dehydrogenases are inhibited to greater or lesser extent by pyrazole depending on their source (Deis and Lester, 1979). However, in view of the interaction of pyrazole with cytochrome P-450 and its inhibition of enzymes other than alcohol dehydrogenase, caution should be used in the interpretation of *in vivo* experiments utilizing this drug.

The effects of pyrazole pretreatment on the metabolism of symmetrically ^{14}C-labeled azoxymethane in F-344 rats were studied by Fiala *et al.* (1978a). Pretreatment with 360 mg/kg pyrazole prior to the administration of 10.5 mg/kg azoxymethane caused a complete inhibition of exhaled $^{14}CO_2$ for approximately 6–8 hr; after this period, metabolism to $^{14}CO_2$ resumed although at a lower rate. Accompanying the inhibition of exhaled $^{14}CO_2$ was a greatly enhanced excretion of nonmetabolized azoxymethane in the urine. At lower doses of pyrazole, exhaled $^{14}CO_2$ was only partially decreased, and increased quantities of methylazoxymethanol (with respect to vehicle pretreated controls) were found in the urine.

These results indicated that pyrazole inhibited at least two steps in the metabolism of the carcinogen. At the lower dose level, alcohol dehydrogenase was inhibited preferentially, in agreement with the results of Zedeck, resulting in greater urinary excretion of methylazoxymethanol. At the higher dose level of pyrazole, the hydroxylation of azoxymethane to methylazoxymethanol was inhibited, resulting in greater excretion of nonmetabolized azoxymethane. Both blocks would be expected to lead to lower $^{14}CO_2$ excretion, as was actually observed. Pyrazole also inhibited the *in vitro* hydroxylation of azoxymethane to methylazoxymethanol by a rat liver microsomal system at concentrations approximately equal to those used in the *in vivo* studies. These results are in agreement with those of Rubin *et al.* (1971), indicating that pyrazole inhibits not only alcohol dehydrogenase enzymes but also microsomal oxygenases.

B. Procarbazine

Procarbazine [N-isopropyl-α-(2-methylhydrazine)-p-toluamide], a hydrazine structurally related to 1,2-dimethylhydrazine, has been used as an antineoplastic agent in advanced Hodgkin's disease and in oat-cell carcinoma of the lung (Carter and Slavik, 1974). The compound itself is carcinogenic in rodents (Kelly *et al.*, 1969; Deckers *et al.*, 1974; National Cancer Institute, 1979b), producing malignant lymphomas, ear duct tumors, mammary adenocarcinomas, and brain tumors in rats and malignant lymphomas or leukemias and olfactory, lung, and uterine tumors in mice. The carcinostatic activity appears to depend on the presence of the methyl group, since the ethyl and N_1-desmethyl analogues are inactive (Schwartz *et al.*, 1967). As in the case of 1,2-dimethylhydrazine and methylazoxymethanol, procarbazine has been demonstrated to methylate DNA *in vivo* (Kreis *et al.*, 1966).

The metabolism of procarbazine in rats and *in vitro* has recently been reinvestigated and, up to a point, appears to follow a course analogous to that of 1,2-dimethylhydrazine (Weinkam and Shiba, 1978; Prough *et al.*, 1979; Dunn *et al.*, 1979) as shown in Fig. 5. Procarbazine (*1* in Fig. 5) is metabolically oxidized to the azo derivative (*2*) which in turn is N-oxidized to

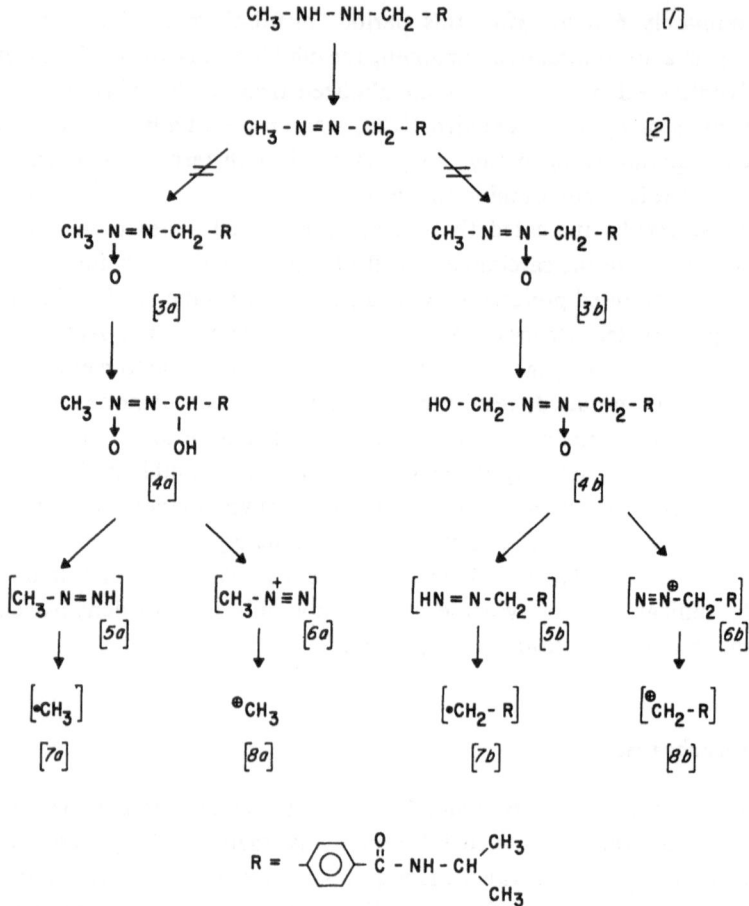

FIGURE 5. Known and postulated metabolic steps in the activation of procarbazine. Note similarity to activation of 1,2-dimethylhydrazine, shown in Fig. 4.

two isomeric azoxy metabolites (*3a* and *3b*). This oxidation can be carried out by rat liver microsomes and is apparently mediated by cytochrome P-450. The *N*-oxidation is sensitive to inhibition by methimazole and metyrapone as well as, in analogy to the *N*-oxidation of azomethane, by disulfiram (Dunn *et al.*, 1979).

Not all of the metabolites shown in Fig. 5 have been conclusively identified, but it would appear that the *N*-oxidation step may be followed by hydroxylation of either the methyl or methylene functions, yielding methyl (*7a* in Fig. 5) and benzylic (*7b*) free radicals and methyl (*8a*) and benzylic (*8b*) carbonium ions as the ultimate reactive species (Weinkam and Shiba, 1978).

Since procarbazine has been found to be converted in part to methane *in vivo* (Schwartz *et al.*, 1967; Dost and Reed, 1967), evidence for the methyl free radical as a metabolite of procarbazine does exist, although such a species may also be formed by pathways other than those in Fig. 5 (Prough *et al.*, 1969).

The effects of disulfiram or other inhibitors on the carcinogenic and/or carcinostatic effects of procarbazine have not as yet been reported in the literature. Such studies may have some merit, since it does not seem impossible that, with an appropriate choice of inhibitors, a preferential enhancement of one or other of the dual biological properties of procarbazine could be effected.

VIII. *N*-Nitrosamines

The chemistry, biochemistry, and carcinogenicity of *N*-nitroso compounds have been comprehensively reviewed by Druckrey *et al.* (1967a), Magee *et al.* (1976), and more recently by Digenis and Issidores (1979). As is the case with the 1,2-dialkylhydrazines, the target organs for the carcinogenicity of *N*-nitrosamines are determined by the nature of the side groups and, presumably, by organ-specific metabolism. In the case of dimethyl-and diethylnitrosamines, the initial activation step involves α-hydroxylation catalyzed by the microsomal cytochrome P-450 system (Czygan *et al.*, 1973; Lotlikar *et al.*, 1975). Metabolism of higher dialkylnitrosamines can involve α-hydroxylation as well as β- or ω-hydroxylation (cf. dibutylnitrosamine discussed in Section VIIIC). Loss of aldehyde from the α-hydroxy metabolite yields an alkyldiazohydroxide which forms the alkylating carbonium ion through the alkyldiazonium ion (Druckrey, 1973; Lijinsky *et al.*, 1968). The activation sequence for dimethylnitrosamine ($R = H$) and diethylnitrosamine ($R = CH_3$) is shown in Fig. 6.

A. Dimethylnitrosamine and Diethylnitrosamine

The effects of disulfiram on the toxicity of various carcinogenic nitrosamines was studied by Schmähl *et al.* (1971, 1976; Schmähl and Krüger, 1972). Pretreatment of mice or rats with disulfiram was found to protect the animals against the acute toxicity of dimethylnitrosamine. Thus, administration of 0.5 g/kg disulfiram by stomach tube 2 hr prior to treatment with

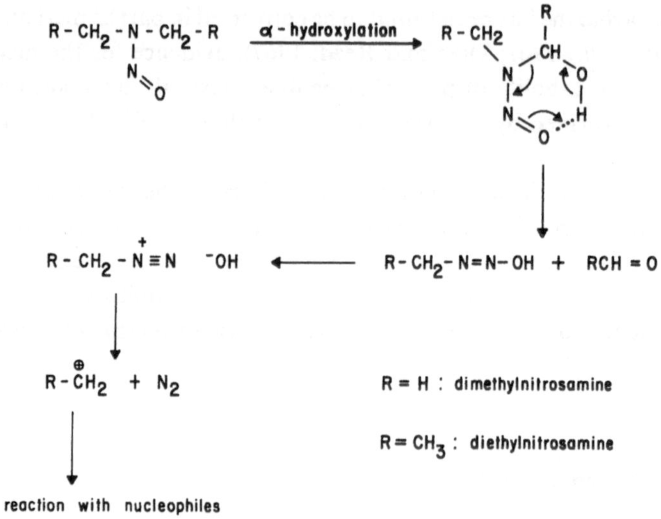

$$R-CH_2-N(N=O)-CH_2-R \xrightarrow{\alpha\text{-hydroxylation}} R-CH_2-N(N=O)-CH(OH)-R$$

$$R-CH_2-\overset{+}{N}\equiv N \quad {}^-OH \longleftarrow R-CH_2-N=N-OH + RCH=O$$

$$R-\overset{\oplus}{CH_2} + N_2$$

$R = H$: dimethylnitrosamine

$R = CH_3$: diethylnitrosamine

reaction with nucleophiles

FIGURE 6. Metabolic activation of dimethylnitrosamine and diethylnitrosamine.

dimethylnitrosamine increased the LD_{50} of the latter from 15 to 27 mg/kg in mice (dimethylnitrosamine given i.p.) and from 63 to 130 mg/kg in rats (dimethylnitrosamine given i.v.). Administration of cysteine had no effect on the toxicity of the carcinogen (Schmähl and Krüger, 1972). Similar toxicity studies with diethyl-, dipropyl-, dibutyl-, and methylpropylnitrosamine and also nitrosomethylurea showed only a slight increase in the LD_{50} of diethylnitrosamine in mice and no effect in rats after pretreatment with disulfiram. No effects of the drug on the toxicity of the other nitrosamines were found.

Using ^{14}C-labeled dimethylnitrosamine, Schmähl and Krüger (1972) found that pretreatment with disulfiram caused a substantial decrease in the amount of ^{14}C incorporated into both RNA and DNA in mouse liver. A decrease in the amount of methylation of guanine at the 7 position was also observed. Thus, these effects paralleled the inhibition of toxicity by disulfiram.

In carcinogenicity studies, Schmähl et al. (1976) found that disulfiram did not decrease the carcinogenicity but, interestingly, changed the organotropy of both dimethyl- and diethylnitrosamine in Sprague–Dawley rats. Repeated weekly administrations of 20 mg/kg diethylnitrosamine alone produced liver tumors in 90% of the rats and malignant carcinomas of the esophagus in 29%. When each administration of the carcinogen was preceded by an intubation of disulfiram (500 mg/kg), 81% of the rats developed predominantly carcinomas of the esophagus and only 31% presented with liver tumors. When dimethylnitrosamine was given at repeated doses of 4 mg/kg per week, 55% of the rats developed liver tumors (mean survival time, 70 weeks). Pretreatment with disulfiram, as in the case of diethylnitrosamine, decreased the number of liver tumors to 3% but curiously produced a high incidence (59%) of squamous cell carcinomas of the paranasal sinus.

In related studies, Abanobi *et al.* (1977) examined the protective effects of diethyldithiocarbamate on liver toxicity and damage to liver DNA in male Wistar rats. As in the experiments of Schmähl and Krüger with disulfiram (Schmähl and Krüger, 1972), Abanobi *et al.* found that pretreatment with diethyldithiocarbamate afforded a temporary protection to rats against liver cell necrosis caused by dimethylnitrosamine (0.14 mmol/kg, i.p.). The carcinogen also caused extensive fragmentation of hepatic DNA, as detected by centrifugation in alkaline sucrose gradients. However, pretreatment with 2.9 mmol/kg diethyldithiocarbamate i.p. 45 min prior to the carcinogen prevented such fragmentation. Pretreatment with diethyldithiocarbamate also resulted in an almost complete inhibition of incorporation of ^{3}H derived from ^{3}H-labeled dimethylnitrosamine into liver DNA. Diethyldithiocarbamate also decreased the clearance of the carcinogen from the blood stream and inhibited its *in vitro* metabolism to formaldehyde by rat liver or hamster microsomes.

In the same series of experiments, Abanobi *et al.* looked for the prevention by diethyldithiocarbamate of strand breakage of liver DNA produced by a variety of other direct and indirect carcinogens. However, in contrast to the results with dimethylnitrosamine, pretreatment with diethyldithiocarbamate had no effect on DNA strand breakage produced by N-hydroxy-2-acetylaminofluorene, 3-hydroxyxanthine, aflatoxin B_1, N-acetoxy-2-acetylaminofluorene, methylmethane sulfonate, methylnitrosourea, or methylazoxymethyl acetate.

The *in vivo* effects of diethyldithiocarbamate were found to be transitory, lasting for approximately 4 hr. For protection longer than 4 hr, multiple administrations of diethyldithiocarbamate were required. Abanobi *et al.* concluded that as long as diethyldithiocarbamate is present in the animal, the metabolic activation of dimethylnitrosamine is inhibited. Coincidently, this inhibition prevents the excretion of the carcinogen and maintains its levels in the rat. Once the levels of diethyldithiocarbamate are decreased through metabolism, the blocks imposed on the activation of the carcinogen are lifted.

The effects of disulfiram, pyrazole, 4-methylpyrazole, and 3-amino-1,2,4-triazole on the metabolism of dimethylnitrosamine, diethylnitrosamine, and N-nitrosopyrrolidine in rats have been extensively studied by Phillips and Lake and associates. With regard to dimethylnitrosamine, Lake *et al.* (1975)

found that this carcinogen was metabolized by rat liver microsomes to methanol in addition to formaldehyde. Although metabolism could be stimulated by phenobarbital pretreatment, conversion to methanol and formaldehyde was significantly inhibited by pyrazole and 3-amino-1,2,4-triazole, known inhibitors of alcohol dehydrogenase and catalase, respectively. Although pyrazole, as discussed previously (Section V.A), exhibits a type II binding spectrum, neither this drug nor 3-amino-1,2,4-triazole inhibited the microsomal metabolism of aniline, a type II compound, or of ethylmorphine, a type I compound.

The observed lack of inhibition of aniline metabolism is not in agreement with the results of Lieber *et al.* (1970). *In vivo* studies from the same laboratory (Phillips *et al.*, 1977) showed that pretreatment with pyrazole, 3-amino-1,2,4-triazole, 4-methylpyrazole, disulfiram, methanol, or ethanol, markedly inhibited the amount of $^{14}CO_2$ exhaled by rats treated with [^{14}C]dimethylnitrosamine. In analogy to the results obtained by Grab and Zedeck (1977) with methylazoxymethyl acetate and pyrazole described above (Section VII.A.3), Phillips *et al.* (1977) found that pretreatment with pyrazole provided significant protection against the lethality of dimethylnitrosamine, increasing the median LD_{50} of the carcinogen and lowering its hepatotoxicity.

Although the *in vitro* effects of these compounds could be ascribed to the inhibition of the dimethylnitrosamine hydroxylase and are similar to our observed inhibition of microsomal azoxymethane hydroxylase (Fiala *et al.*, 1978a) by pyrazole and disulfiram, the *in vivo* effects are more difficult to interpret, since the inhibitors could also be blocking the further oxidation of methanol and formaldehyde to CO_2. The effects of the pyrazoles alone or in conjunction with disulfiram on the carcinogenicity of dimethylnitrosamine could provide additional information on the mechanism of these agents.

B. *N*-Nitrosopyrrolidine

The metabolic activation of *N*-nitrosopyrrolidine, a powerful hepato-

carcinogen in rats has been described by Hecht *et al.* (1978) who demonstrated α-hydroxylation of the carcinogen as an activation pathway by rat liver microsomes and also *in vivo*. With regard to metabolism *in vivo*, Cottrell *et al.* (1979) showed that the metabolism of N-nitroso-[2,5-^{14}C]pyrrolidine to $^{14}CO_2$ in the rat was considerably inhibited by pretreatment with disulfiram, pyrazole, 3-methylpyrazole (a poor inhibitor of alcohol dehydrogenase), iminazole (a monoamine oxidase inhibitor and, like pyrazole, a type II binding compound), and tranylcypromine (a potent monoamine oxidase inhibitor). Iminazole, pyrazole, and disulfiram, in that order, were also effective in prolonging the half-life of the carcinogen in rat blood. The effects of these inhibitors on the carcinogenicity of N-nitrosopyrrolidine have not as yet been determined.

C. N-n-Butyl-N-(4-hydroxybutyl)nitrosamine

The selective carcinogenicity of di-n-butylnitrosamine (DBN) and N-n-butyl-N-(4-hydroxybutyl)nitrosamine (BBN) for the rat bladder was discovered by Druckrey *et al.* (1964). The metabolism of these compounds has been extensively studied by Okada and co-workers (Okada and Ishidata, 1977; Okada and Suzuki, 1972). A major metabolite of both DBN and BBN in the rat is N-n-butyl-N-(3-carboxypropyl)nitrosamine (BCPN). The latter is a strong urinary bladder carcinogen as well as a mutagen in *S. typhimurium* TA 1535 without S-9 activation (Okada and Ishidate, 1977) and thus may represent the proximate carcinogen. A partial scheme for the metabolism of DBN is shown in Fig. 7.

Disulfiram was found by Irving *et al.* (1979) to be a potent inhibitor of the carcinogenicity of BBN for the rat urinary bladder. In these experiments, male Wistar rats were given 0.025% BBN in the drinking water, with or without 0.5% disulfiram in the diet, for 15 weeks. Twenty-five weeks after the initial exposure to BBN, 27 of 27 rats treated with BBN alone presented with bladder cancer, whereas 0 of 27 rats treated with BBN and disulfiram were so affected. At 32–42 weeks after initial exposure to BBN, 57 of 57 rats on BBN alone had bladder cancer, whereas the incidence for the BBN-plus-disulfiram group was only 7 of 55. No tumors were found in rats treated with disulfiram alone. In common with the findings of others (cf. National Cancer Institute 1979a,b), disulfiram in the diet caused a significant initial weight loss. This transitory weight loss was followed by a nearly normal weight gain after a few weeks and a more rapid gain once disulfiram was removed from the diet.

The exact mechanism whereby disulfiram inhibits the carcinogenicity of BBN is unknown, but several possibilities were suggested by Irving *et al.*

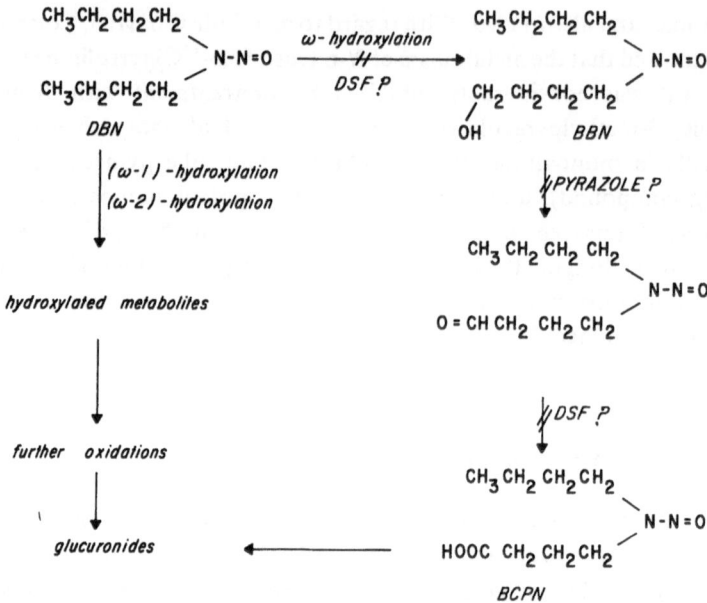

FIGURE 7. Partial scheme for metabolic activation of di-*n*-butylnitrosamine (DBN). Pathways which, in theory, might be inhibited by disulfiram (DSF) and pyrazole are indicated. BBN, *N-n*-butyl-*N*-(4-hydroxybutyl)nitrosamine; BCPN, *N-n*-butyl-*N*-(3-carboxypropyl)nitrosamine.

(1979). Since disulfiram is known to inhibit the enzymatic oxidation of acetaldehyde, it could be that the drug also inhibits the activation of BBN to BCPN by analogous enzymes. On the other hand, the detoxication of BBN or its further metabolites could be enhanced by disulfiram, since this drug is known (Marselos *et al.*, 1976) to increase the levels of several enzymes involved in the glucuronidation pathway. Obviously, these possibilities are not mutually exclusive. Since the activation of BBN to BCPN presumably proceeds by way of an alcohol dehydrogenase-catalyzed reaction through an aldehyde intermediate, it would be of interest to determine whether pyrazole or 4-methylpyrazole would block the metabolism and carcinogenicity of BBN as might be expected.

IX. Arylamines

A. 2-Acetylaminofluorene

The carcinogenicity of 2-acetylaminofluorene (AAF) and other arylamines has been extensively reviewed by Clayson and Garner (1976). The chemical induces tumors mainly of the liver, ear duct, and mammary gland in the rat. As shown in Fig. 8, the first step in the activation of this compound or its deacetylated metabolite is N-hydroxylation (Cramer *et al.*, 1960; Irving, 1962; Weisburger and Weisburger, 1973), a microsomal cytochrome P-450-catalyzed reaction (Thorgeirsson *et al.*, 1973; Lotlikar *et al.*, 1974). Further activation may proceed through the formation of nitroxide free radicals, catalyzed by one-electron oxidants such as H_2O_2-peroxidase, which undergo dismutation to yield the highly reactive N-acetoxy-AAF (Bartsch *et al.*, 1972). Alternatively or additionally, esterification of the N-hydroxy group with acetate, sulfate, or glucuronate yields products reacting directly with nucleic acids and proteins (reviewed by Irving, 1970). Detoxication reactions consist of C-hydroxylations of both AAF and the free amine followed by conjugation.

The effects of disulfiram on the carcinogenicity of AAF were studied by Malejka-Giganti *et al.* (1980) who found that disulfiram at 0.9% in the diet reduced the carcinogenicity of AAF (0.1 mmol/kg i.p., three times a week for 4 weeks) for the mammary gland in female Sprague–Dawley rats. The same treatment had no effect on the carcinogenicity of N-hydroxy-AAF. This

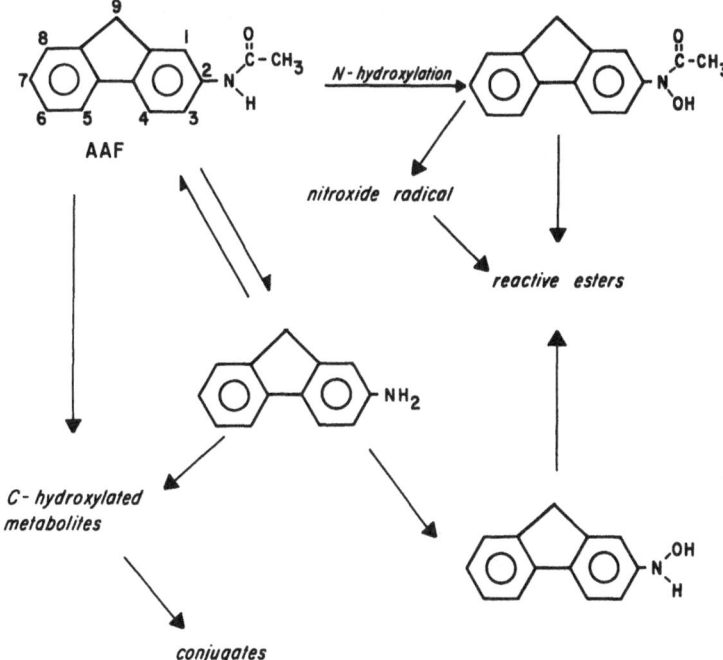

FIGURE 8. Partial scheme for metabolic activation of 2-acetylaminofluorene (AAF).

suggested that disulfiram inhibited the metabolism of AAF to N-hydroxy-AAF. Indeed, liver microsomes obtained from disulfiram-fed rats showed a markedly reduced capacity to N-hydroxylate AAF, as did microsomes obtained from control animals but preincubated with disulfiram. On the other hand, in these studies the cytochrome P-450 levels of the liver microsomes were found to be unaffected by disulfiram, which contrasts with the findings of others (Hunter and Neal, 1975; Zemaitis and Greene, 1976; Lang et al., 1976). Both disulfiram and AAF were found to have a type I cytochrome P-450-binding spectrum; thus, disulfiram may alter the metabolism of AAF through competitive binding with cytochrome P-450.

B. 3,2'-Dimethyl-4-aminobiphenyl

The carcinogenicity of this chemical (DMAB) has been extensively studied by Walpole et al. (1952), Spjut and Noall (1970), and Spjut and Spratt (1965). The compound induces a wide variety of neoplasms including small intestinal and colon tumors in male and female rats and mammary tumors in female rats. In contrast to the colon carcinogen 1,2-dimethylhydrazine, evidence exists that the active metabolite of DMAB is transported to the intestine by the bile and acts directly on the intestinal mucosa (Cleveland et al., 1967).

We studied the effects of disulfiram on the carcinogenicity of DMAB in male F-344 rats (Fiala et al., 1978b). Groups of 30 rats were maintained on powdered chow plus 2.5 g/kg disulfiram for the first 9 weeks, whereupon the level of disulfiram was decreased to 1 g/kg for the next 33 weeks because of large losses in body weights. DMAB was given weekly at 20 mg/kg, s.c., in corn oil, for a total of 40 weeks beginning 2 weeks after the rats were placed on the disulfiram diet. The distribution of selected tumors in rats on control and disulfiram diets autopsied 22 weeks after the last injection of the carcinogen is shown in Table 2. In contrast to the findings of Wattenberg with 1,2-dimethylhydrazine and disulfiram in mice (Wattenberg, 1975), we saw no significant reduction in the multiplicity or incidence of DMAB-induced colon tumors in the disulfiram-treated animals. However, a trend toward a lower incidence of duodenal, skin, salivary, and testicular tumors was observed. The

TABLE 2. Distribution of DMAB-Induced Tumors in Control and Disulfiram-Treated F-344 Rats

Site	Number of tumors[a]			Number of rats with tumors[a]		
	DMAB	DMAB + DSF	DSF	DMAB	DMAB + DSF	DSF
Sm intestine, carcinoma	7	3	—	7	2	—
Sm intestine, adenoma	2	0	—	2	0	—
Sm intestine, total	9	3	—	8	2	—
Colon, carcinomaa	5	3	—	5	3	—
Colon, adenoma	6	7	—	5	6	—
Colon, total	11	10	—	8	9	—
Skin	12	5[d]	—	9	5	—
Salivary gland	7[b]	2	—	7	2	—
Ear duct	2	5[b]	—	2	5	—
Preputial gland	2	2	—	2	2	—
Lung	3	3	1	3	3	1
Subcutaneous	1	1	—	1	1	—
Leukemia[c]	1	3	—	1	3	—
Heart[d]	0	1	—	0	1	—
Urinary bladder	0	1	—	0	1	—
Testis	8	1	2	8	1	2
Total	56	37	3	25	23	3
Total excl. testis	48	36	1	23	23	1

[a] 30 rats each in DMAB and DMAB + DSF groups; 15 rats in DSF group.
[b] One pulmonary metastasis.
[c] Includes leukemias of spleen, liver, lung.
[d] Fibroma (mamartoma).

latter occur "spontaneously" in aging male F-344 rats. The number of ear duct tumors appeared to be increased in the disulfiram group.

In preliminary studies, we have obtained evidence that DMAB is activated through N-hydroxylation and that the glucuronide of the N-hydroxy metabolite is excreted in the bile (Fiala et al., 1980). The metabolite, a strong mutagen in *Salmonella typhimurium* strain TA-100 without S-9 activation, could be responsible for the intestinal tumors. If the N-hydroxylation of DMAB were inhibited by disulfiram, as was observed by Malejka-Giganti for AAF, this might explain the decreased carcinogenicity in the small intestine. The lack of effect on the colon is not explainable in this way, and it is obvious that more work in this area is required.

X. Azo Dyes: 3′-Methyl-4-dimethylaminoazobenzene

The hepatocarcinogenicity of 3′-methyl-4-dimethylaminoazobenzene (3′-Me-DAB) and other azo dyes has been comprehensively reviewed by

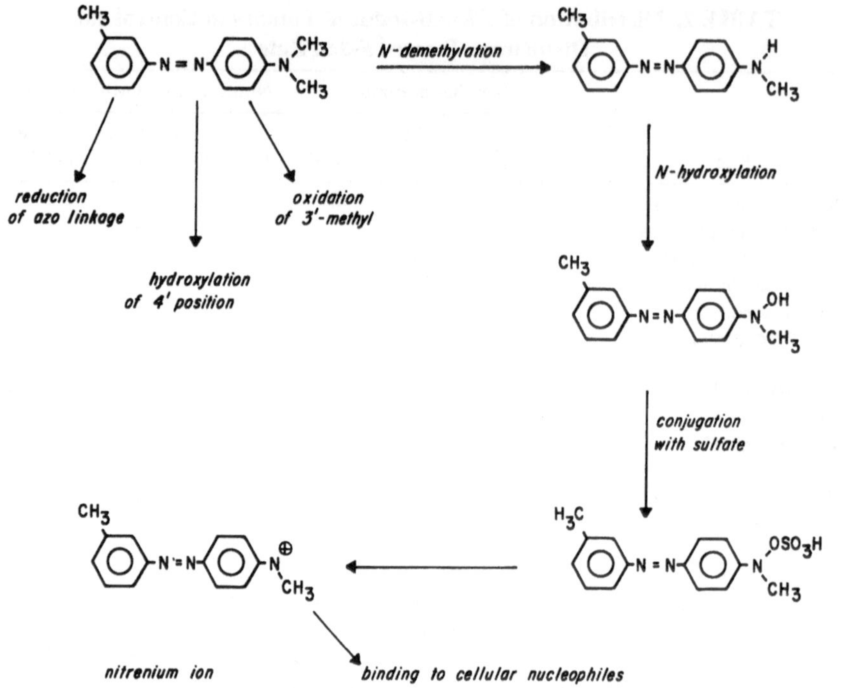

FIGURE 9. Partial scheme for metabolic activation of 3'-methyl-4-dimethylaminoazobenzene.

Miller and Miller (1953) and Terayama (1967). The probable metabolism of this carcinogen is presented in Fig. 9.

Although metabolism via the reduction of the azo linkage, C-hydroxylation, oxidation of the 3' methyl group, and N-demethylation has actually been demonstrated with 3'-Me-DAB (Mori et al., 1979a,b), the activation pathway involving N-hydroxylation and subsequent formation of the unstable sulfate ester and the nitrenium ion have been shown, thus far, only with the closely related N-methyl-4-aminoazobenzene (Kadlubar et al., 1976a,b; Miller et al., 1979). The pathway in Fig. 9 assumes that the activation sequences for 3'-Me-DAB and N-methyl-4-aminoazobenzene are identical even though the former is the stronger hepatocarcinogen. It is of interest that whereas an N-hydroxylation step is required for the activation of both AAF and N-methyl-4-aminoazobenzene in the case of the latter, the reaction is catalyzed not by a cytochrome P-450-dependent system but, rather, by a flavoprotein amine oxidase (Kudlubar et al., 1976a,b).

The inhibition of the hepatocarcinogenicity of 3'-Me-DAB in male Sprague–Dawley rats by disulfiram was described by S. Fiala et al. (1980). Whereas feeding of 3'-Me-DAB at 0.06% produced visible neoplastic nodules in rat livers at about 11 weeks and incipient tumors at 12–14 weeks, the feeding of 0.06% 3′-Me-DAB plus 1% disulfiram produced no neoplastic nodules or tumors even after 27 weeks. Interestingly, in rats fed 3′-Me-DAB plus disulfiram, the hepatic levels of the enzyme γ-glutamyl transferase, a widely used marker for chemically induced carcinogenesis (S. Fiala and A. Fiala, 1969, 1973), increased for the first 50 days at the same rate as did the levels of the enzyme in rats fed 3′-Me-DAB alone. After this time, γ-glutamyl transferase activity leveled off in the livers of rats on disulfiram plus 3′-Me-DAB but continued to rise in the livers of rats on 3′-Me-DAB alone. When, after approximately 80 days on a diet of 3′-Me-DAB or 3′-Me-DAB plus disulfiram, the rats were placed on normal diet, γ-glutamyl transferase continued to increase in the former group but gradually decreased to near basal levels in the latter. Thus, disulfiram appears to prevent some form of an irreversible change that leads to malignant transformation and which is also reflected in an ever-increasing level of γ-glutamyl transferase. The observation that disulfiram does not prevent the initial reversible increase in the level of the marker enzyme was interpreted by the authors to mean that disulfiram inhibits the neoplastic but not the preneoplastic stage of 3′-Me-DAB-induced hepatocarcinogenesis.

XI. Ultraviolet Light

The effects of dietary glutathione (0.1%), phenobarbital (0.05%), butylated hydroxytoluene (0.5%), and disulfiram (0.2%) on protection against u.v. light carcinogenesis in female hairless mice were described by Black *et al.* (1978). Although glutathione afforded no protection, significant inhibition of both initiation and development of actinic lesions was observed with phenobarbital, butylated hydroxytoluene, and disulfiram. The mechanism of protection by these three chemically unrelated compounds is not understood; however, an "umbrageous" effect caused by accumulation of the compounds in the skin with consequent absorption of u.v. light was apparently ruled out, at least in the case of phenobarbital and butylated hydroxytoluene.

XII. Spontaneous Tumors

Both disulfiram and sodium diethyldithiocarbamate were examined for carcinogenicity in the Carcinogenesis Testing Program conducted by the National Cancer Institute (1979a,b,c). In these assays, disulfiram was given in the diet at 300 ppm or 600 ppm for 107 weeks to both male and female F-344 rats and at levels of 500 ppm or 2000 ppm to male B6C3F1 mice and 100 or 500 ppm to female B6C3F1 mice. Similarly, sodium diethyldithiocarbamate was given at levels of 1250 or 2500 ppm for 104 weeks to male and female F-344 rats and 500 or 4000 ppm to male and female B6C3F1 mice for 108–109 weeks.

Although no tumors occurred in the rats or mice of either sex at incidences that were significantly higher in the dosed groups than in matched control groups, examination of the data on the pathology of all animals revealed that the incidence of spontaneous pituitary tumors in male and female rats and the incidence of spontaneous mammary tumors in female rats on diets containing either disulfiram or diethyldithiocarbamate were significantly lower than the incidence of these tumors in the matched control groups. No differences attributed to the thiono sulfur compounds were noted with respect to spontaneous testicular tumors in male rats. Also, the incidence of various spontaneous tumors in mice of either sex was not altered by these compounds. These data are summarized in Tables 3 and 4. It is rather too tempting to speculate that because of the disulfiram and diethyldithiocarbamate inhibition these "spontaneous" tumors could actually be caused by an endogenously produced carcinogen whose activation is inhibited. However, because of the endocrine nature of these tumors and the known inhibition by both compounds of dopamine-β-hydroxylase (cf. Sections II and III) leading to decreased catecholamine synthesis, it is possible that a complex mechanism involving hormonal factors may be involved.

TABLE 3. Incidence of Spontaneous Tumors in Rats Fed Control and Disulfiram-Containing Diets

Tumor	Control	Low dose[a]	High dose[b]
Male F344 rats			
Pituitary:			
chromophobe adenoma	13/20 (65%)	11/46 (24%)	7/45 (16%)
chromophobe carcinoma	0	0	1/45 (2%)
Testis: interstitial-cell tumor	13/20 (65%)	41/50 (82%)	33/50 (69%)
Female F344 rats			
Pituitary:			
chromophobe adenoma	16/20 (80%)	12/49 (24%)	20/48 (42%)
Mammary gland:			
adenocarcinoma	1/20 (5%)	0	0
fibroadenoma	3/20 (15%)	3/50 (6%)	0

[a] Low dose, 300 ppm in diet.
[b] High dose, 600 ppm in diet.

TABLE 4. Incidence of Spontaneous Tumors in Rats Fed Control
and Sodium Diethyldithiocarbamate-Containing Diets

Tumor	Control	Low dose[a]	High dose[b]
Male F344 rats			
Pituitary: adenoma (NOS)	5/16 (31%)	7/50 (14%)	6/48 (13%)
Pancreatic islets: islet cell adenoma	3/16 (19%)	2/49 (4%)	1/48 (2%)
Testis: interstitial-cell tumor	14/16 (88%)	42/50 (84%)	44/50 (88%)
Female F344 rats			
Pituitary: adenoma (NOS)	9/20 (45%)	9/50 (18%)	16/50 (32%)
Mammary gland: fibroadenoma	3/20 (15%)	3/50 (6%)	0

[a] Low dose, 1250 ppm in diet.
[b] High dose, 2500 ppm in diet.

XIII. Other Effects of Thiono Sulfur Compounds

Disulfiram was reported to significantly increase the acute hepatotoxicity of vinyl chloride monomer, $ClCH=CH_2$, in Arochor 1254-pretreated rats (Jaeger et al., 1977). The effect was ascribed to the inhibition of aldehyde dehydrogenase, resulting in accumulation of chloroacetaldehyde, a metabolite of vinyl chloride. In contrast, both disulfiram and diethyldithiocarbamate were found to decrease the acute lethal and hepatotoxic effects of inhaled vinylidene chloride, $Cl_2C=CH_2$, in mice (Short et al., 1977), and inhibition of metabolism together with an increase in detoxication were suggested as possible explanations for this effect. As in the case of vinyl chloride monomer, disulfiram treatment was found to enhance the toxicity of 1,2-dibromoethane during chronic inhalation studies in Sprague–Dawley rats, producing a higher incidence of hepatocellular dysplasia, splenic atrophy, and testicular atrophy (Winston et al., 1979).

Diethyldithiocarbamate was reported to decrease the hepatotoxicity of carbon tetrachloride in rats and mice (Sakaguchi et al., 1966; Popp et al., 1978). While Popp et al. suggested that such protective effect may result from the trapping of the free radicals produced during the metabolism of carbon tetrachloride, evidence for inhibition of the metabolism of the compound was obtained by Siegers et al. (1978) who observed prolonged half-life and decreased clearance of carbon tetrachloride in rats and mice treated with diethyldithiocarbamate. These authors also observed decreased binding of $^{14}CCl_4$ metabolites to liver microsomes incubated in the presence of the inhibitor.

ACKNOWLEDGMENTS. Supported in part by N.C.I. Grant CA-15400 through the National Large Bowel Cancer Project and by N.C.I. Grant CA-17613. The excellent secretarial assistance of Elaine Harvey in the preparation of this manuscript is gratefully acknowledged.

References

Abanobi, S. E., Popp, J. A., Chang, S. K., Harrington, G. W., Lotlikar, P. D., Hadjiolov, D., Levitt, M., Rajalakshmi, S., and Sarma, D. S. R., 1977, Inhibition of dimethylnitrosamine-induced strand breaks in liver DNA and liver cell necrosis by diethyldithiocarbamate, *J. Natl. Cancer Inst.* 58:263.
Abeles, R. H., and Lee, H. A., Jr., 1960, The dismutation of formaldehyde by liver alcohol dehydrogenase, *J. Biol. Chem.* 235:1499.
Abelin, I., Herren, C., and Berli, N., 1958, Über die erregende Wirkung des Alkohols auf den Adrenalin und Noradrenalinhaushalt des menschlichen Organismus, *Helv. Med. Acta* 25:591.
Aebi, H., Dewald, B., and Suter, H., 1965, Autoxydation N2-substitutierter Methylhydrazin: Beinflussung der Cu and Fe-Katalyse durch Proteine, Deoxyribonucleinsäure und EDTA, *Helv. Chim. Acta* 48:656.
Ames, B. N., McCann, J., and Yamasaki, E., 1975, Methods for detecting carcinogens and mutagens with the *Salmonella* mammalian-microsome mutagenicity test, *Mutation Res.* 31:347.
Bartsch, H., Miller, J. A., and Miller, E. C., 1972, *N*-Acetoxy-*N*-acetylaminoarenes and nitrosoarenes. One-electron nonenzymatic and enzymatic oxidation products of various carcinogenic aromatic acethydroxamic acids, *Biochim. Biophys. Acta* 273:40.
Benn, M. H., and Kazmaier, P., 1972, Methylation with (Z)-methyl-ONN-azoxymethanol: The nature of the reactive species, *J. Chem. Soc. [Chem. Commun.]* 1972:887.
Biancifiori, C., Giorneiil-Santilli, F. E., Milia, U., and Severi, L., 1966, Pulmonary tumors in rats induced by oral hydrazine sulphate, *Nature* 212:414.
Bigger, C. A. H., Tomaszewski, J. E., Andrews, A. W., and Dipple, A., 1980, Evaluation of metabolic activation of 7,12-dimethylbenz[*a*]anthracene *in vitro* by Aroclor 1254-induced rat liver S-9 fraction, *Cancer Res.* 40:655.
Black, H. S., Chan, J. T., and Brown, G. E., 1978, Effects of dietary constituents on ultraviolet light-mediated carcinogenesis, *Cancer Res.* 38:1384.
Bond, E. J., and De Matteis, F., 1969, Biochemical changes in rat liver after administration of carbon disulphide, with particular reference to microsomal changes, *Biochem. Pharmacol.* 18:2531.
Borchert, P., and Wattenberg, L. W., 1976, Inhibition of macromolecular binding of benzo-[*a*]pyrene and inhibition of neoplasia by disulfiram, *J. Natl. Cancer Inst.* 57:173.
Campbell, R. L., Singh, D. V., and Nigro, N. D., 1975, Importance of the fecal stream on the induction of colon tumors by azoxymethane in rats, *Cancer Res.* 35:1369.
Campbell, R. L., Suppnick, J. D., Hettrick, J. M., and Nigro, N. D., 1978, Rat liver microsome-mediated *N*-demethylation and mutagenicity of azoxymethane, *Cancer Res.* 38:4585.
Carlsson, A., Henning, M., Lindberg, P., Martinson, P., Trolin, G., Waldeck, B., and Wickberg, B., 1978, On the disulfiramlike effect of coprine, the pharmacologically active principle of *Coprinus atramentarius, Acta Pharmacol. Toxicol.* 42:292.
Carter, S. K., and Slavik, M., 1974, Chemotherapy of cancer, *Rev. Pharmacol.* 14:157.

Child, G. P., and Crump, M., 1952, The toxicity of tetraethylthiuram disulphide (Antabuse) to mouse, rat, rabbit and dog, *Acta Pharmacol. Toxicol.* **8**:305.

Clay, K. L., Watkins, W. D., and Murphy, R. C., 1977, Metabolism of pyrazole. Structure elucidation of urinary metabolites, *Drug Metab. Disp.* **5**:149.

Clayson, D. B., and Garner, R. C., 1976, Carcinogenic aromatic amines and related compounds, in: *Chemical Carcinogenesis* (C. E. Searle, ed.), pp. 366–461, ACS Monograph 173, American Chemical Society, Washington.

Cleveland, J. C., Litvak, S., and Cole, J. W., 1967, Identification of the route of action of carcinogen 3,2'-dimethyl-4-aminobiphenyl in the induction of intestinal neoplasia, *Cancer Res.* **27**:708.

Cooper, H. K., Buecheler, J., and Kleihues, P., 1978, DNA alkylation in mice with genetically different susceptibility to 1,2-dimethylhydrazine-induced colon carcinogenesis, *Cancer Res.* **38**:3063.

Cottrell, R. C., Young, P. J., Walters, D. G., Phillips, J. C., Lake, B. G., and Gangolli, S. D., 1979, Studies of the metabolism of N-nitrosopyrrolidine in the rat, *Toxicol. Appl. Pharmacol.* **51**:101.

Cramer, J. W., Miller, J. A., and Miller, E. C., 1960, N-Hydroxylation: A new metabolic reaction observed in the rat with the carcinogen 2-acetylaminofluorene, *J. Biol. Chem.* **235**:885.

Czygan, P., Greim, H., Garro, A. J., Hutterer, F., Schaffner, F., Popper, H., Rosenthal, O., and Cooper, D. Y., 1973, Microsomal metabolism of dimethylnitrosamine and the cytochrome P-450 dependency of its activation to a mutagen, *Cancer Res.* **33**:2983.

Dalvi, R. R., and Neal, R. A., 1978, Metabolism *in vivo* of carbon disulfide to carbonyl sulfide and carbon dioxide, *Biochem. Pharmacol.* **27**:1608.

Dalvi, R. R., Poore, R. E., and Neal, R. A., 1975, Toxicological implications of the mixed function oxidase catalyzed metabolism of carbon disulfide, *Chem. Biol. Interact.* **10**:347.

Deckers, C., Deckers-Passau, L., Maisin, J., Gauthier, J. M., and Mace, F., 1974, Carcinogenicity of procarbazine, *Z. Krebsforsch.* **81**:79.

Deis, F. H., and Lester, D., 1979, Biochemical pharmacology of pyrazoles, in: *Biochemistry and Pharmacology of Ethanol*, Vol. 2 (E. Majchrowicz and E. P. Noble, eds.), pp. 303–323, Plenum Press, New York.

Deitrich, R. A., and Erwin, V. G., 1971, Mechanism of the inhibition of aldehyde dehydrogenase *in vivo* by disulfiram and diethyldithiocarbamate, *Mol. Pharmacol.* **7**:301.

De Matteis, F., 1973, Drug-induced destruction of cytochrome P-450, *Drug Metab. Disp.* **1**:267.

De Matteis, F., 1974, Covalent binding of sulfur to microsomes and loss of cytochrome P-450 during the oxidative desulfuration of several chemicals, *Mol. Pharmacol.* **10**:849.

De Matteis, F., and Seawright, A. A., 1973, Oxidative metabolism of carbon disulphide in the rat. Effect of treatments which modify the liver toxicity of carbon disulphide, *Chem. Biol. Interact.* **7**:375.

de Saint-Blanquat, G., and Derache, R., 1976, Mecanisme d'action des substances anti-alcool dépendantes (Disulfirame), *J. Pharmacol. (Paris)* **7**:393.

Digenis, G. A., and Issidores, C. H., 1979, Some biochemical aspects of N-nitroso compounds, *Bioorg. Chem.* **8**:97.

Dipple, A., 1976, Polynuclear aromatic hydrocarbons, in: *Chemical Carcinogenesis* (C. E. Searle, ed.), ACS Monograph 173, American Chemical Society, Washington.

Dost, F. N., and Reed, D. J., 1967, Methane formation *in vivo* from N-isopropyl-α(2-methylhydrazino)-p-toluamide hydrochloride, a tumor inhibiting methylhydrazine derivative, *Biochem. Pharmacol.* **16**:1741.

Druckrey, H., 1969, Krebserzeugung durch chemische Substanzen, in: *Fortschritte der Krebsforschung* (C. G. Schmidt and O. Wetter, eds.), pp. 37–65, F. K. Schattauer Verlag, Stuttgart.

Druckrey, H., 1970, Production of colonic carcinomas by 1,2-dialkylhydrazines and azoxyalkanes, in *Carcinoma of the Colon and Antecedent Epithelium* (W. J. Burdette, ed.), pp. 267–279, C. C. Thomas, Springfield, Illinois.

Druckrey, H., 1973, Specific carcinogenic and teratogenic effects of 'indirect' alkylating methyl and ethyl compounds and their dependency on stages of ontogenic developments, *Xenobiotica* 3:271.

Druckrey, H., Preussmann, R., Ivankovic, S., Schmidt, C. H., Mennel, H. D., and Stahl, K. W., 1964, Selektive Erzeugung von Blasenkrebs an Ratten durch Bibutyl- und N-Butyl-N-butanol-(4)-nitrosamin, *Z. Krebsforsch.* 66:280.

Druckrey, H., Preussmann, R., Matzkies, R., and Ivankovic, S., 1966, Carcinogene Wirkung von 1,2-Diäthylhydrazin an Ratten, *Naturwissenschaften* 53:557.

Druckrey, H., Preussmann, R., Ivankovic, S., and Schmähl, D., 1967a, Organotrope carcinogene Wirkungen bei 65 verschiedenen N-Nitroso-Verbindungen an BD-Ratten, *Z. Krebsforsch.* 69:103.

Druckrey, H., Preussmann, R., Matzkies, F., and Ivankovic, S., 1967b, Selektive Erzeugung von Darmkrebs bei Ratten durch 1,2-Dimethylhydrazin, *Naturwissenschaften* 54:285.

Dunn, D. L., Lubet, R. A., and Prough, R. A., 1979, Oxidative metabolism of N-isopropyl-α-(2 methylhydrazino)-p-toluamide hydrochloride (Procarbazine) by rat liver microsomes, *Cancer Res.* 39:4555.

Faiman, M. D., 1979, Biochemical pharmacology of disulfiram, in: *Biochemistry and Pharmacology of Ethanol*, Vol. 2 (E. Majchrowicz and E. P. Noble, eds.), pp. 325–348, Plenum Press, New York.

Faiman, M. D., Haya, K., and Artman, L., 1978, Distribution of radioactivity in rats after i.p. and oral S^{35} disulfiram (DSF) administration, *Alcohol Clin. Exp. Res.* 2:217.

Ferguson, J. K. W., 1956, A new drug for alcoholism treatment, *Can. Med. Assoc. J.* 74:793.

Feytmans, E., Morales, M. N., and Leighton, F., 1973, Effects of pyrazole and 3-amino-1,2,4-triazole on methanol and ethanol metabolism by the rat, *Biochem. Pharmacol.* 22:349.

Fiala, E. S., 1977, Investigations into the metabolism and mechanism of action of the colon carcinogens 1,2-dimethylhydrazine and azoxymethane, *Cancer* 40:2436.

Fiala, E. S., 1980, The formation of azoxymethane, a colon carcinogen during the chemical oxidation of methylamine, *Carcinogenesis* 1:57.

Fiala, E. S., and Weisburger, J. H., 1975, Metabolism of 1,2-dimethylhydrazine-^{14}C, *Proc. Am. Assoc. Cancer Res.* 16:15.

Fiala, E. S., Bobotas, G., Kulakis, C., and Weisburger, J. H., 1976a, Separation of 1,2-dimethylhydrazine metabolites by high-pressure liquid chromatography, *J. Chromatogr.* 117:181.

Fiala, E. S., Kulakis, C., Bobotas, G., and Weisburger, J. H., 1976b, Detection and estimation of azomethane in expired air of 1,2-dimethylhydrazine-treated rats, *J. Natl. Cancer Inst.* 56:1271.

Fiala, E. S., Bobotas, G., Kulakis, C., Wattenberg, L. W., and Weisburger, J. H., 1977a, Effects of disulfiram and related compounds on the metabolism *in vivo* of the colon carcinogen 1,2-dimethylhydrazine, *Biochem. Pharmacol.* 26:1763.

Fiala, E. S., Kulakis, C., Christiansen, G., and Weisburger, J. H., 1977b, *In vivo* and *in vitro* metabolism of the colon carcinogen azoxymethane (AOM), *Proc. Am. Assoc. Cancer Res.* 18:105.

Fiala, E. S., Kulakis, C., Christiansen, G., and Weisburger, J. H., 1978a, Inhibition of the metabolism of the colon carcinogen, azoxymethane, by pyrazole, *Cancer Res.* 38:4515.

Fiala, E. S., Son, O. S., and Weisburger, J. H., 1978b, The effects of disulfiram (DSF) on the carcinogenicity of 3,2'-dimethyl-4-aminobiphenyl (DMAB), *Proc. Am. Assoc. Cancer Res.* 19:66.

Fiala, E. S., Nussbaum, M., and Weisburger, J. H., 1980, Biliary metabolites of 3,2'-dimethyl-4-aminobiphenyl in the F344 rat, *Proc. Am. Assoc. Cancer Res.* **21**:119.

Fiala, S., and Fiala, A. E., 1969, Activation of glutathionase in rat liver during carcinogenesis, *Naturwissenschaften* **56**: 565.

Fiala, S., and Fiala, E. S., 1973, Activation by chemical carcinogens of γ-glutamyl transpeptidase in rat and mouse liver, *J. Natl. Cancer Inst.* **51**:151.

Fiala, S., Trout, E. C., Ostrander, H., and Fiala, A. E., 1980, γ-Glutamyltransferase and the inhibition of azodye-produced neoplasia by concomitant administration of disulfiram, *J. Natl. Cancer Inst.* **64**:267.

Fishbein, L., 1976, Environmental health aspects of fungicides. 1. Dithiocarbamates, *J. Toxicol. Environ. Health* **1**:713.

Freundt, K. J., Kuttner, P., and Dreher, W., 1976, Specificity and sensitivity of the inhibition of drug metabolism following inhalation of carbon disulphide-air mixtures, *Arzneim. Forsch.* **26**:793.

Gelboin, H. V., and Ts'O, P. O. P. (eds.), 1978, *Polycyclic Hydrocarbons and Cancer*, Vols. 1 and 2, Academic Press, New York.

Gessner, T., and Jakubowski, M., 1972, Diethyldithiocarbamic acid methyl ester, a metabolite of disulfiram, *Biochem. Pharmacol.* **21**:219.

Goldstein, M., Anagnoste, B., Lauber, E., and McKereghan, M. R., 1964, Inhibition of dopamine β-hydroxylase by disulfiram, *Life Sci.* **3**:763.

Grab, D. J., and Zedeck, M. S., 1977, Organ-specific effects of the carcinogen methylazoxymethanol related to metabolism by nicotinamide adenine dinucleotide-dependent dehydrogenases, *Cancer Res.* **37**:4182.

Hald, J., and Jacobsen, E., 1948a, A drug sensitizing the organism to ethyl alcohol, *Lancet* **2**:1001.

Hald, J., and Jacobsen, E., 1948b, The formation of acetaldehyde in the organism after ingestion of Antabuse (tetraethylthiuram-disulfide) and alcohol, *Acta Pharmacol. Toxicol.* **4**:305.

Haley, T. J., 1979, Disulfiram (tetraethylthioperoxydicarbonic diamide): A reappraisal of its toxicity and therapeutic application, *Drug Metab. Rev.* **9**:319.

Hawks, A., and Magee, P. N., 1974, The alkylation of nucleic acids of rat and mouse *in vivo* by the carcinogen, 1,2-dimethylhydrazine, *Br. J. Cancer* **30**:440.

Hecht, S. S., Chen, C. B., and Hoffmann, D., 1978, Evidence for metabolic α-hydroxylation of N-nitrosopyrrolidine, *Cancer Res.* **38**:215.

Heikkila, R. E., Cabbat, F. S., and Cohen, G., 1976, *In vivo* inhibition of superoxide dismutase in mice by diethyldithiocarbamate, *J. Biol. Chem.* **251**:2182.

Hernberg, S., Tolonen, M., and Nurminen, M., 1976, Eight-year follow-up of viscose rayon workers exposed to carbon disulfide, *Scand. J. Work Environ. Health* **2**:27.

Holck, H. G., Lish, P. M., Sjogren, D. W., Westerfield, N. W., and Malone, M. H., 1970, Effects of disulfiram on growth, longevity and reproduction of the albino rat, *J. Pharm. Sci.* **59**:1267.

Horisberger, M., and Matsumoto, H., 1968, Studies of methylazoxymethanol. Synthesis of ^{14}C and ^{3}H labelled methylazoxymethylacetate, *J. Labelled Cmpds.* **4**:164.

Hunter, A. L., and Neal, R. A., 1975, Inhibition of hepatic mixed function oxidase activity *in vitro* and *in vivo* by various thiono-sulfur-containing compounds, *Biochem. Pharmacol.* **24**:2199.

International Agency for Research on Cancer, 1976, *Some Carbamates, Thiocarbamates and Carbazides*, IARC Monograph Vol. 12, p. 186, International Agency for Research on Cancer, Lyon.

Irving, C. C., 1962, N-Hydroxylation of the carcinogen 2-acetylaminofluorene by rabbit-liver microsomes, *Biochim. Biophys. Acta* **65**:564.

Irving, C. C., 1970, Conjugates of N-hydroxy compounds, in: *Metabolic Conjugation and Metabolic Hydrolysis*, Vol. 1 (W. H. Fishman, ed.), pp. 53–119, Academic Press, New York.

Irving, C. C., Tice, A. J., and Murphy, W. M., 1979, Inhibition of N-n-butyl-N-(4-hydroxybutyl) nitrosamine induced urinary bladder cancer in rats by administration of disulfiram in the diet, *Cancer Res.* **39**:3040.

Jaeger, R. J., Murphy, S. D., Reynolds, E. S., Szabo, S., and Moslen, M. T., 1977, Chemical modification of acute hepatotoxicity of vinyl chloride monomer in rats, *Toxicol. Appl. Pharmacol.* **41**:597.

Kadlubar, F. F., Miller, J. A., and Miller, E. C., 1976a, Microsomal N-oxidation of the hepatocarcinogen N-methyl-4-aminoazobenzene and the reactivity of N-hydroxy-N-methyl-4-aminoazobenzene, *Cancer Res.* **36**:1196.

Kadlubar, F. F., Miller, J. A., and Miller, E. C., 1976b, Hepatic metabolism of N-hydroxy-N-methyl-4-aminoazobenzene and other N-hydroxy arylamines to reactive sulfuric acid esters, *Cancer Res.* **36**:2350.

Kaslander, J., 1963, Formation of an S-glucuronide from tetraethylthiuram disulphide (Antabuse) in man, *Biochim. Biophys. Acta* **71**:730.

Kelly, M. G., O'Gara, R. W., Yancy, S. T., Gadekar, K., Botkin, C., and Oliverio, V. T., 1969, Comparative carcinogenicity of N-isopropyl-α-(2-methylhydrazino)-p-toluamide · HCl (procarbazine hydrochloride), its degradation products, other hydrazines, and isonicotinic acid hydrazide, *J. Natl. Cancer Inst.* **42**:337.

Kitson, T. M., 1976, The effects of some analogues of disulfiram on the aldehyde dehydrogenases of sheep liver, *Biochem. J.* **155**:445.

Kitson, T. M., 1977, The disulfiram–ethanol reaction. A review, *J. Stud. Alcohol* **38**:96.

Kreis, W., Piepho, S. B., and Bernhard, H. W., 1966, Studies on the metabolic fate of the C-14 labeled methyl group of a methyl hydrazine derivative in P815 mouse leukemia, *Experientia* **22**:431.

Kromer, W., and Freundt, K. J., 1976, Hemmung der oxidativen N-Demethylierung *in vitro* durch Schwefelkohlenstoff, *Arzneim. Forsch.* **26**:189.

Kwentus, J., and Major, L. F., 1979, Disulfiram in the treatment of alcoholism, *J. Stud. Alcohol* **40**:428.

Lake, B. G., Minski, M. J., Phillips, J. C., Gangolli, S. D., and Lloyd, A. G., 1975, Investigations into the hepatic metabolism of dimethylnitrosamine in the rat, *Life Sci.* **17**:1599.

Lang, M., Marselos, M., and Törrönen, R., 1976, Modifications of drug metabolism by disulfiram and diethyldithiocarbamate I. Mixed function oxidase, *Chem. Biol. Interact.* **15**:267.

Laqueur, G. L. and Spatz, M., 1975, Oncogenicity of cycasin and methylazoxymethanol, *Gann Monogr. Cancer Res.* **17**:189.

Lacqueur, G. L., McDaniel, E. G., and Matsumoto, H., 1967, Tumor induction in germfree rats with methylazoxymethanol (MAM) and synthetic MAMAcetate, *J. Natl. Cancer Inst.* **39**:355.

Lee, C.-C., Russell, J. Q., and Minor, J. L., 1978, Oral toxicity of ferric demethyldithiocarbamate (Ferbam) and tetramethylthiuram disulfide (Thiram) in rodents, *J. Toxicol. Environ. Health* **4**:93.

Levin, W., Wood, A. W., Lu, A. Y. H., Ryan, D., West, S., Donney, A. H., Thakker, D. R., Yagi, H., and Jerina, D. M., 1977, Role of purified cytochrome P-448 and epoxide hydrase in the activation and detoxification of benzo[a]pyrene, in: *Drug Metabolism Concepts* (D. M. Jerina, ed.), ACS Symposium Series 44, American Chemical Society, Washington.

Lieber, C. S., Rubin, E., DeCarli, L. M., Misra, P., and Gang, H., 1970, Effects of pyrazole on hepatic function and structure, *Lab. Invest.* **22**:615.

Lijinsky, W., Lee, J., and Ross, A. E., 1968, Mechanism of alkylation of nucleic acids by nitrosomethylamine, *Nature* **218**:1174.

Likhachev, A. J., Margison, G. P., and Montesano, R., 1977, Alkylated purines in the DNA of various rat tissues after administration of 1,2-dimethylhydrazine, *Chem. Biol. Interact.* **18**:235.

Likhachev, A. Ya., Petrov, A. S., Prvanova, L. G., and Pozharisski, K. M. 1978. Mechanism of methylation of DNA bases by symmetrical dimethylhydrazine, *Bull. Exp. Biol. Med. (Engl. Trans.)* **86**:679.

Linderholm, H., and Berg, K., 1951, Method for determination of tetraethylthiuram disulphide (Antabuse, Abstinyl) and diethyldithiocarbamate in blood and urine. Some studies on metabolism of tetraethylthiuramdisulphide, *Scand. J. Clin. Lab. Invest.* **3**:96.

Lotlikar, P. D., Luha, L., and Zaleski, K., 1974, Reconstituted hamster liver microsomal enzyme system for N-hydroxylation of the carcinogen 2-acetylaminofluorene, *Biochem. Biophys. Res. Commun.* **59**:1349.

Lotlikar, P. D., Baldy, W. J., Jr., and Dwyer, E. N., 1975, Dimethylnitrosamine demethylation by reconstituted microsomal cytochrome P-450 enzyme system, *Biochem. J.* **152**:705.

Magee, P. N., Montesano, R., and Preussmann, R., 1976, N-Nitroso compounds and related carcinogens, in: *Chemical Carcinogenesis* (C. E. Searle, ed.), ACS Monograph 173, American Chemical Society, Washington.

Malejka-Giganti, D., McIver, R. C., and Rydell, R. E., 1980, Inhibitory effect of disulfiram on mammary tumor induction by N-2-fluorenylacetamide and on its metabolic conversion to N-hydroxy-N-2-fluorenylacetamide, *J. Natl. Cancer Inst.* **64**:1471.

Marselos, M., Lang, M., and Törrönen, R., 1976, Modifications of drug metabolism by disulfiram and diethyldithiocarbamate II. D-Glucuronic acid pathway, *Chem. Biol. Interact.* **15**:277.

Martin, M.-S., Martin, F., Justrabo, E., Knopf, J.-F., Bastien, H., and Knobel, S., 1974, Induction de cancers coliques chez le rat par injection unique de 1,2-diméthylhydrazine, *Biol. Gastroenterol. (Paris)* **7**:37.

Matsubara, N., Mori, H., and Hirono, I., 1978, Effect of colostomy on intestinal carcinogenesis by methylazoxymethanol acetate in rats, *J. Natl. Cancer Inst.* **61**:1161.

Matsumoto, H., and Higa, H., 1966, Studies on methylazoxymethanol, the aglycone of cycasin: Methylation of nucleic acids *in vitro*, *Biochem. J.* **98**:20C.

Matsumoto, H., and Strong, F. L., 1963, The occurrence of methylazoxymethanol in *Cycas circinalis* L., *Arch. Biochem. Biophys.* **101**:299.

Matsumoto, H., Takata, R. H., and Komeiji, D. Y., 1979, Synthesis of the glucuronic acid conjugate of methylazoxymethanol, *Cancer Res.* **39**:3070.

Mazel, P., Henderson, J. F., and Axelrod, J., 1964, S-Demethylation by microsomal enzymes, *J. Pharmacol. Exp. Ther.* **143**:1.

McKenna, M. J., and Di Stefano, V., 1977, Carbon disulfide. II. A proposed mechanism for the action of carbon disulfide on dopamine-β-hydroxylase, *J. Pharmacol. Exp. Ther.* **202**:253.

Miller, E. C., Kadlubar, F. F., Miller, J. A., Pitot, H. C., and Drinkwater, N. D., 1979, The N-hydroxy metabolites of N-methyl-4-aminoazobenzene and related dyes as proximate carcinogens in the rat and mouse, *Cancer Res.* **39**:3411.

Miller, J. A., 1970, Carcinogenesis by chemicals: An overview—G. H. A. Clowes Memorial Lecture, *Cancer Res.* **30**:559.

Miller, J. A., and Miller, E. C., 1953, The carcinogenic aminoazodyes, *Adv. Cancer Res.* **1**:339.

Mori, Y., Hori, T., and Toyoshi, K., 1979a, Carcinogenic azo dyes. XII. Detection of new metabolites of aminoazo dyes by rat liver, *Chem. Pharm. Bull. (Tokyo)* **27**:235.

Mori, Y., Yamamoto, T., and Toyoshi, K., 1979b, Carcinogenic azo dyes. XI. Analysis of biliary and urinary metabolites of 3'-methyl-4-(methylamino)azobenzene in rat, *Chem. Pharm. Bull. (Tokyo)* **27**:379.

Moriya, M., Kato, K., Ohta, T., Watanabe, K., Watanabe, Y., and Shirasu, Y., 1978, Detection of mutagenicity of the colon carcinogen 1,2-dimethylhydrazine by the host-mediated assay and its correlation to carcinogenicity, *J. Natl. Cancer Inst.* **61**:457.

Moriya, M., Ohta, T., Watanabe, K., Watanabe, Y., Sugiyama, F., Meyazawa, T., and Shirasu, Y., 1979, Inhibitors for the mutagenicities of colon carcinogens, 1,2-dimethylhydrazine and azoxymethane, in the host-mediated assay, *Cancer Lett.* **7**:325.

Nagasawa, H. T., Shirota, F. N., and Matsumoto, H., 1976, Decomposition of methylazoxymethanol, the aglycone of cycasin, in D_2O, *Nature* **236**:234.

National Cancer Institute, 1979a, *Bioassay of Sodium Diethyldithiocarbamate for Possible Carcinogenicity*, NCI Technical Report Series No. 172, U.S. Dept. Health, Education and Welfare, Public Health Service, National Institute of Health, Washington.

National Cancer Institute, 1979b, *Bioassay of Procarbazine for Possible Carcinogenicity*, NCI Technical Report Series No. 19, U.S. Dept. Health, Education and Welfare, Public Health Service, National Institute of Health, Washington.

National Cancer Institute, 1979c, *Bioassay of Tetraethylthiuram Disulfide for Possible Carcinogenicity*, NCI Technical Report Series No. 166, U.S. Dept. Health, Education and Welfare, Public Health Service, National Institute of Health, Washington.

Neims, A. H., Coffey, D. S., and Hellerman, L., 1966a, Interaction between tetraethylthiuram disulfide and the sulfhydryl group of D-amino acid oxidase, *J. Biol. Chem.* **241**:5941.

Neims, A. H., Coffey, D. S., and Hellerman, L., 1966b, A sensitive radioassay for sulfhydryl groups with tetraethylthiuram disulfide, *J. Biol. Chem.* **241**:3036.

Nigro, N. D., and Campbell, R. L., 1978, Inhibition of azoxymethane-induced intestinal cancer by disulfiram, *Cancer Lett.* **5**:91.

Okada, M., and Ishidate, M., 1977, Metabolic fate of N-n-butyl-N-(4-hydroxybutyl)-nitrosamine and its analogues. Selective induction of urinary bladder tumors in the rat, *Xenobiotica* **7**:11.

Okada, M., and Suzuki, E., 1972, Metabolism of butyl-(4-hydroxybutyl)nitrosamine in rats, *Gann* **63**:391.

Oswald, H., and Krüger, F. W., 1969, Die cancerogene Wirkung von 1,2-Dimethylhydrazin beim Goldhamster, *Arzneim. Forsch.* **19**:1891.

Pegg, A. E., 1978, Inhibition of the alkylation of nucleic acids and of the metabolism of 1,2-dimethylhydrazine by aminoacetonitrile, *Chem. Biol. Interact.* **23**:273.

Phillips, J. C., Lake, B. G., Gangolli, S. D., Grasso, P., and Lloyd, A. G., 1977, Effects of pyrazole and 3-amino-1,2,4-triazole on the metabolism and toxicity of dimethylnitrosamine in the rat, *J. Natl. Cancer Inst.* **58**:629.

Popp, J. A., Shinozuka, H., and Farber, E., 1978, The protective effects of diethyldithiocarbamate and cycloheximide on the multiple hepatic lesions induced by carbon tetrachloride in the rat, *Toxicol. Appl. Pharmacol.* **45**:549.

Poynter, R. W., Ball, C. R., Goodban, J., and Thackrah, T., 1971/72, The influence of physostigmine on the activation of methylazoxymethanol acetate, a potent carcinogen, by a serum factor *in vitro*, *Chem. Biol. Interact.* **4**:139.

Pozharisski, K. M., Likhachev, A. J., Klimashevski, V. F., and Shaposhnikov, J. D., 1979, Experimental intestinal cancer research with special reference to human pathology, *Adv. Cancer Res.* **30**:165.

Preussmann, R., Druckrey, H., Ivankovic, S., and v. Hodenberg, A., 1969, Chemical structure and carcinogenicity of aliphatic hydrazo, azo, and azoxy compounds and of triazenes, potential *in vivo* alkylating agents, *Ann. N. Y. Acad. Sci.* **163**:697.

Prough, R. A., Wittkop, J. A., and Reed, D. J., 1969, Evidence for the hepatic metabolism of some monoalkylhydrazines, *Arch. Biochem. Biophys.* **131**:369.

Prough, R. A., Lubet, R. A., Wiebkin, P., and Dunn, D. L., 1979, The role of cytochrome P-450 in the metabolism of the therapeutic 1-benzyl-2-methylhydrazine derivative, procarbazine, *Proc. Am. Assoc. Cancer Res.* **20**:151.

Rogers, K. J., and Pegg, A. E., 1977, Formation of O^6-methylguanine by alkylation of rat liver, colon, and kidney DNA following administration of 1,2-dimethylhydrazine, *Cancer Res.* **37**:4082.

Rosin, M. P., and Stich, H. F., 1979, Assessment of the use of the *Salmonella* mutagenesis assay to determine the influence of antioxidants on carcinogen-induced mutagenesis, *Int. J. Cancer* **23**:722.

Rouach, H., Ribiere, C., Nordmann, J., and Nordmann, R., 1976, Effects of pyrazole on rat liver tryptophan oxygenase, *Life Sci.* **19**:505.

Rubin, E., Gang, H., and Lieber, C. S., 1971, Interaction of ethanol and pyrazole with hepatic microsomes, *Biochem. Biophys. Res. Commun.* **42**:1.

Rublo, C. A., Nylander, G., and Santos, M., 1980, Experimental colon cancer in the absence of intestinal contents in Sprague-Dawley rats, *J. Natl. Cancer Inst.* **64**:569.

Sakaguchi, T., Nishimura, H., Masuda, K., Tsuge, I., Onishi, K., and Tatsumi, H., 1966, The relationship between chemical structure and protective effect of dithiocarbamate derivatives against experimental hepatic injury induced by carbon tetrachloride administration in rats, *Biochem. Pharmacol.* **15**:756.

Schmähl, D., and Krüger, F. W., 1972, Influence of disulfiram (tetraethylthiuramdisulfide) on the biological actions of *N*-nitrosamines, in: *Topics in Chemical Carcinogenesis* (W. Nakahara, S. Takayame, T. Sugimura, and S. Odashima, eds.), pp. 199-210, University Park Press, Baltimore.

Schmähl, D., Krüger, F. W., Ivankovic, S., and Preissler, P., 1971, Verminderung der Toxität von Dimethylnitrosamin bei Ratten und Mäusen nach Behandlung mit Disulfiram, *Arzneim. Forsch.* **21**:1560.

Schmähl, D., Krüger, F. W., Hales, M., and Diehl, B., 1976, Influence of disulfiram on the organotropy of the carcinogenic effect of dimethylnitrosamine and diethylnitrosamine in rats, *Z. Krebsforsch.* **85**:271.

Schoental, R., 1973, The mechanisms of action of the carcinogenic nitroso and related compounds, *Br. J. Cancer* **28**:436.

Schurr, A., Ho, B. T., and Schoolar, J. C., 1978, The effects of disulfiram on rat liver mitochondrial monoamine oxidase, *Life Sci.* **22**:1979.

Schwartz, D. E., Brubacher, G. B., and Vecchi, M., 1967, Metabolic formation of methane from *N*-methyl-substituted hydrazine compounds and carcinostatic activity, in: *International Conference on Radioactive Isotopes in Pharmacology* (P. G. Waser and B. Glasson, eds.), p. 351, Wiley, Interscience, New York.

Short, R. D., Winston, J. M., Minor, J. L., Seifter, J., and Lee, C.-C., 1977, Effect of various treatments on toxicity of inhaled vinylidene chloride, *Environ. Health Perspect.* **21**:125.

Siegers, C.-P., Filser, J. G., and Bolt, H. M., 1978, Effect of dithiocarb on metabolism and covalent binding of carbon tetrachloride, *Toxicol. Appl. Pharmacol.* **46**:709.

Souček, B., and Mádlo, Z., 1953, Absorption, metabolism and excretion of carbon disulfide in the organism. VI. Chromatographic proof of the reaction of CS_2 and amino acids in the blood [in Czech], *Prac. Lek.* **5**:309.

Spjut, H. J., and Noall, M. W., 1970, Colonic neoplasm induced by 3,2'-dimethyl-4-aminobiphenyl, in: *Carcinoma of the Colon and Antecedent Epithelium* (N. J. Burdette, ed.), pp. 280-288, C. C. Thomas, Springfield, Illinois.

Spjut, H. J., and Spratt, J. S., 1965, Endemic and morphologic similarities existing between spontaneous colonic neoplasms in man and 3:2'-dimethyl-4-aminobiphenyl induced colonic neoplasms in rats, *Ann. Surg.* **161**:309.

Stanford Research Institute, 1978, *Chemical Economics Handbook,* Stanford Research Institute, Stanford, California.

Strömme, J. H., 1963, Inhibition of hexokinase by disulfiram and diethyldithiocarbamate, *Biochem. Pharmacol.* **12**:157.

Strömme, J. H., 1965a, Metabolism of disulfiram and diethyldithiocarbamate in rats with demonstration of an *in vivo* ethanol-induced inhibition of glucuronic acid conjunction of the thiol, *Biochem. Pharmacol.* **14**:393.

Strömme, J. H., 1965b, Interactions of disulfiram and diethyldithiocarbamate with serum proteins studied by means of a gel-filtration technique, *Biochem. Pharmacol.* **14**:381.

Strömme, J. H., 1966, Distribution and chemical forms of diethyldithiocarbamate and tetraethylthiuram disulphide (disulfiram) in mice in relation to radioprotection, *Biochem. Pharmacol.* **15**:287.

Sunderman, F. W., 1967, Diethyldithiocarbamate therapy of thallotoxicosis, *Am. J. Med. Sci.* **253**:107.

Swenberg, J. A., Cooper, H. K., Bucheler, J., and Kleihues, P., 1979, 1,2-Dimethylhydrazine-induced methylation of DNA bases in various rat organs and the effect of pretreatment with disulfiram, *Cancer Res.* **39**:465.

Szabo, S., Horvath, E., Kovacs, K., and Larsen, P. R., 1978, Pyrazole-induced thyroid necrosis: A distinct organ lesion, *Science* **199**:1209.

Terayama, H., 1967, Aminoazo carcinogenesis—methods and biochemical problems, in: *Methods in Cancer Research*, Vol. 1 (H. Busch, ed.), pp. 399–449, Academic Press, New York.

Theorell, H., and Yonetani, T., 1963, Liver alcohol dehydrogenase–DPN–pyrazole complex. A model of a ternary intermediate in the enzyme reaction, *Biochem. Z.* **338**:537.

Thorgeirsson, S. S., Jollow, D. J., Sasame, H. A., Green, I., and Mitchell, J. R., 1973, The role of cytochrome P-450 in *N*-hydroxylation of 2-acetylaminofluorene, *Mol. Pharmacol.* **9**:398.

Thurnherr, N., Deschner, E. E., Stonehill, E. H., and Lipkin, M., 1973, Induction of adenocarcinoma of the colon in mice by weekly injections of 1,2-dimethylhydrazine, *Cancer Res.* **33**:940.

Toth, B., 1969, Lung tumor induction and inhibition of breast adenocarcinomas by hydrazine sulfate in mice, *J. Natl. Cancer Inst.* **42**:469.

Toth, B., 1973, 1,1-Dimethylhydrazine (unsymmetrical) carcinogenesis in mice. Light microscopic and ultrastructural studies on neoplastic blood vessels, *J. Natl. Cancer Inst.* **50**:181.

Toth, B., and Shimizu, H., 1973, Methylhydrazine tumorigenesis in Syrian golden hamsters and the morphology of malignant histiocytomas, *Cancer Res.* **33**:2744.

Truitt, E. B., Jr., and Walsh, M. J., 1971, The role of acetaldehyde in the actions of ethanol, in: *The Biology of Alcoholism*, Vol. 1 (B. Kissin and H. Begleiter, eds.), pp. 161–195, Plenum Press, New York.

Walpole, H. L., Williams, H. M. C., and Roberts, D. C., 1952, The carcinogenic action of 4-aminobiphenyl and 3:2′-dimethyl-4-aminobiphenyl, *Br. J. Indust. Med.* **9**:255.

Ward, J. M., 1975, Dose response to a single injection of azoxymethane in rats, *Vet. Pathol.* **12**:165.

Wattenberg, L. W., 1974, Inhibition of carcinogenic and toxic effects of polycyclic hydrocarbons by several sulfur-containing compounds, *J. Natl. Cancer Inst.* **52**:1583.

Wattenberg, L. W., 1975, Inhibition of dimethylhydrazine-induced neoplasia of the large intestine by disulfiram, *J. Natl. Cancer Inst.* **54**:1005.

Wattenberg, L. W., 1977, Inhibition of carcinogenic and toxic effects of polycyclic hydrocarbons by benzyl isothiocyanate and related compounds, *J. Natl. Cancer Inst.* **58**:395.

Wattenberg, L. W., 1978a, Inhibitors of chemical carcinogenesis, *Adv. Cancer Res.* **26**:197.

Wattenberg, L. W., 1978b, Inhibition of chemical carcinogenesis, *J. Natl. Cancer Inst.* **60**:11.

Wattenberg, L. W., and Fiala, E. S., 1978, Inhibition of 1,2-dimethylhydrazine-induced neoplasia of the large intestine in female CF_1 mice by carbon disulfide, *J. Natl. Cancer Inst.* **60**:1515.

Wattenberg, L. W., Lam, L. K. T., Fladmoe, A. V., and Borchert, P., 1977, Inhibitors of colon carcinogenesis, *Cancer* **40**:2432.

Weinkam, R. J., and Shiba, D. A., 1978, Metabolic activation of procarbazine, *Life Sci.* **22**:937.
Weisburger, J. H., 1971, Colon carcinogens: Their metabolism and mode of action, *Cancer* **28**:60.
Weisburger, J. H., and Weisburger, E. K., 1973, Biochemical formation and pharmacological, toxicological and pathological properties of hydroxylamines and hydroxamic acids, *Pharmacol. Rev.* **25**:1.
West, B., and Sunderman, F. W., 1958, Nickel poisoning. VII. The therapeutic effectiveness of alkyl dithiocarbamates in experimental animals exposed to nickel carbonyl, *Am. J. Med. Sci.* **236**:15.
Winston, J. M., Hong, C. B., Lee, C. C., and Wong, L. C. K., 1979, Effect of 3- or 6-month inhalation of 1,2-dibromoethane in rats treated with disulfiram, *Toxicol. Appl. Pharmacol.* **48**:A25.
Wiseman, J. S., and Abeles, R. H., 1979, Mechanism of inhibition of aldehyde dehydrogenase by cyclopropanone hydrate and the mushroom toxin, coprine, *Biochemistry* **18**:427.
Wittig, G., Wildner, G. P., and Ziebarth, D., 1971, Der Einfluss der Ingesta auf die Kanzerisierung des Rattendarms durch Dimethylhydrazin, *Arch. Geschwulstforsch.* **37**:105.
Zedeck, M. S., and Brown, G. B., 1977, Methylation of intestinal and hepatic DNA in rats with methylazoxymethanol acetate, *Cancer* **40**:2580.
Zedeck, M. S., and Sternberg, S. S., 1974, A model system for studies of colon carcinogenesis: Tumor induction by a single injection of methylazoxymethanol acetate, *J. Natl. Cancer Inst.* **53**:1419.
Zedeck, M. S., and Tan, Q. H., 1978, Effect of pyrazole on tumor induction by methylazoxymethanol (MAM) acetate: Relationship to metabolism of MAM, *Pharmacologist* **20**:174.
Zedeck, M. S., Frank, N., and Wiessler, M., 1979, Metabolism of the colon carcinogen methylazoxymethanol acetate, in: *Frontiers of Gastrointestinal Research*, Vol. 4 (L. van der Reis, ed.), pp. 32–37, Karger, Basel.
Zemaitis, M. A., and Greene, F. E., 1976, Impairment of hepatic microsomal drug metabolism in the rat during daily disulfiram administration, *Biochem. Pharmacol.* **25**:1355.
Zemaitis, M. A., and Greene, F. E., 1979, *In vivo* and *in vitro* effects of thiuram disulfides and dithiocarbamates on hepatic microsomal drug metabolism in the rat, *Toxicol. Appl. Pharmacol.* **48**:343.

3

Retinoids and Chemoprevention of Cancer

MICHAEL B. SPORN and
DIANNE L. NEWTON

I. Introduction

The role of retinol and its esters in determining normal epithelial cell differentiation has been known for over 50 years since the classical studies of Wolbach and Howe (1925) who observed the differentiated cells of various specialized epithelia throughout the body were replaced by squamous, keratinizing cells during retinoid* deficiency.

In their remarkable paper, the authors also made another highly significant observation that clearly indicated that the study of retinoids would some day be of definite importance with respect to the problem of cancer. Wolbach and Howe noted that

> growth activity of [retinoid-deficient] epithelium is not diminished. On the contrary, there is convincing evidence that it is greatly augmented. In [some of the retinoid-deficient] animals, the behavior of the replacing epithelium in respect to numbers of mitotic figures and response on the part of the connective tissue and blood vessels suggests the acquisition of neoplastic properties. . . . It is highly probable that the epithelium of gland ducts, respiratory mucosa, and genitourinary

---

*We have defined the new word, "retinoid," to include the entire set of molecules comprised of both natural and synthetic analogues of vitamin A (retinol); see Sporn *et al.* (1976b). The word retinoid is a generic term similar to the word steroid or carotenoid and should not be used as the name of a specific substance.

MICHAEL B. SPORN and DIANNE L. NEWTON • Laboratory of Chemoprevention, National Cancer Institute, Bethesda, Maryland 20205.

> tract have secretory functions, so that we conclude that the [retinoid] deficiency results in loss of specific chemical functions of the epitheliums concerned, while the power of growth becomes augmented.

This remarkable insight into the fundamental nature of the neoplastic process still serves today as a useful guide for understanding the role of retinoids in control of neoplastic development. We are still far from understanding the molecular mechanisms whereby retinoid deficiency or excess can enhance or suppress the develpment of neoplasia. However, it is clear at present that retinoids can play an important role in this process. In this chapter, we shall highlight some recent advances in chemoprevention of cancer with retinoids, although we shall not attempt a comprehensive review. For the latter purpose, several other reviews are suggested (Boutwell, 1979; Lotan, 1980; Frolik and Roller, 1981). Moreover, we shall not deal with recent developments relating to retinoids and cancer treatment. There have been major new advances in this area that have shown that retinoids can control the differentiation or proliferation of certain malignant cells of either animal or human origin (Lotan and Nicolson, 1977; Lotan *et al.*, 1978, 1980; Strickland and Mahdavi, 1978; Dion *et al.*, 1978; Lotan, 1979; Meyskens and Salmon, 1979; Lacroix and Lippman, 1980; Breitman *et al.*, 1980), and this topic is now worthy of a review in itself. Since our own interests have been concentrated in studies of structure–function relationships of retinoids with respect to control of epithelial cell differentiation, we shall give particular emphasis to this last topic.

II. Retinoids and Epithelial Cell Differentiation

The rationale for the use of retinoids (the entire set of molecules comprised of both natural and synthetic analogues of vitamin A) for cancer prevention rests primarily on their ability to control normal differentiation of many epithelial tissues, much as if the retinoids were functioning as steroid hormones that control differentiation in target organs. Most, if not all, epithelial tissues throughout the body are totally dependent on retinoids for their proper differentiation and growth. In many epithelia, normal cell differentiation and growth do not occur in the absence of retinoids. Instead, either a potentially premalignant lesion (squamous metaplasia) occurs with replacement of functional, differentiated epithelial cells by keratinized squamous cells (as in the case of tracheobronchial epithelium, Wong and Buck, 1971; Harris *et al.*, 1972) or the number of mature, differentiated epithelial cells diminishes (as in the case of intestinal epithelium, De Luca *et al.*, 1969; Rojanapo *et al.*, 1980).

Epithelial tissues that depend on retinoids for normal cellular differentiation account for the majority of primary human cancers; the organ and tissue sites include bronchi and trachea, mammary gland, intestine, stomach, prostate, pancreatic ducts, uterus, kidney, bladder, testis, and skin (Wolbach and Howe, 1925; Moore, 1957). This tissue requirement of retinoids for normal cellular differentiation provides the basis for an extremely sensitive assay which we have routinely used for measurement of biological activity of new synthetic retinoids. In the absence of retinoids, tracheal organ cultures lose their normal columnar ciliated and mucus cells, with replacement by keratinized squamous cells. Addition of biologically active retinoids (at concentrations as low as 10^{-11} M) to the organ cultures reverses the process of keratinization and leads to regeneration of a normal mucociliary epithelium (Clamon *et al.*, 1974; Sporn *et al.*, 1976a). The application of this assay to studies of structure–function relationships of retinoids will be discussed in detail in Section VI.

III. Suppression of Malignant Transformation and Tumor Promotion by Retinoids

From a mechanistic point of view, the critical phenomenon with respect to retinoids and cancer prevention is their ability to act directly on cells in organ culture, monolayer culture, or suspension culture to suppress the process of malignant transformation. This phenomenon has been known since Lasnitzki (1955) first reported that premalignant epithelial lesions in organ cultures of mouse prostate glands could be suppressed by addition of nontoxic levels of retinyl acetate. This organ culture system has subsequently been used as a means to correlate structure and function of various retinoids (Chopra and Wilkoff, 1977), although it is considerably more difficult and definitely less sensitive than the tracheal organ culture system. It is of importance to note that effects of retinoids on suppression of malignant transformation can occur after the application of carcinogen and after the initial molecular damage caused by the carcinogen has occurred. In this prostatic system, then, the retinoids are not causing an "antiinitiating" effect but rather an "antipromoting" effect during the "progression" phase of carcinogenesis. An electron-microscopic analysis of the effects of retinoids on prostatic organ cultures that have been exposed to chemical carcinogens has been published recently (Müller-Salamin et al., 1979).

Although the suppressive effects of retinoids on malignant transformation were first reported in organ culture studies, such systems have major liabilities for studies on the biochemical mechanism of action of retinoids, particularly because of the heterogeneity of cell types in an organ culture and because of the difficulty in sampling aliquots of cells at various times during an experiment.

Thus, a major advance occurred with the original monolayer cell culture studies by Merriman and Bertram (1979) who reported that retinol, retinyl acetate, and retinal all were effective in suppressing the transformation of 10T1/2 cells (a nonneoplastic, cloned mouse fibroblastic cell line growing in monolayer culture) caused by 3-methylcholanthrene. In their experiments, treatment with retinoids did not begin until at least 7 days after carcinogen exposure; retinoids were effective in suppressing transformation even when their application was delayed for as long as 21 days after carcinogen treatment of the 10T1/2 cells. Dose–response studies definitely showed that the effects of the retinoids in suppressing transformation were not mediated by a cytotoxic mechanism, since activity of retinyl acetate was found at concentrations as low as the 10^{-8} to 10^{-7} M range. This system has also been subsequently used (Bertram, 1980) for structure–function analysis of retinoids.

In view of the relative ease with which many aspects of malignant transformation can be studied in this classical monolayer cell culture system, it no doubt will be intensively used in the future for further mechanistic studies of suppression of malignant transformation. It should be emphasized that the suppressive effect of the retinoids requires their continued presence and that on their removal from the cell culture dish, phenotypic expression of the transformed state occurs. Monolayer cell culture studies have also shown that retinoids can suppress phenotypic expression of malignant transformation induced by γ-irradiation of 10T1/2 cells (Harisiadis et al., 1978). In these studies, the retinoids were present in the cultures during the time when the cells were irradiated, so that they may also have had an "antiinitiating" effect in this experimental system.

Understanding of the biochemical mechanism of suppression of malignant transformation by retinoids has been furthered with the report that retinoids block phenotypic cell transformation caused by sarcoma growth factor (SGF) (Todaro et al., 1978). Sarcoma growth factor is a heat-stable, acid-stable polypeptide (molecular weight 6,000–12,000) (De Larco and Todaro, 1978) and is a member of a class of polypeptides that have been called "transforming growth factors" (TGFs) (Sporn et al., 1981). These TGFs are all acid-stable polypeptides of relatively low molecular weight that are direct (although reversible) effectors of cell transformation, if cell morphology and anchorage-independent growth are taken as indices of the transformed phenotype.

If one wishes to assay the effects of TGFs, the nonneoplastic normal rat kidney (NRK) fibroblastic cell line may be used. Normal rat kidney cells, when grown in monolayer culture, have an orderly growth pattern and are subject to density-dependent inhibition of cell growth. Furthermore, NRK cells will not form progressively growing colonies in soft agar; they show anchorage dependence. In the presence of nanogram quantities of SGF, NRK cells have a disorderly growth pattern in monolayer culture, are no longer subject to density-dependent inhibition of growth, and will form progressively growing colonies in soft agar (anchorage independence) (De Larco and Todaro, 1978). All of these properties are believed to be significantly correlated with the neoplastic behavior of cells. When NRK cells were treated simultaneously with SGF and nanomolar levels of retinoids (including, in separate experiments, retinyl acetate, retinoic acid, retinyl methyl ether, and retinylidene dimedone), the phenotypic transforming effects of the sarcoma growth factor were inhibited. In control experiments, it could be shown that the effects of the retinoids were not mediated by a cytotoxic mechanism, since they did not inhibit the growth of NRK cells that were not exposed to SGF, nor was there any inhibition of the ability of rat or mouse cells that had been genotypically transformed by Moloney sarcoma virus to grow in soft agar (Todaro et al., 1978). We shall again refer to the above experiments, which show an antagonism between retinoids and a proliferative polypeptide hormone-like substance (SGF), in our discussion of mechanism of action of retinoids in Section VIII.

The suppression of tumor promotion by retinoids has been another area of carcinogenesis studies in which major advances have recently been made. The most striking data have been obtained in studies in which retinoids have been shown to antagonize the proliferative, tumor-promoting effects of phorbol esters, which are the active principles of croton oil. Biochemical studies have shown that active retinoids are potent inhibitors of the induction of the enzyme, ornithine decarboxylase, which undergoes an immense increase in mouse skin treated with active phorbol esters (Verma et al., 1978). Antagonistic effects between retinoids and phorbol esters have been shown in a large number of systems, both *in vivo* and *in vitro*, and have been well reviewed in other articles (Verma et al., 1979; Boutwell and Verma, 1979).

Another important promoting agent that causes proliferative effects that are antagonized by retinoids is asbestos. Studies with tracheal organ cultures have shown that retinyl methyl ether will diminish the hyperplastic effects of both amosite and crocidolite asbestos as well as lessen the degree of cellular atypia caused by these agents (Mossman et al., 1980). As an increasing amount of interest is now being devoted to the importance of promoting effects in human carcinogenesis, it would appear that there will be an increasing amount of investigation devoted to the use of retinoids as agents that block the proliferative effects of various promoters.

IV. Retinoid Deficiency and Carcinogenesis

If retinoids are of intrinsic importance for the maintenance of normal epithelial cell differentiation, and if they are also natural suppressors of malignant transformation and tumor promotion, then retinoid deficiency should be a state of enhanced risk for development of cancer. This is indeed the case and has been shown experimentally in animals and epidemiologically in man.

Recent studies in rats exposed to chemical carcinogens have shown that in three different organ systems, lung (Nettesheim and Williams, 1976), bladder (Cohen et al., 1976), and colon (Newberne and Rogers, 1973; Rogers et al., 1973), there is a markedly enhanced risk for development of malignancy if the animals are vitamin A deficient. The chemical carcinogens used have been as diverse as 3-methylcholanthrene (Nettesheim and Williams, 1976), N-[4-(5-nitro-2-furyl)-2-thiazolyl]formamide (FANFT) (Cohen et al., 1976), dimethylhydrazine (Rogers et al., 1973), and aflatoxin B_1 (Newberne and Rogers, 1973).

Similarly, there is now a wealth of data from retrospective human epidemiologic studies that leads to a similar conclusion, although with considerably less precision. Several of these epidemiologic studies have correlated low dietary intake of β-carotene (based on questionnaire evaluation of food habits) with an increased susceptibility to development of cancer of the lung (Bjelke, 1975; Mettlin et al., 1979), stomach (Hirayama, 1979), or bladder (Mettlin and Graham, 1979). There has recently been an increasing interest in prospective studies, which unfortunately are also expensive and difficult, to obtain further data in this area. As results of these studies become available, they should add further valuable information on this important nutritional problem.

V. Natural Retinoids and Prevention of Carcinogenesis

The well-known facts that squamous, metaplastic, dedifferentiated lesions occur in retinoid-deficient epithelial tissues and that these lesions often resemble those seen in the same tissues during early stages of carcinogenesis have led to a wealth of experimental studies to determine if retinoids might be useful agents for the prevention of cancer. We have summarized these studies in our previous reviews (Sporn *et al.*, 1976b; Sporn and Newton, 1979) and shall not discuss them in detail here.

In the first studies that were performed, investigators were limited to the use of the natural retinoids, retinyl palmitate and retinyl acetate (vitamin A palmitate and acetate). Some of these studies showed significant protection in rats and hamsters against the development of cancer of the stomach, vagina, uterine cervix, and respiratory tract, although conflicting results have been obtained by many investigators. These conflicting results include failure to achieve protection against chemically induced tumors, and in some cases in which very high doses of retinyl palmitate have been applied directly to epithelial tissues (e.g., the hamster cheek pouch), an enhancement of carcinogenesis has been reported. Such enhancement of carcinogenesis is

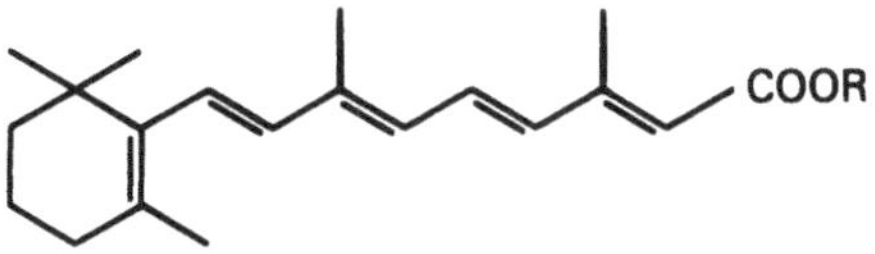

Structure, R =	Trivial Name	Source	ED_{50}, M	(Number of Cultures)
H	Retinoic acid, Tretinoin	b, g	3×10^{-11}	(1853)
CH_3	Retinoic acid methyl ester	g	3×10^{-10}	(139)
C_2H_5	Retinoic acid ethyl ester	g	5×10^{-10}	(124)

FIGURE 1. Structure and activity of all-*trans*-retinoic acid and its esters. Sources of retinoids in this and subsequent figures were as follows: *a*, Nancy Acton and Arnold Brossi, National Institute of Arthritis, Metabolism and Digestive Diseases, Bethesda, Maryland; *b*, BASF Aktiengesellschaft, Ludwigshafen am Rhein, Germany; *c*, Ralph S. Becker, University of Houston, Houston, Texas; *d*, F. Ivy Carroll, Research Triangle Institute, Research Triangle Park, North Carolina; *e*, Marcia I. Dawson, SRI International, Menlo Park, California; *f*, Clayton H. Heathcock, University of California, Berkeley, California; *g*, Hoffmann-La Roche Inc., Nutley, New Jersey and F. Hoffmann-La Roche & Co., A.G., Basel, Switzerland; *h*, Johnson & Johnson, New Brunswick, New Jersey; *i*, Koji Nakanishi, Columbia University, New York, New York; *j*, Y. Fulmer Shealy, Southern Research Institute, Birmingham, Alabama; *k*, Steven C. Welch, University of Houston, Houston, Texas.

usually a manifestation of retinoid toxicity. The inherent toxicity of high doses of retinoids is best shown in the experiments of Levij and Polliack (1968; Levij et al., 1969) in which 10% solution of retinyl palmitate in paraffin was topically applied to the hamster cheek pouch, resulting in an enhancement of the carcinogenicity of 7,12-dimethylbenzanthracene at this site. In these experiments, the retinoid appears to act as a promoting agent, resembling croton oil.

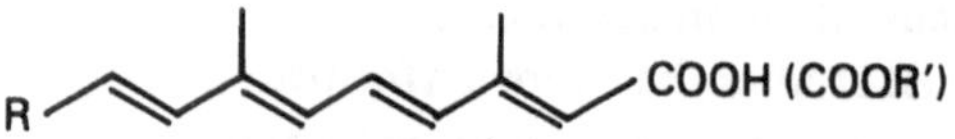

Structure, R =	Trivial Name	Source	ED_{50}, M	(Number of Cultures)
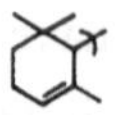	alpha-Retinoic acid	g	$<1 \times 10^{-8}$	(63)
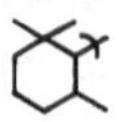	5,6-Dihydroretinoic acid	g	$<1 \times 10^{-9}$	(45)
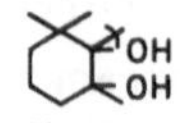 R' = Me	5,6-Dihydroxyretinoic acid methyl ester	g	2×10^{-7}	(12)
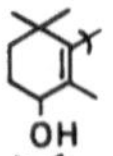	4-Hydroxyretinoic acid	g	7×10^{-10}	(43)
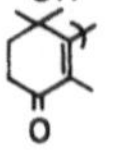	4-Ketoretinoic acid	g	7×10^{-10}	(35)
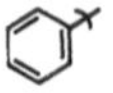	Phenyl analog of retinoic Acid	g	1×10^{-6}	(29)
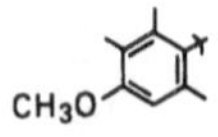 CH_3O	4-Methoxy-2,3,6-trimethylphenyl analog of retinoic acid; TMMP analog of retinoic acid	g	5×10^{-9}	(228)
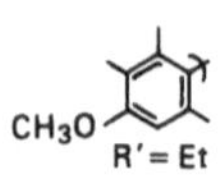 CH_3O, R' = Et	4-Methoxy-2,3,6-trimethylphenyl analog of retinoic acid ethyl ester; TMMP analog of retinoic acid ethyl ester; Etretinate	g	2×10^{-8}	(92)
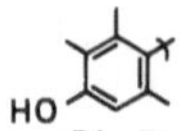 HO, R' = Et	4-Hydroxy-2,3,6-trimethylphenyl analog of retinoic acid ethyl ester	g	Inactive, 12/13 cultures, 1×10^{-7}	(22)
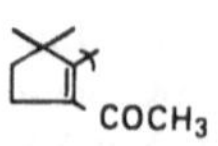 $COCH_3$	Dimethylacetyl cyclopentenyl analog of retinoic acid	g	5×10^{-10}	(103)

FIGURE 2. Structure and activity of ring-modified analogues of all-*trans*-retinoic acid and its esters.

Structure, R =	Trivial Name	Source	ED_{50}, M	(Number of Cultures)
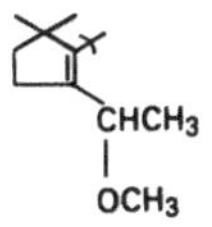 [structure with CHCH₃, OCH₃]	Dimethylmethoxyethyl cyclopentenyl analog of retinoic acid	g	2×10^{-10}	(81)
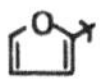 [furyl structure]	2-Furyl analog of retinoic acid	g	Inactive, 10/13 cultures, 1×10^{-6}	(27)
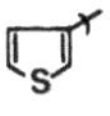 [thienyl structure]	3-Thienyl analog of retinoic acid	b	$>1 \times 10^{-8}$	(23)
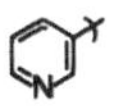 [pyridyl structure]	3-Pyridyl analog of retinoic acid	g	3×10^{-7}	(22)

FIGURE 2. (*Continued*)

Since it is well known that high local doses of retinoids can cause irritating toxic effects on tissue, in part because of their ability to disrupt lysosomes (Fell *et al.*, 1962; Goodman *et al.*, 1974), these results are hardly surprising. In all experiments performed with natural retinoids, problems of toxicity and of achieving adequate tissue distribution have always been major. It is well known that feeding of retinyl acetate or retinyl palmitate does not result in a useful elevation of serum retinoid until immense amounts of retinoid have been deposited in the liver (mostly as retinyl palmitate), at which point toxic manifestations may be seen. These toxic effects may include damage to the liver itself or generalized damage to membrane systems in organs throughout the body (Moore, 1967). Thus, feeding of the natural retinyl esters has not been a particularly useful method of influencing experimental carcinogenesis with the exception of prevention of mammary carcinogenesis.

In the case of the mammary gland, it has been shown that oral administration of retinyl acetate will elevate mammary tissue levels of retinoids, and retinyl acetate has been successfully used to prevent experimental breast cancer in the rat (Moon *et al.*, 1977). However, the dosage level must be very carefully monitored to avoid problems of toxicity. In addition to esters of retinol, its carboxylic acid metabolite, all-*trans*-retinoic acid, has been used to prevent skin carcinogenesis in the mouse (Bollag, 1972; Verma *et al.*, 1979), and an extensive literature has been developed on the mechanism of this phenomenon (Verma *et al.*, 1978; Boutwell and Verma, 1979). However, problems of toxicity have precluded further extensive oral use of all-*trans*-retinoic acid in man.

In summary, although under some circumstances natural retinoids can prevent the development of epithelial cancer, they have limited usefulness as agents for chemoprevention of cancer in both animals and man because of inadequate pharmacokinetic properties or their ability to produce undesirable toxic effects. Unless these undesirable properties of natural retinoids can be

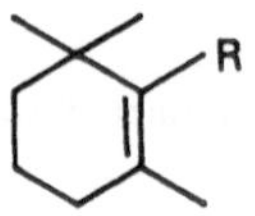

Structure, R =	Trivial Name	Source	ED_{50}, M	(Number of Cultures)
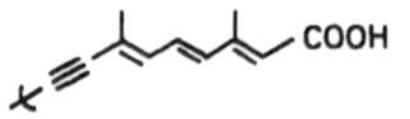 COOH (7,8-dehydro)	7,8-Dehydroretinoic acid	b	5×10^{-10}	(26)
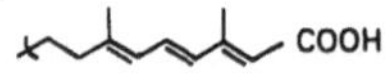 COOH	7,8-Dihydroretinoic acid	g	1×10^{-8}	(53)
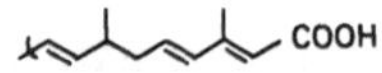 COOH	9,10-Dihydroretinoic acid	g	1×10^{-7}	(53)
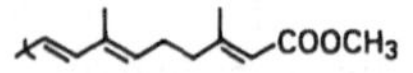 $COOCH_3$	11,12-Dihydroretinoic acid methyl ester	g	4×10^{-8}	(40)
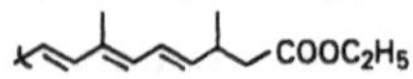 $COOC_2H_5$	13,14-Dihydroretinoic acid ethyl ester	g	3×10^{-8}	(47)
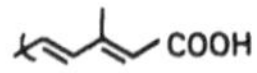 COOH	C_{15} analog of retinoic acid	g	Inactive, 7/7 cultures, 1×10^{-6} M	(13)
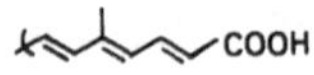 COOH	C_{17} analog of retinoic acid	f	Inactive, 6/6 cultures, 1×10^{-8} M	(12)
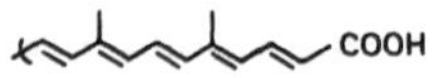 COOH	C_{22} analog of retinoic acid	c, g	3×10^{-9}	(17)
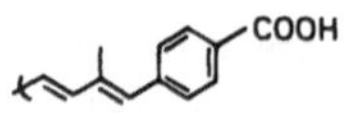 COOH (aryltriene trans)	Aryltriene analog of retinoic acid *(trans)*	e	2×10^{-10}	(24)
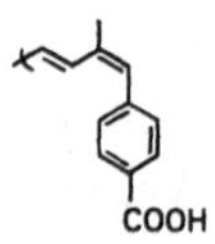 COOH (aryltriene cis)	Aryltriene analog of retinoic acid *(cis)*	e	$>1 \times 10^{-9}$	(11)

FIGURE 3. Structure and activity of side chain-modified analogues of all-*trans*-retinoic acid and its esters.

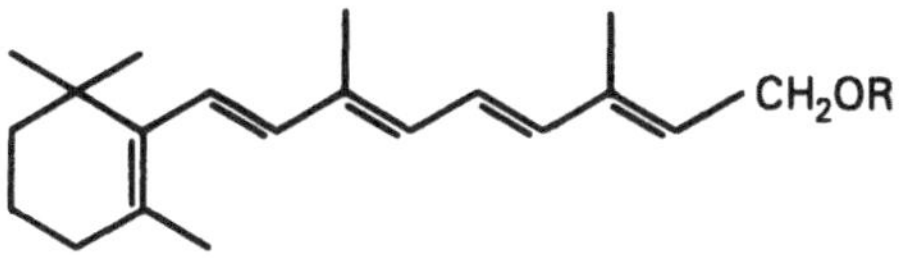

FIGURE 4. Structure and activity of all-*trans*-retinol, retinyl esters, and retinyl ethers.

Structure, R =	Trivial Name	Source	ED_{50}, M	(Number of Cultures)
H	Retinol	b, g	7×10^{-10}	(83)
$COCH_3$	Retinyl acetate	b, g	1×10^{-9}	(152)
CH_3	Retinyl methyl ether	b, g	3×10^{-9}	(134)
C_4H_9	Retinyl butyl ether	b, g	3×10^{-8}	(71)
C_6H_5	Retinyl phenyl ether	g	8×10^{-8}	(31)

successfully modified by the organic chemist, retinoids will remain an impractical means for prevention of human cancer. The concept of synthetic modification of natural hormones to yield useful, more specific, and less toxic new drugs is a very fundamental one in modern pharmacology, and this is indeed the approach that will be required if retinoids are to achieve their potential promise for prevention of cancer in man.

VI. Structure–Activity Relationships of New Synthetic Retinoids*

We have repeatedly stressed that the future of retinoids in cancer prevention rests on the development of new synthetic analogues and that it is essential to abandon the obsolete concept that large doses of natural "vitamin A" (a chemical misnomer in modern terms) should be used for cancer prevention in men and women. Synthetic retinoid chemistry is now a highly developed field, and excellent reviews exist (Mayer and Isler, 1971; Frolik and Roller, 1981). More than a thousand retinoid analogues have been synthesized, and many of these are described in the patent literature as well as in chemical journals. The range of synthetic modifications that have been made is very broad. The basic structure of the ring, side chain, and polar terminus of the retinoid molecule can all be modified to yield biologically active analogues. A major screening problem for cancer prevention is the initial testing of newly synthesized retinoids. Although the eventual goal may

*This section and all figures discussed in this section have been previously published (Newton *et al.*, 1980) and are reprinted with permission from *Cancer Research*.

be cancer prevention, initial *in vivo* screening for this purpose is prohibitively expensive in addition to requiring a prolonged period of time before results of these tests become available. We have therefore stressed the utilization of an *in vitro* screen for the preliminary evaluation of the biological activity of new retinoids.

Since the tracheal organ culture assay (Clamon *et al.*, 1974; Sporn *et al.*, 1976a) measures the intrinsic ability of retinoids to control epithelial cell differentiation, it is believed to have significant predictive value for the potential use of a new retinoid for prevention of epithelial cancer. Obviously any *in vitro* test has dangerous liabilities for prediction of *in vivo* activity. In spite of these limitations, however, the tracheal organ culture assay is a most valuable procedure for initial evaluation of the biological activity of a new retinoid. It is an extremely sensitive assay and has been used routinely to evaluate activity of new retinoids, the concentration of which may be as low as 10^{-10} to 10^{-11} M during the assay procedure. Thus, it is possible to measure biological activity with less than a milligram of a new retinoid; with radioactively labeled retinoid metabolites, assays have been performed with only a few micrograms of material. The length of assay is relatively brief, and test results may be evaluated within a month after beginning the assay. This section provides data on 87 retinoids from a total set of over 30,000 hamster tracheas that have been used for assays at the National Cancer Institute. Each trachea has come from a separate animal that has been raised on a vitamin A-deficient diet. From each hamster, the trachea has been removed under sterile conditions and maintained in organ culture *in vitro* for 3–10 days, as

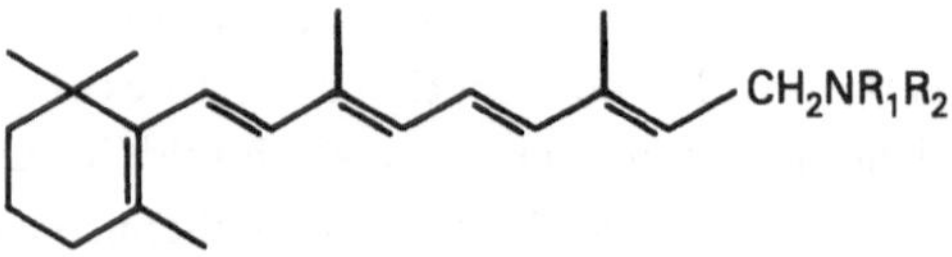

Structure, $R_1 =$, $R_2 =$	Trivial Name	Source	ED_{50}, M	(Number of Cultures)
H, $COCH_3$	*N*-Acetyl retinyl amine	b,g	9×10^{-9}	(113)
H, COC_6H_5	*N*-Benzoyl retinyl amine	b	2×10^{-9}	(61)
CH_3, $COCH_3$	*N*-Methyl *N*-acetyl retinyl amine	d	$>1 \times 10^{-9}$	(35)
CH_3, COC_6H_5	N-Methyl *N*-benzoyl retinyl amine	d	1×10^{-9}	(30)

FIGURE 5. Structure and activity of all-*trans*-retinyl amine derivatives.

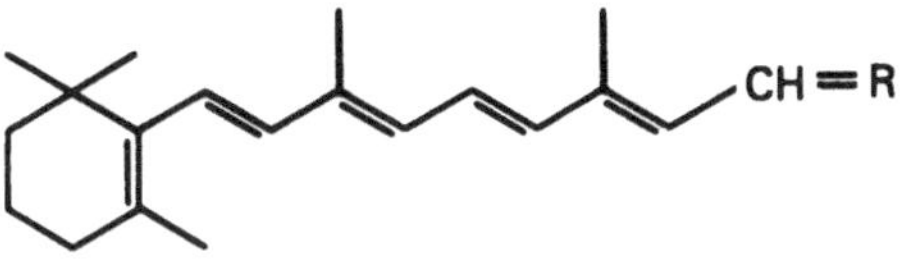

Retinoids and Chemoprevention of Cancer

[Structure of all-trans-retinal with CH=R terminal group]

Structure, R =	Trivial Name	Source	ED_{50}, M	(Number of Cultures)
O	Retinal	b,g	3×10^{-10}	(98)
NNHCOCH$_3$	Retinal acetylhydrazone	g	4×10^{-10}	(54)
NOH	Retinal oxime	g	1×10^{-8}	(61)
C(COCH$_3$)$_2$	3-Retinylidene-2,4-pentanedione; retinylidene acetylacetone	a	2×10^{-9}	(86)
C(COCH$_2$CH$_3$)$_2$	4-Retinylidene-3,5-heptanedione	a	4×10^{-9}	(12)
C(COCH$_2$CH$_2$CH$_3$)$_2$	5-Retinylidene-4,6-nonanedione	a	Inactive, 6/7 cultures 1×10^{-8} M	(14)
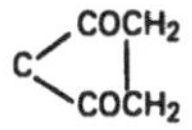 C(COCH$_2$)$_2$ (cyclopentane ring)	2-Retinylidene-1,3-cyclopentanedione	a	Inactive, 16/17 cultures 1×10^{-8} M	(29)
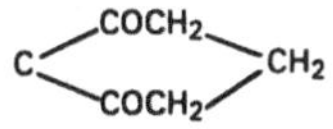 C(COCH$_2$)$_2$CH$_2$ (cyclohexane ring)	2-Retinylidene-1,3-cyclohexanedione	a	1×10^{-10}	(107)
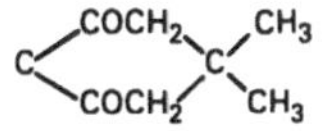 C(COCH$_2$)$_2$C(CH$_3$)$_2$	2-Retinylidene-5,5-dimethyl-1,3-cyclohexanedione; Retinylidene dimedone	a	2×10^{-10}	(150)
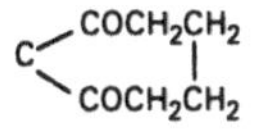 C(COCH$_2$CH$_2$)$_2$	2-Retinylidene-1,3-cycloheptanedione	a	4×10^{-10}	(51)
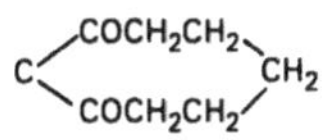 C(COCH$_2$CH$_2$)$_2$CH$_2$	2-Retinylidene-1,3-cyclooctanedione	a	2×10^{-10}	(37)
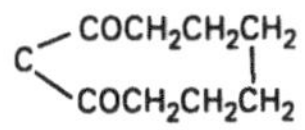 C(COCH$_2$CH$_2$CH$_2$)$_2$	2-Retinylidene-1,3-cyclononanedione	a	2×10^{-10}	(36)

FIGURE 6. Structure and activity of all-*trans*-retinal and derivatives.

described below. Data are shown for retinoids in which the ring, side chain, and polar terminal group of the basic molecule have been modified.

The standard assay that has been used measures the ability of retinoids to reverse keratinization in a defined *in vitro* system (Clamon *et al.*, 1974; Sporn *et al.*, 1976a). Tracheas were taken from hamsters that were in very early stages of vitamin A deficiency (Clamon *et al.*, 1975) and placed in organ culture. At the time of the culture, the animals were 29–31 days old (they had been weaned at 21 days) and were still gaining some weight, with an average weight of 47–52 g. Their tracheal epithelium was generally low columnar or cuboidal, with only occasional patches of squamous metaplasia. Each trachea was opened from the larynx to the carina along the membranous dorsal wall and cultured in a serum-free medium (CMRL-1066; with crystalline bovine insulin, 1.0 μg/ml; hydrocortisone hemisuccinate, 0.1 μg/ml; glutamine, 2

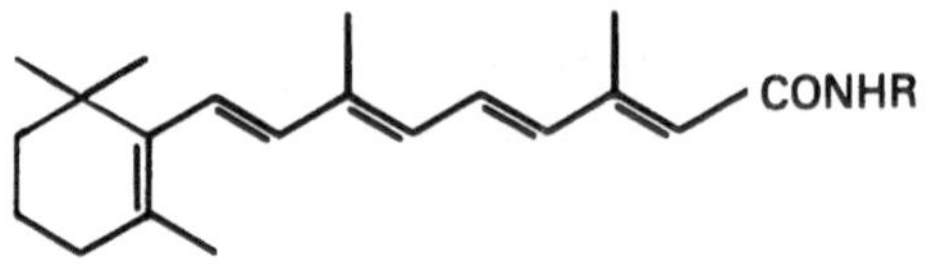

Structure, R =	Trivial Name	Source	ED_{50}, M	(Number of Cultures)
C_2H_5	N-Ethyl retinamide	g	1×10^{-9}	(86)
n-C_3H_7	N-Propyl retinamide	g, h	2×10^{-10}	(62)
n-C_4H_9	N-n-Butyl retinamide	g, h	7×10^{-10}	(39)
t-C_4H_9	N-t-Butyl retinamide	h	$> 1 \times 10^{-8}$	(22)
2-C_2H_4OH	N-2-Hydroxyethyl retinamide	g, h	1×10^{-10}	(68)
2-C_3H_6OH	N-2-Hydroxypropyl retinamide	b	3×10^{-10}	(22)
3-C_3H_6OH	N-3-Hydroxypropyl retinamide	b	2×10^{-10}	(21)
2,3-C_3H_5(OH)$_2$	N-2,3-Dihydroxypropyl retinamide	b	2×10^{-10}	(22)
CH(CH$_3$)CH$_2$CH$_2$OH	N-1-Methyl-3-hydroxypropyl retinamide	b	$> 1 \times 10^{-9}$	(40)
4-n-C_4H_8OH	N-4-Hydroxybutyl retinamide	b	2×10^{-10}	(41)
C_6H_5	N-Phenyl retinamide	g, h	4×10^{-10}	(31)
2-C_6H_4OH	N-2-Hydroxyphenyl retinamide	h	1×10^{-9}	(60)
3-C_6H_4OH	N-3-Hydroxyphenyl retinamide	h	3×10^{-10}	(55)
4-C_6H_4OH	N-4-Hydroxyphenyl retinamide	h	3×10^{-10}	(77)
4-C_6H_4OCOC$_4H_9$	N-4-Pivaloyloxyphenyl retinamide	h	2×10^{-10}	(41)

FIGURE 7. Structure and activity of all-*trans*-retinoic acid amides.

Structure, R =	Trivial Name	Source	ED_{50}·M	(Number of Cultures)
2-C_6H_4COOH	N-2 Carboxyphenyl retinamide	b	$< 1 \times 10^{-10}$	(57)
3-C_6H_4COOH	N-3-Carboxyphenyl retinamide	b	1×10^{-10}	(42)
4-C_6H_4COOH	N-4-Carboxyphenyl retinamide	b	1×10^{-10}	(70)
CN_4H	N-5-Tetrazolyl retinamide	b	$< 1 \times 10^{-10}$	(65)
$CH_2CH_2OSO_3Na$	N-2-Retinamidoethyl sodium sulfate	e	2×10^{-10}	(14)

FIGURE 7. (*Continued*)

mM; penicillin, 100 units/ml; and streptomycin, 100 μg/ml, added). Cultures were gassed with 50% oxygen, 45% nitrogen, and 5% CO_2. The culture dishes were rocked at 35.5–36.0 degrees to allow the tracheas contact with both gas and medium. All tracheas were grown in medium containing no retinoid for the first 3 days. At the end of 3 days some tracheas were harvested; almost all of these tracheas had significant squamous metaplasia: in a set of several thousand such cultures, approximately 60% had keratinized lesions.

The remaining tracheas were then divided into different groups that were then treated with either (1) retinoid dissolved in spectro grade dimethylsulfoxide (DMSO) (final concentrations of DMSO in culture medium was never greater than 0.1%) or (2) an equivalent amount of DMSO alone. Culture medium was changed three times a week, and all of the remaining tracheas were harvested at the end of 10 days in culture. Tracheas were fixed in 10% buffered formalin and embedded in paraffin. Cross sections of 5 μm were made through the midportion, stained with hematoxylin and eosin, and then scored with a microscope for the presence of keratin and keratohyaline granules, both of which were found in approximately 90% of control cultures (in a set of several thousand such cultures) that had received no retinoid for the entire 10-day culture period.

Analogues were scored as "inactive" if both keratin and keratohyaline granules were seen; they were scored as "active" if neither keratin nor keratohyaline granules were seen. Retinoids were received in sealed ampules under argon or nitrogen. These sealed ampules were stored at −20°C or below. Once opened, ampules were stored in a vapor-phase nitrogen freezer. Stock solutions of retinoids were made in DMSO at 0.1–1.0 mg/ml, and vials were stored in a vapor-phase nitrogen freezer. After thawing, contents of a given vial were used only once and then discarded. All work with retinoids were performed under subdued light or in rooms with "gold" fluorescent lamps.

Figures 1–11 show the activity of 87 retinoids in the hamster tracheal organ culture assay. Dose–response curves (Sporn et al., 1976a) were made for each retinoid, and the values derived for the dose effective in suppressing keratinization in half the cultures have been tabulated. All-*trans*-retinoic acid ($ED_{50} = 3 \times 10^{-11}$ M in a total of 1853 cultures, see Fig. 1) has been used as the reference substance. Most of the analogues in which the ring (Fig. 2) or the side chain (Fig. 3) has been modified are significantly less active in the tracheal organ culture assay. Retinol, retinyl acetate, and retinyl ethers (Fig. 4) are all less active than retinoic acid, as are retinyl amine derivatives (Fig. 5). A large number of retinal derivatives have been made, some of which have been useful in various biological studies (Todaro et al., 1978; Dickens et al., 1979; Bertram, 1980), but none are as active as retinoic acid in tracheal organ culture (Fig. 6).

In view of their relative ease of synthesis from either retinoyl chloride or retinoyl imidazole and the appropriate amine, a particularly large number of amide derivatives have been synthesized and tested (Fig. 7). Derivatization of the polar terminus of the retinoid molecule to form amides offers the possibility of synthesizing a set of compounds with an especially wide range of

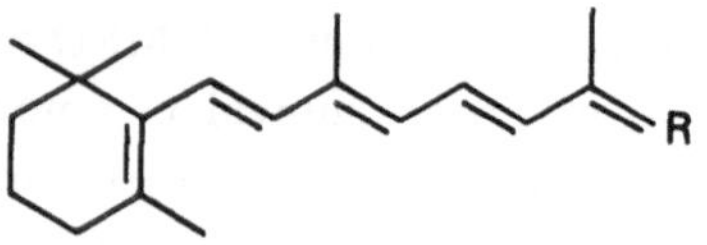

Structure, R =	Trivial Name	Source	ED_{50}, M	(Number of Cultures)
CHCH$_3$	Axerophthene	b	2×10^{-9}	(86)
CHCH$_2$CH$_3$	Retinyl methane; 15-Methyl axerophthene	b	$>1 \times 10^{-8}$	(11)
C(CH$_3$)$_2$	14-Methyl axerophthene	b	$>1 \times 10^{-8}$	(12)
CHCOCH$_3$	Methyl retinone	l	2×10^{-7}	(37)
CHC(CH$_3$)$_2$OH	15-Dimethyl retinol	a	$>1 \times 10^{-8}$	(9)
CHCH$_2$SCOCH$_3$	Retinyl thioacetate	k	$>1 \times 10^{-8}$	(13)
O	C$_{18}$ Ketone	c	Inactive, 8/8 cultures, 1×10^{-8} M	(8)

FIGURE 8. Structure and activity of additional modifications of the polar terminus of the retinoid molecule.

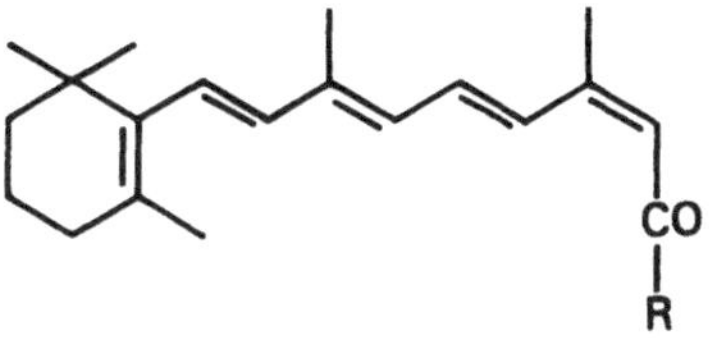

FIGURE 9. Structure and activity of 13-cis-retinoic acid and derivatives.

Structure, R =	Trivial Name	Source	ED_{50}, M	(Number of Cultures)
OH	13-cis-Retinoic acid; Isotretinoin	b, g	3×10^{-11}	(69)
$NH(C_2H_5)$	N-Ethyl 13-cis-retinamide	j	3×10^{-10}	(37)
$NH(2\text{-}C_2H_4OH)$	N-2-Hydroxyethyl 13-cis-retinamide	j	3×10^{-10}	(40)
$NH(2,3\text{-}C_3H_5[OH]_2)$	N-2,3-Dihydroxypropyl 13-cis-retinamide	b	1×10^{-10}	(29)
$NH(4\text{-}C_6H_4OH)$	N-4-Hydroxyphenyl 13-cis-retinamide	j	$>1 \times 10^{-9}$	(88)
$NH(CN_4H)$	N-5-Tetrazolyl 13-cis-retinamide	b	2×10^{-10}	(63)

chemical properties, including derivatives that have the interesting property of being soluble in both water and chloroform, as in the case of 2-retinamidoethyl sodium sulfate (Fig. 7). Most of these compounds have appreciable activity in the 10^{-9} to 10^{-10} M range, with the notable exception of sterically hindered amides such as *t*-butyl retinamide or 1-methyl-3-hydroxypropyl retinamide, suggesting that, as a class, the amides must be hydrolyzed to retinoic acid before exerting their biological activity. Several of the retinamides have been reported to be significantly less toxic than all-*trans*-retinoic acid and to be useful for inhibition of carcinogenesis in experimental animals (Hixson and Denine, 1979; Moon *et al.*, 1979; Thompson and Becci, 1979). Other modifications of the polar terminus (Fig. 8), particularly the addition of one or two carbon atoms, have led to analogues in which activity has been significantly diminished.

13-*cis*-Retinoic acid and several of its amide derivatives (Fig. 9) are highly active in tracheal organ culture. It has recently been suggested (Frolik *et al.*, 1980) that isomerization of all-*trans*-retinoic acid to the 13-*cis*-isomer may occur during physiological action of all-*trans*-retinoic acid. Newly synthesized 13-*cis*-retinamides (Fig. 9) are currently in initial stages of evaluation to determine if they will be more useful than all-*trans*-retinamides

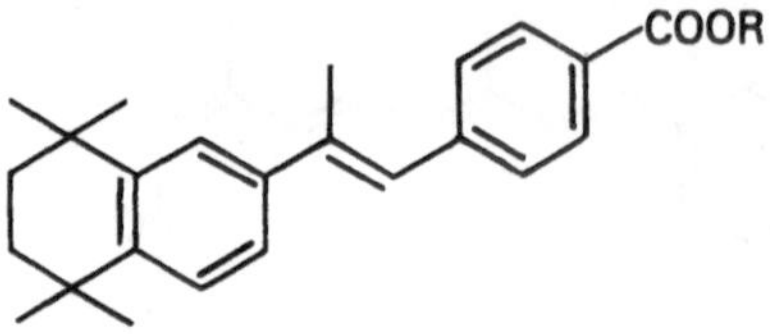

Structure, R =	Trivial Name	Source	ED_{50}, M	(Number of Cultures)
H	Ro 13-7410	g	1×10^{-11}	(50)
C_2H_5	Ro 13-6298	g	1×10^{-11}	(80)

FIGURE 10. Structure and activity of ring- and side-chain-modified analogues of all-*trans*-retinoic acid and its esters.

as inhibitors of carcinogenesis. Figure 10 shows two new structures in which both the ring and side chain of the retinoid molecule have been modified. In these retinoids, a *gem*-dimethyl group has been inserted at position 4 of the cyclohexenyl ring, and two aromatic rings have been introduced into the side chain; these new structures are intensely active. In view of the suggestion that 5,6-epoxyretinoic acid might be an activated form of retinoic acid McCormick *et al.*, 1978; Wertz *et al.*, 1979), this compound as well as three related analogues (5,6-epoxyretinoic acid methyl ester, 5,6-epoxyretinyl acetate, and the 5,6-epoxy analogue of retinylidene dimedone) were tested (Fig. 11). All of the epoxides are significantly less active in the tracheal organ culture assay than their respective parent compounds.

The tracheal organ culture assay is highly specific for retinoid structures. A wide variety of other terpenoid and related structures have been tested and been found to be inactive (data not shown); these compounds include juvenile hormones I, II, and III, mycophenolic acid, and abscisic acid. Although β-ionone has not been tested, it is apparent that the side chain is of major importance for biological activity, since the C_{15} and C_{17} analogues of retinoic acid (Fig. 3) are almost totally inactive, and each of the four isomeric dihydroretinoic acid analogues (Fig. 3) are markedly less active than all-*trans*-retinoic acid or its methyl and ethyl esters. Similarly, the C_{18} ketone (Fig. 8) was totally inactive at 1×10^{-8} M.

The data shown in Figs. 1–11 indicate that a very wide range of modifications in the ring, side chain, or polar terminus of the retinoid molecule can be made and still allow expression of biological activity. However, it is noteworthy that few analogues have been made that are more active than either all-*trans*- or 13-*cis*-retinoic acid. In particular, we find no evidence that a 5,6-epoxide is an activated form (McCormick *et al.*, 1978;

Wertz et al., 1979), although such a molecule might require synthesis *in situ* in a cell in order to demonstrate enhanced biological activity. Similarly, both 4-hydroxy- and 4-ketoretinoic acids, which are early products of oxidative metabolism of retinoic acid (Frolik et al., 1979), were found to be markedly less active than all-*trans*-retinoic acid. The possibility that retinoic acid might also be activated by epoxidation at the 9,10 or 11,12 double bonds cannot presently be ruled out, since these compounds have not yet been definitively synthesized and tested for biological activity. However, there is little or no evidence at present that any natural, known retinoid metabolite is more active in the tracheal organ culture assay than either all-*trans*- or 13-*cis*-retinoic acid. It is interesting that in many other *in vitro* test systems retinoic acid has been consistently more active than retinol, retinyl esters, or retinal (Wilkoff et al., 1976; Chopra and Wilkoff, 1977; Strickland and Mahdavi, 1978; Verma et al., 1978, 1979; Lotan et al., 1980).

The correlations of activity of retinoids in this tracheal system with many other in vitro test systems are excellent. Such test systems include reversal of changes induced by carcinogens in mouse prostate organ cultures (Lasnitzki and Goodman, 1974; Chopra and Wilkoff, 1977), suppression of keratinization in chick skin organ cultures (Wilkoff et al., 1976), inhibition of induction of ornithine decarboxylase in mouse skin (Verma et al., 1979), inhibition of growth of murine melanoma cells (Lotan et al., 1978, 1980), enhancement of adhesion of transformed mouse fibroblasts (Adamo et al., 1979), and suppression of malignant transformation in a cloned mouse fibroblast cell line (Bertram, 1980). It is of interest that the present tracheal assay system gives a broader range of positive results than some of the other test systems,

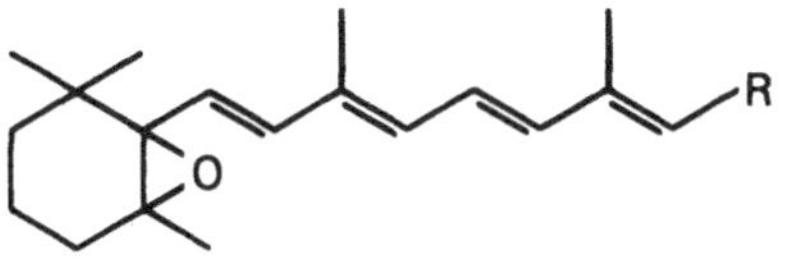

Structure, R =	Trivial Name	Source	ED_{50}, M	(Number of Cultures)
COOH	5,6-Epoxyretinoic acid	g	2×10^{-9}	(44)
COOCH$_3$	5,6-Epoxyretinoic acid methyl ester	k	3×10^{-9}	(45)
CH$_2$OCOCH$_3$	5,6-Epoxyretinyl acetate	k	4×10^{-9}	(35)
CH (C$_8$H$_{10}$O$_2$)	5,6-Epoxide of retinylidene dimedone	a	3×10^{-9}	(46)

FIGURE 11. Structure and activity of 5,6-all-*trans*-epoxyretinoids.

particularly with amide derivatives which show rather low activity in several other assays (Wilkoff et al., 1976; Strickland and Mahdavi, 1978; Adamo et al., 1979; Verma et al., 1979; Lotan et al., 1980). Presumably the tracheal system has the necessary enzymes to hydrolyze retinamides; the low activity of a sterically hindered amide such as t-butyl retinamide is again noteworthy in this context.

Finally, the intense activity of the two retinoids in Fig. 10 suggests that chemical synthesis can provide new molecules that may have a stronger interaction with a receptor molecule or site than all-*trans*-retinoic acid in a manner analogous to the enhanced binding of 9-α-fluoroglucocorticoids to hydrocortisone receptors. It remains to be determined whether the best approach to cancer prevention with new synthetic retinoids will involve a further increase in their intrinsic biological activity (as can be measured with the tracheal organ culture assay) or perhaps will involve a further decrease in their intrinsic toxicity, as we have suggested elsewhere (Sporn et al., 1979).

VII. Prevention of Cancer in Experimental Animals with New Synthetic Retinoids

With the increased availability of biologically active synthetic retinoids, there has been an increased testing of these compounds in long-term animal tests for prevention of carcinogenesis. Most of the experimental designs have involved testing the retinoids as "antipromoting" agents. A number of organ-specific animal models now exist in which initiation may be rapidly completed in a defined period by the administration of a small number of doses (or even a single dose) of carcinogen. One then can study the effect of retinoids in blocking further promotion or progression of carcinogenesis during the latency period when cells are still in a preneoplastic state and before invasive malignancy is histologically detectable.

This approach has recently been used quite extensively in the prevention of experimental bladder and breast cancer, and several synthetic retinoids have been shown to be effective. Since both human (Farrow et al., 1976) and experimental (Squire et al., 1977) studies have shown that the severity of preneoplastic lesions of the bladder can be evaluated on a semiquantitative basis, bladder carcinogenesis has been a particularly useful area for assessing the ability of retinoids to arrest tumor promotion and progression.

The retinoid that has undergone the most extensive testing has been 13-*cis*-retinoic acid. This compound has been effective in arresting neoplastic progression in the following bladder carcinogenesis systems: (1) Wistar–Lewis rats dosed by direct application of N-methyl-N-nitrosourea to the bladder (Squire et al., 1977); (2) Fischer rats dosed orally with N-butyl-N-4-hydroxybutylnitrosamine (HO-BBN) (Grubbs et al., 1977b); (3) C57 BL/6 mice dosed orally with HO-BBN (Becci et al., 1978); and (4) B6D2F$_1$ hydrid mice dosed orally with HO-BBN (Becci et al., 1981). These different animal models provide a spectrum of both transitional cell and squamous cell carcinoma of the bladder that closely resembles various stages of the human disease. In experiments performed with HO-BBN in rats, it was found that even if treatment with 13-cis-retinoic acid was delayed for 2 months after carcinogen treatment was completed, there was a substantial protective effect (Becci et al., 1979). Very recent studies have shown that the two amide derivatives, ethyl retinamide and 2-hydroxyethyl retinamide, both inhibit bladder carcinogenesis induced by HO-BBN in Fischer rats (Thompson et al., 1981), and B6D2F$_1$ hybrid mice (Becci et al., 1980).

Since breast cancer is also a disease characterized by a prolonged series of premalignant epithelial changes before development of invasive malignancy, and since excellent animal models are available, the effect of retinoids in prevention of this disease has also been extensively studied. The first synthetic retinoid shown to be effective was retinyl methyl ether in experiments using 7,12-dimethylbenzanthracene as the carcinogen (Grubbs et al., 1977a). More recent studies have employed N-methyl-N-nitrosourea as the carcinogen, since the cancers induced by this agent more closely resemble human breast cancer (Gullino et al., 1975). The most notable protective effect was obtained with 4-hydroxyphenyl retinamide which, at nontoxic doses, can provide a marked extension of the latency period before appearance of palpable cancers (Moon et al., 1979). In these studies, whole mounts of the rat mammary gland made after chronic feeding of the retinoid indicated that 4-hydroxyphenyl retinamide had a strong antiproliferative effect on mammary epithelium that apparently is not the result of suppression of ovarian function. Retinyl acetate also was found to have a very strong preventive effect on mammary carcinogenesis induced by methyl nitrosourea (Moon et al., 1977, 1979), but the toxic effects of high doses of this retinoid on the liver were very pronounced (Moon et al., 1979) and emphasize the need for further development of synthetic analogues.

Many new retinoids have been screened for prevention of skin papillomas and carcinomas in mice, and these studies have been summarized in detail elsewhere (Mayer et al., 1978; Verma et al., 1979). Particularly noteworthy have been the synergistic effects of retinoids and steroids (Weeks *et al.*, 1979) as well as retinoids and protease inhibitors (Verma *et al.*, 1980) in prevention of skin carcinogenesis. Attempts to prevent epithelial carcinogenesis at other organ sites have not yet given as definitive results as the studies on bladder, breast, and skin. Results of new studies on attempted prevention of pancreatic, prostatic, esophageal, and colon carcinogenesis will be awaited with much interest. At present, there are no clear pharmacokinetic principles for selection of a new retinoid for prevention of cancer at these target sites. However, given the fundamental mechanistic similarities of many types of epithelial carcinogenesis, one may anticipate that use of new synthetic retinoids might eventually prove to be valuable in modulating carcinogenesis at these additional target sites.

VIII. Mechanism of Action of Retinoids in Chemoprevention of Cancer

The successful use of retinoids in chemoprevention of cancer has raised further questions about their mechanism of action, both cellular and molecular. Many of these questions remain unanswered and are the basis for much of the current significant research in this area. At the cellular level, retinoids may be regarded as agents that modulate the processes of proliferation and differentiation as was first noted by Wolbach and Howe in 1925. An overall discussion of the total problem of the control of cell proliferation and differentiation is beyond the scope of this chapter. However, with respect to the role of retinoids in controlling cellular proliferation during carcinogenesis, it appears that retinoids are modulating the effects of specific polypeptide hormones that enhance cell division in specific epithelial target organs such as the proliferative effect of prolactin on mammary epithelium.

Whole mounts of the mammary gland of rats fed 4-hydroxyphenyl retinamide clearly indicate that this retinoid has a potent antiproliferative effect on mammary epithelium (Moon *et al.*, 1979); there was markedly decreased ductal branching and end bud proliferation in animals fed this retinoid. The structure of the mammary gland of animals fed the retinoid resembled that of animals treated with a suppressor of pituitary prolactin release such as the ergot derivative, 2-bromoergocryptine (Welsch, 1976). Furthermore, in recent studies (Welsch *et al.*, 1980), a marked synergism has been found between retinoids and 2-bromoergocryptine in prevention of mammary cancer induced in rats by nitrosomethylurea; the combined modality was far superior to either treatment alone. It should be emphasized, however, that there is no evidence at present for a direct molecular interaction at a receptor site between retinoids and prolactin. The available information only suggests that retinoids suppress the overall biological effects of prolactin on mammary epithelium.

Studies in cell culture have allowed a more direct demonstration of the ability of retinoids to modulate the effects of a polypeptide that has the ability to enhance cellular proliferation. This has been shown in studies, referred to earlier (Section III), in which very low, noncytotoxic concentrations of retinoids antagonize the effects of the polypeptide, sarcoma growth factor, which causes both cell multiplication and anchorage-independent growth of cells that otherwise would not grow in soft agar (Todaro et al., 1978). Details of these experiments are shown in Tables 1 and 2. It should again be emphasized that there is no evidence at present for a direct molecular interaction at a receptor site between retinoids and sarcoma growth factor.

In summary, the retinoids appear to have significant biological interactions with polypeptide hormones that cause cell proliferation including those that may be involved in the expression of the malignant phenotype. Since it has been suggested that the development of malignancy involves the expression of transforming polypeptides (transforming growth factors), (Todaro and De Larco, 1978), and since retinoids can suppress the effects of these TGFs (by molecular interactions yet to be elucidated), a new tentative mechanism whereby retinoids suppress the development of cancer may now be postulated. Undoubtedly the molecular aspects of this entire problem will

TABLE 1. Effect of SGF and Retinyl Acetate on the final Cell Density of Rat Fibroblast Cell Cultures[a]

Treatment	Cells per plate (10^{-6})	
	Experiment 1	Experiment 2
Untreated control	1.2	1.0
+ Retinyl acetate (1.9×10^{-8} M)	1.3	1.1
SGF-treated ($10 \mu g\ ml^{-1}$)	3.6	2.6
+ Retinyl acetate (1.9×10^{-8} M)	1.4	0.9
+ DMSO (1 : 1000)	3.3	2.5

[a] A subclone (536-7) of a normal rat fibroblast cell clone, NRK 49F, susceptible to the growth-stimulating effect of SGF was seeded at 2×10^5 cells per plate in 60-mm plastic Petri dishes. The cells were treated at the time of inoculation and refed with medium (Dulbecco's modified medium with 1% fetal calf serum) containing the additions shown every third day. Cell counts were made 10 days after seeding. The SGF came from supernatants of MSV-transformed mouse NIH/3T3 cells. Retinyl acetate was dissolved in dimethyl sulfoxide (DMSO). The final concentration of DMSO in all experiments was 0.1%. Neither retinyl acetate nor DMSO alone showed any effect on the growth, final cell density, or cloning efficiency of the normal rat fibroblasts at the concentrations used. Reprinted with permission from Todaro et al. (1978).

TABLE 2. Effect of SGF and Various Retinoids on the Colony-Forming Ability of Rat Fibroblasts Plated in Soft Agar[a]

Treatment	Colonies per plate		
	Experiment 1	Experiment 2	Experiment 3
Untreated controls	0	0	0
+ Retinyl acetate (1.9×10^{-8} M)	0	0	0
+ Retinoic acid (2.0×10^{-8} M)	NT	0	NT
+ Retinylidene dimedone (1.5×10^{-8} M)	NT	NT	0
+ Retinyl methyl ether (2.0×10^{-8} M)	NT	NT	0
SGF-treated ($10\mu g\ ml^{-1}$)	44.5	39.0	49.5
+ Retinyl acetate (1.9×10^{-8} M)	2.5	1.5	8.0
+ Retinoic acid (2.0×10^{-8} M)	NT	3.2	NT
+ Retinylidene dimedone (1.5×10^{-8} M)	NT	NT	0.5
+ Retinyl methyl ether (2.0×10^{-8} M)	NT	NT	14.5

[a] On day 0, 1×10^5 rat fibroblast cells, clone 536-7, were treated in monolayer cultures using Dulbecco's modified medium with 1% fetal calf serum as described in the legend to Table 1. On day 2, they were seeded at 1×10^4 cells per plate in 0.3% soft agar containing the additions shown. All cells not treated with SGF (whether treated with retinoid or not) remained as single cells with occasional (<10%) small colonies of 2–4 cells. Colonies with greater than 20 cells after 2 weeks in agar were scored as positive. NT, not tested. Reprinted with permission from Todaro et al. (1978).

require further study and likely will involve further consideration of biochemical mechanisms whereby retinoids interact with the genome as well as participate in determining the structure of cell membranes.

IX. Mechanism of Toxicity of Retinoids

The well-known toxicity syndrome, often called "hypervitaminosis A" (which is actually a misnomer, since the toxic effects of retinoids are not an accentuation of their normal effects), has been described in many reviews (Moore, 1957, 1967; Mayer et al., 1978). A better general term would be "retinoid toxicity" (Harrison et al., 1977), since the toxicity of retinoids can indeed be dissociated from the intrinsic effects that retinoids have on cellular differentiation (Bollag, 1974; Sporn et al., 1976a). The detailed molecular mechanism of retinoid toxicity is still unknown, although it has been known for a long time that retinoids can destabilize cellular membranes, particularly those of lysosomes (Fell *et al.,* 1962; Goodman *et al.,* 1974).

Recent studies strongly implicate involvement of the prostaglandins in the mechanism of retinoid toxicity. Elevated levels of prostaglandins have been found in cultures of dog kidney cells that have been exposed to high concentrations of some of the more toxic retinoids (Levine and Ohuchi, 1978). Conversely, inhibitors of prostaglandin synthesis such as aspirin (Harrison *et al.,* 1977) or several of the nonsteroidal antiinflammatory agents (Hixson and Denine, 1978) have been shown to protect mice from lethal and other toxic effects of all-*trans*-retinoic acid. All retinoids do not increase synthesis of prostaglandins; the important finding has recently been made that the relatively nontoxic analogue, 4-hydroxyphenyl retinamide, is a potent inhibitor of prostaglandin synthesis (Levine, 1980). These results suggest that studies of the effects of retinoids on prostaglandin synthesis may be useful predictors of retinoid toxicity as well as offer a mechanism for understanding the undesirable effects of these agents.

X. Combination Chemoprevention with Retinoids

Although there have been numerous studies of prevention of experimental cancer with retinoids, if the extent of carcinogenic exposure is high enough, the retinoids are not effective in blocking the development of malignancy. In addition, as we have noted, effective doses of retinoids may often cause highly undesirable toxicity. The possibility of using retinoids synergistically with other chemopreventive agents thus has been considered as a means both to increase desired potency and to decrease undesired toxicity. The first study to demonstrate such synergism utilized retinoids and fluorinated glucocorticoids to inhibit skin carcinogenesis in mice, and a markedly useful synergism was found (Weeks *et al.,* 1979); these results have been confirmed by others (Verma *et al.,* 1980). Subsequently, strongly synergistic chemopreventive effects between retinoids and protease inhibitors have been reported in the same skin carcinogenesis system (Verma *et al.,* 1980). Retinoids and a suppressor of prolactin release from the pituitary (2-bromoergocryptine) have also been shown to be strongly synergistic in preventing mammary cancer in the rat (Welsch *et al.,* 1980).

These studies on "combination chemoprevention" with retinoids have just begun in the field of carcinogenesis studies but already show promise of leading to developments that may have practical implications for prevention of human cancer. The use of combination chemotherapy employing several cytotoxic drugs is a well established discipline in the pharmacological approach to cancer treatment. It remains to be seen whether a similar approach of using several noncytotoxic drugs that suppress malignant transformation by different molecular mechanisms will be of equivalent usefulness in the field of cancer prevention.

ACKNOWLEDGMENTS. We thank Ellen Friedman for expert assistance with the manuscript. Retinoids have been generously provided to our experimental program by BASF Aktiengesellschaft, Hoffmann-LaRoche, Inc., and Johnson & Johnson.

References

Adamo, S., De Luca, L. M., Akalovsky, I., and Bhat, P. V., 1979, Retinoid-induced adhesion in cultured, transformed mouse fibroblasts, *J. Natl. Cancer Inst.* **62**:1473.

Becci, P. J., Thompson, H. J., Grubbs, C. G., Squire, R. A., Brown, C. C., Sporn, M. B., and Moon, R. C., 1978, Inhibitory effect of 13-cis-retinoic acid on urinary bladder carcinogenesis induced in C57BL/6 mice by N-butyl-N-(4-hydroxybutyl)nitrosamine, *Cancer Res.* **38**:4463.

Becci, P. J., Thompson, C. J., Grubbs, C. J., Brown, C. C., and Moon, R. C., 1979, Effect of delay in administration of 13-cis-retinoic acid on the inhibition of urinary bladder carcinogenesis in the rat, *Cancer Res.* **39**:3141.

Becci, P. J., Thompson, H. J., Sporn, M. B., and Moon, R. C., 1980, Retinoid inhibition of highly invasive urinary bladder carcinomas induced in mice by N-butyl-N-(4-hydroxybutyl)nitrosamine (OH-BBN), *Proc. Am. Assoc. Cancer Res.* **21**:88.

Becci, P. J., Thompson, H. J., Strum, J. M., Brown, C. C., Sporn, M. B., and Moon, R. C., 1981, N-Butyl-N-(4-hydroxybutyl)nitrosamine-induced urinary bladder cancer in C57BL/6 × DBA/2-F_1 mice, a useful model for study of chemoprevention of cancer with retinoids, *Cancer Res.* **41**:927.

Bertram, J. S., 1980, Structure–activity relationships among various retinoids and their ability to inhibit neoplastic transformation and to increase cell adhesion in the C3H10T1/2 CL8 cell line, *Cancer Res.* **40**:3141.

Bjelke, E., 1975, Dietary vitamin A and human lung cancer, *Int. J. Cancer* **15**:561.

Bollag, W., 1972, Prophylaxis of chemically induced benign and malignant epithelial tumors by vitamin A (retinoic acid), *Eur. J. Cancer* **8**:689.

Bollag, W., 1974, Therapeutic effects of an aromatic retinoic acid analog on chemically induced skin papillomas and carcinomas of mice, *Eur. J. Cancer* **10**:731.

Boutwell, R. K., 1979, Selected abstracts on vitamin A in cancer biology, International Cancer Research Data Bank (ICRDB), National Cancer Institute, Bethesda, Maryland.

Boutwell, R. K., and Verma, A., 1979, Effects of vitamin A and related retinoids on the biochemical processes linked to carcinogenesis, *Pure Appl. Chem.* **51**:857.

Breitman, T. R., Selonick, S. E., and Collins, S. J., 1980, Induction of differentiation of the human promyelocytic leukemia cell line (HL-60) by retinoic acid, *Proc. Natl. Acad. Sci. USA* **77**:2936.

Chopra, D. P., and Wilkoff, L. J., 1977, Reversal by vitamin A analogues of hyperplasia induced by N-methyl-N'-nitro-N-nitrosoguanidine in mouse prostate organ cultures, *J. Natl. Cancer Inst.* **58**:923.

Clamon, G. H., Sporn, M. B., Smith, J. M., and Saffiotti, U., 1974, α- and β-retinyl acetate reverse metaplasias of vitamin A deficiency in hamster trachea in organ culture, *Nature* **250**:64.

Clamon, G. H., Sporn, M. B., Smith, J. M., and Henderson, W. R., 1975, Effect of α-retinyl acetate on growth of hamsters fed vitamin A-deficient diets, *J. Nutr.* **105**:215.

Cohen, S. M., Wittenberg, J. F., and Bryan, G. T., 1976, Effect of avitaminosis A and hypervitaminosis A on urinary bladder carcinogenicity of N-[4-(5-nitro-2-furyl)-2-thiazolyl] formamide, *Cancer Res.* **36**:2334.

De Larco, J. E., and Todaro, G. J., 1978, Growth factors from murine sarcoma virus-transformed cells, *Proc. Natl. Acad. Sci. USA* **75**:4001.

De Luca, L., Little, E. P., and Wolf, G., 1969, Vitamin A and protein synthesis by rat intestinal mucosa, *J. Biol. Chem.* **244**:701.

Dickens, M. S., Custer, R. P., and Sorof, S., 1979, Retinoid prevents mammary gland transformation by carcinogenic hydrocarbon in whole-organ culture, *Proc. Natl. Acad. Sci. USA* **76**:5891.

Dion, L. D., Blalock, J. E., and Gifford, G. E., 1978, Retinoic acid and the restoration of anchorage dependent growth to transformed mammalian cells, *Exp. Cell Res.* **117**:15.

Farrow, G. M., Utz, D. C., and Rife, C. C., 1976, Morphological and clinical observations of patients with early bladder cancer treated with total cystectomy, *Cancer Res.* **36**:2495.

Fell, H. B., Dingle, J. T., and Webb, M., 1962, Studies on the mode of action of excess of vitamin A. The specificity of the effect on embryonic chick-limb cartilage in culture and on isolated rat liver lysosomes, *Biochem. J.* **83**:63.

Frolik, C. A., and Roller, P. P., 1981, The role of retinoids (vitamin A and its analogs) in the prevention of epithelial cancer, in: *Antitumor Compounds of Natural Origin* (A. Aszalos, ed.), CRC Press, Boca Raton, Fla., in press.

Frolik, C. A., Roberts, A. B., Tavela, T. E., Roller, P. P., Newton, D. L., and Sporn, M. B., 1979, Isolation and identification of 4-hydroxy- and 4-oxoretinoic acid, *in vitro* metabolites of all-*trans*-retinoic acid in hamster trachea and liver, *Biochemistry* **18**:2092.

Frolik, C. A., Roller, P. P., Roberts, A. B., and Sporn, M. B., 1980, In vitro and *in vivo* metabolism of all-*trans*- and 13-*cis*-retinoic acid in hamsters. Identification of 13-*cis*-4-oxoretinoic acid, *J. Biol. Chem.* **255**:8057.

Goodman, D. S., Smith, J. E., Hembry, R. M., and Dingle, J. T., 1974, Comparison of the effects of vitamin A and its analogs upon rabbit ear cartilage in organ culture and upon growth of the vitamin A-deficient rat, *J. Lipid Res.* **15**:406.

Grubbs, C. J., Moon, R. C., Sporn, M. B., and Newton, D. L., 1977a, Inhibition of mammary cancer with retinyl methyl ether, *Cancer Res.* **37**:599.

Grubbs, C. J., Moon, R. C., Squire, R. A., Farrow, G. M., Stinson, S. F., Goodman, D. G., Brown, C. C., and Sporn, M. B., 1977b, 13-*cis*-Retinoic acid: Inhibition of bladder carcinogenesis induced in rats by N-butyl-N-(4-hydroxybutyl)nitrosamine, *Science* **198**:743.

Gullino, P. M., Pettigrew, H. M., and Grantham, F. H., 1975, N-Nitrosomethylurea as mammary gland carcinogen in rats, *J. Natl. Cancer Inst.* **54**:401.

Harisiadis, L., Miller, R. C., Hall, E. J., and Borek, C., 1978, A vitamin A analogue inhibits radiation-induced oncogenic transformation, *Nature* **274**:486.

Harris, C. C., Sporn, M. B., Kaufman, D. G., Smith, J. M., Jackson, F. E., and Saffiotti, U., 1972, Histogenesis of squamous metaplasia in the hamster tracheal epithelium caused by vitamin A deficiency or benzo(a)pyrene–ferric oxide, *J. Natl. Cancer Inst.* **48**:743.

Harrison, S. D., Jr., Hixson, E. J., Burdeshaw, J. A., and Denine, E. P., 1977, Effect of aspirin administration on retinoic acid toxicity in mice, *Nature* **269**:511.

Hirayama, T., 1979, Diet and cancer, *Nutr. Cancer* **1**(3):67.

Hixson, E. J., and Denine, E. P., 1978, Effect of non-steroidal antiinflammatory agents on toxicity of retinoic acid in mice, *Toxicol. Appl. Pharmacol.* **45**:317.

Hixson, E. J., and Denine, E. P., 1979, Comparative subacute toxicity of retinyl acetate and three synthetic retinamides in Swiss mice, *J. Natl. Cancer Inst.* **63:**1359.

Lacroix, A., and Lippman, M. E., 1980, Binding of retinoids to human breast cancer cell lines and their effects on cell growth, *J. Clin. Invest.* **65:**586.

Lasnitzki, I., 1955, The influence of A hypervitaminosis on the effect of 20-methylcholanthrene on mouse prostate glands grown *in vitro, Br. J. Cancer* **9:**434.

Lasnitzki, I., and Goodman, D. S., 1974, Inhibition of the effects of methylcholanthrene on mouse prostate in organ culture by vitamin A and its analogs, *Cancer Res.* **34:**1564.

Levij, I. S., and Polliack, A., 1968, Potentiating effect of vitamin A on 9,10-dimethylbenzanthracene carcinogenesis in the hamster cheek pouch, *Cancer* **22:**300.

Levij, I. S., Rwomushana, J. W., and Polliack, A., 1969, Enhancement of chemical carcinogenesis in the hamster cheek pouch by prior topical application of vitamin A palmitate, *J. Invest. Dermatol.* **53:**228.

Levine, L., 1980, *N*-(4-Hydroxyphenyl) retinamide: A synthetic analog of vitamin A that is a potent inhibitor of prostaglandin biosynthesis, *Prostagland. Med.* **4:**285.

Levine, L., and Ohuchi, K., 1978, Retinoids as well as tumor promoters enhance deacylation of cellular lipids in MDCK cells, *Nature* **276:**274.

Lotan, R., 1979, Different susceptibilities of human melanoma and breast carcinoma cell lines to retinoic acid-induced growth inhibition, *Cancer Res.* **39:**1014.

Lotan, R., 1980, Effects of vitamin A and its analogs (retinoids) on normal and neoplastic cells, *Biochim. Biophys. Acta* **605:**33.

Lotan, R., and Nicolson, G. L., 1977, Inhibitory effects of retinoic acid or retinyl acetate on the growth of untransformed, transformed, and tumor cells *in vitro, J. Natl. Cancer Inst.* **59:**1717.

Lotan, R., Giotta, G., Nork, E., and Nicolson, G. L., 1978, Characterization of the inhibitory effects of retinoids on the *in vitro* growth of two malignant murine melanomas, *J. Natl. Cancer Inst.* **60:**1035.

Lotan, R., Neumann, G., and Lotan, D., 1980, Relationships among retinoid structure, inhibition of growth, and cellular retinoic acid-binding protein in cultured S91 melanoma cells, *Cancer Res.* **40:**1097.

Mayer, H., and Isler, O., 1971, Total synthesis, in: *Carotenoids* (O. Isler, ed.), pp. 325–575, Birkhauser, Basel.

Mayer, H., Bollag, W., Hänni, R., and Rüegg, R., 1978, Retinoids, a new class of compounds with prophylactic and therapeutic activities in oncology and dermatology, *Experientia* **34:**1105.

McCormick, A. M., Napoli, L., Schnoes, H. K., and DeLuca, H. F., 1978, Isolation and identification of 5,6-epoxyretinoic acid: A biologically active metabolite of retinoic acid, *Biochemistry* **17:**4085.

Merriman, R. L., and Bertram, J. S., 1979, Reversible inhibition by retinoids of 3-methylcholanthrene-induced neoplastic transformation in C3H/10T1/2 CL8 cells, *Cancer Res.* **39:**1661.

Mettlin, C., and Graham, S., 1979, Dietary risk factors in human bladder cancer, *Am. J. Epidemiol.* **110:**255.

Mettlin, C., Graham, S., and Swanson, M., 1979, Vitamin A and lung cancer, *J. Natl. Cancer Inst.* **62:**1435.

Meyskens, F. L., and Salmon, S. E., 1979, Inhibition of human melanoma colony formation by retinoids, *Cancer Res.* **39:**4055.

Moon, R. C., Grubbs, C. J., Sporn, M. B., and Goodman, D. G., 1977, Retinyl acetate inhibits mammary carcinogenesis induced by *N*-methyl-*N*-nitrosourea, *Nature* **267:**620.

Moon, R. C., Thompson, H. J., Becci, P. J., Grubbs, C. J., Gander, R. J., Newton, D. L., Smith, J. M., Phillips, S. L., Henderson, W. R., Mullen, L. T., Brown, C. C., and Sporn, M. B.,

1979, N-(4-Hydroxyphenyl)retinamide, a new retinoid for prevention of breast cancer in the rat, *Cancer Res.* **39**:1339.
Moore, T., 1957, *Vitamin A*, Elsevier, Amsterdam.
Moore, T., 1967, Pharmacology and toxicology of vitamin A, in: *The Vitamins*, Second Edition, Vol. I (W. H. Sebrell and R. S. Harris, eds.), pp. 280–294, Academic Press, New York.
Mossman, B. T., Craighead, J. E., and MacPherson, B. V., 1980, Asbestos-induced ephithelial changes in organ cultures of hamster trachea: Inhibition by retinyl methyl ether, *Science* **207**:311.
Müller-Salamin, L., Matter, A., and Lasnitzki, I., 1979, Interaction of retinoic acid and 3-methylcholanthrene on the fine structure of mouse prostate epithelium *in vitro*, *J. Natl. Cancer Inst.* **63**:485.
Nettesheim, P., and Williams, M. L., 1976, The influence of vitamin A on susceptibility of the rat lung to 3-methylcholanthrene, *Int. J. Cancer* **17**:351.
Newberne, P. M., and Rogers, A. E., 1973, Rat colon carcinomas associated with aflatoxin and marginal vitamin A, *J. Natl. Cancer Inst.* **50**:439.
Newton, D. L., Henderson, W. R., and Sporn, M. B., 1980, Structure–activity relationships of retinoids, *Cancer Res.* **40**:3413.
Rogers, A. E., Herndon, B. J., and Newberne, P. M., 1973, Induction by dimethylhydrazine of intestinal carcinoma in normal rats fed high or low levels of vitamin A, *Cancer Res* **33**:1003.
Rojanapo, W., Lamb, A. J., and Olson, J. A., 1980, The prevalance, metabolism, and migration of goblet cells in rat intestine following the induction of rapid synchronous vitamin A deficiency, *J. Nutr.* **110**:178.
Sporn, M. B., and Newton, D. L., 1979, Chemoprevention of cancer with retinoids, *Fed. Proc.* **38**:2528.
Sporn, M. B., Dunlop, N. M., Newton, D. L., and Henderson, W. R., 1976a, Relationships between structure and activity of retinoids, *Nature* **263**:110.
Sporn, M. B., Dunlop, N. M., Newton, D. L., and Smith, J. M., 1976b, Prevention of chemical carcinogenesis by vitamin A and its synthetic analogs, *Fed. Proc.* **35**:1332.
Sporn, M. B., Newton, D. L., Smith, J. M., Acton, N., Jacobson, A. R., Brossi, A., 1979, Retinoids and cancer prevention: The importance of the terminal group of the retinoid molecule in modifying activity and toxicity, in: *Carcinogens: Identification and Mechanism of Action* (A. C. Griffin and C. R. Shaw, eds.), pp. 441–453, Raven Press, New York.
Sporn, M. B., Newton, D. L., Roberts, A. B., De Larco, J. E., and Todaro, G. J., 1981. Retinoids and the suppression of the effects of polypeptide transforming factors—a new molecular approach to chemoprevention of cancer, in: *Molecular Action and Targets for Cancer Chemotherapeutic Agents* (A. C. Sartorelli, J. R. Bertino, and J. S. Lazo, eds.), pp. 541–554, Academic Press, New York.
Squire, R. A., Sporn, M. B., Brown, C. C., Smith, J. M., Wenk, M. L., and Springer, S., 1977, Histopathological evaluation of the inhibition of rat bladder carcinogenesis by 13-*cis*-retinoic acid, *Cancer Res.* **37**:2930.
Strickland, S., and Mahdavi, V., 1978, The induction of differentiation in teratocarcinoma stem cells by retinoic acid, *Cell* **15**:393.
Thompson, H. J., Becci, P. J., Grubbs, C. J., Shealy, Y. F., Stanek, E. J., Brown, C. C., Sporn, M. B., and Moon, R. C., 1981, Inhibition of urinary bladder cancer by N-(ethyl)-all-*trans* retinamide and N-(2-hydroxyethyl)-all-*trans*-retinamide in rats and mice, *Cancer Res.* **41**:933.
Todaro, G. J., and De Larco, J. E., 1978, Growth factors produced by sarcoma virus-transformed cells, *Cancer Res.* **38**:4147.
Todaro, G. J., De Larco, J. E., and Sporn, M. B., 1978, Retinoids block phenotypic cell transformation produced by sarcoma growth factor, *Nature* **276**:272.
Verma, A. K., Rice, H. M., Shapas, B. G., and Boutwell, R. K., 1978, Inhibition of 12-*O*-

tetradecanoylphorbol-13-acetate-induced ornithine decarboxylase activity in mouse epidermis by vitamin A analogs (retinoids), *Cancer Res.* **38**:793.

Verma, A. K., Shapas, B. G., Rice, H. M., and Boutwell, R. K. 1979, Correlation of the inhibition by retinoids of tumor promoter-induced mouse epidermal ornithine decarboxylase activity and of skin tumor promotion, *Cancer Res.* **39**:419.

Verma, A. K., Conrad, E. A., and Boutwell, R. K., 1980, Inhibition of mouse skin carcinogenesis by a retinoid, steroid, and protease inhibitor, *Proc. Am. Assoc. Cancer Res.* **21**:93.

Weeks, C. E., Slaga, T. J., Hennings, H., Gleason, G. L., and Bracken, W. M., 1979, Inhibition of phorbol ester-induced tumor promotion in mice by vitamin A analog and anti-inflammatory steroid, *J. Natl. Cancer Inst.* **63**:401.

Welsch, C. W., 1976, Prophylaxis of early preneoplastic lesions of the mammary gland, *Cancer Res.* **36**:2621.

Welsch, C. W., Brown, C. K., Goodrich-Smith, M., and Moon, R. C., 1980, Chronic prolactin suppression and retinoid treatment in the prophylaxis of NMU-induced mammary carcinogenesis in female rats: A comparison, *Proc. Am. Assoc. Cancer Res.* **21**:58.

Wertz, P. W., Kensler, T. W., Mueller, G. C., Verma, A. K., and Boutwell, R. K., 1979, 5,6-Epoxyretinoic acid opposes the effects of 12-*O*-tetradecanoyl-phorbol-13-acetate in bovine lymphocytes, *Nature* **277**:227.

Wilkoff, L. J., Peckham, H. J., Dulmadge, E. A., Mowry, R. W., and Chopra, D. P., 1976, Evaluation of vitamin A analogs in modulating epithelial differentiation of 13-day chick embryo metatarsal skin explants, *Cancer Res.* **36**:964.

Wolbach, S. B., and Howe, P. R., 1925, Tissue changes following deprivation of fat-soluble A vitamin, *J. Exp. Med.* **42**:753.

Wong, Y., and Buck, R., 1971, An electron microscopic study of metaplasia of the rat tracheal epithelium in vitamin A deficiency, *Lab Invest.* **24**:55.

4

Ascorbic Acid Inhibition of N-Nitroso Compound Formation in Chemical, Food, and Biological Systems

SIDNEY S. MIRVISH

I. Introduction

Cameron *et al.* (1979) have reviewed the effect of ascorbic acid (ASC) on tumor growth and progression and on carcinogenesis in general. Five years ago (Mirvish, 1975a), I reviewed the subject of this chapter, and the present review covers reports up to the middle of 1979.

II. *In Vitro* Studies

A. Studies in Acidic Aqueous Solutions

Most N-nitroso (NNO) compounds, including both nitrosamines and nitrosamides, are carcinogenic in experimental animals, and these compounds could be responsible for certain human cancers if there were a significant human exposure. Such exposure could take place because NNO compounds occurred in the environment or because these compounds were produced from their precursors (nitrite and amines or amides) *in vivo*. The acidic stomach

---

SIDNEY S. MIRVISH • Eppley Institute for Research in Cancer, University of Nebraska Medical Center, Omaha, Nebraska 68105.

contents form a likely site of *in vivo* nitrosation, because an acidic pH favors the formation of NNO compounds (*N*-nitrosation) from nitrite.

Since 1968, we and others have been investigating the kinetics of NNO compound formation from nitrite and amines or amides with regard to the occurrence of this process in the environment and *in vivo* (Mirvish, 1975b). The basic work in this area had been done earlier by physical chemists (Ridd, 1961). The kinetics are important because they disclose the ease with which different nitrogen compounds are nitrosated and the dependency of the nitrosation on nitrite concentration and pH. There are 200,000-fold ranges in the ease of nitrosation of different secondary amines and of different *N*-substituted amides. The ease of nitrosation of secondary amines tends to increase as the basicity of the amine decreases. Nitrosation of moderately and strongly basic amines proceeds with an optimum rate at pH 3.0–3.4, and this is related to the fact that the acidic dissociation constant (pK_a) of nitrous acid (HNO_2) is 3.4. Nitrosation of very weakly basic amines, e.g., aminopyrine, and of certain amino acids shows an optimum pH around 2.0. Amide nitrosation proceeds ten times faster for each 1-unit drop in pH, without an optimum pH. Amine nitrosation is proportional to nitrite concentration squared, whereas amide nitrosation is proportional simply to nitrite concentration. Nitrosation can be catalyzed by thiocyanate (which occurs in saliva), halides, formaldehyde, and complexes of certain transition-metal ions. The kinetics of the catalyzed reactions differ from those for the uncatalyzed reactions.

In 1972, Dr. Michael Eagen in my laboratory was trying unsuccessfully to reproduce the finding by Lijinsky *et al.* (1972) that the antibiotic tertiary amine oxytetracycline yields dimethylnitrosamine (DMN) when treated with nitrite. This reaction was considered unusual, since secondary amines were the only amines widely known to yield nitrosamines. With help from Dr. L. Wallcave, Dr. Eagen traced his failure to the fact that we were using a commercial sample of oxytetracycline containing large amounts of ASC added as an antioxidant. Dr. P. Shubik, Director of the Eppley Institute, strongly encouraged the work, since he was intrigued by the possibility that ASC could be used to inhibit nitrosamine formation. Accordingly, we studied the effect of ASC in blocking the formation of NNO compounds in simple chemical systems (Mirvish *et al.*, 1972a). As an example of our results, Table 1 compares the inhibition of morpholine nitrosation by ASC, urea, and ammonium sulfamate.

In all cases, a solution of nitrite was mixed with a solution containing amine and inhibitor, so that the inhibitor and amine competed for the nitrite. From the results for morpholine, other amines, and methylurea, it was clear

TABLE 1. Inhibition of Morpholine Nitrosation[a]

		Yield without inhibitor (%)	Percent inhibition by		
pH	Time (min)		ASC	Urea	Ammonium sulfamate
1	45	7	—	95	100
2	30	20	98	24	100
3	30	65	100	2	99
4	30	34	100	—	71

[a] Conditions: 25 mM morpholine, 50 mM nitrite, 100 mM inhibitor, 25°C. Data are from Mirvish et al. (1972a). Reprinted from Mirvish (1981) with permission of the publisher.

that ASC inhibited nitrosation effectively from pH 1 to pH 4. (Above this pH, nitrosation becomes very slow.) In contrast, urea and ammonium sulfamate were more or less effective at pH 1 and 2 but were relatively ineffective at pH 3 and 4. The mechanism is simply that ASC removes the nitrite by reacting with it and, for the inhibition to work, sufficient ASC has to be added for most of the nitrite to be consumed. (The ASC : nitrite ratio was generally 2 : 1) The inhibition was effective for slowly nitrosated amines such as dimethylamine (except under one condition where very little DMN was formed) and for amines nitrosated at moderate speeds, e.g., morpholine and piperazine. Inhibition was incomplete for the very rapidly nitrosated N-methylaniline, because ASC competes rather poorly with this amine for nitrite.

The chemical reaction involved is nitrite reduction to nitric oxide (NO) linked to the oxidation of ASC to dehydroascorbic acid. The kinetics of this reaction was studied by Dahn et al. (1960). Ascorbic acid and ascorbate anion react with N_2O_3, the active form of nitrous acid (Fig. 1).

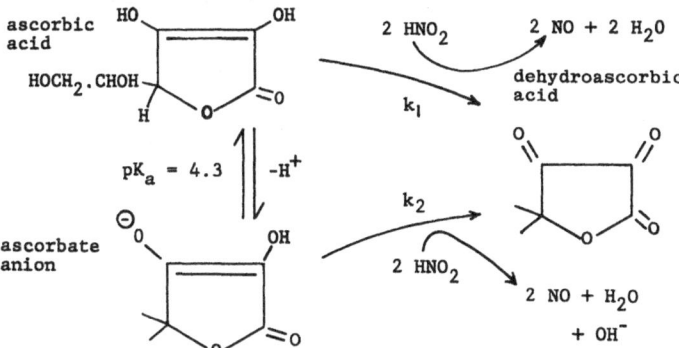

FIGURE 1. Oxidation of ascorbic acid and ascorbate anion by nitrous acid to give dehydroascorbic acid. The k_2/k_1 ratio is 230:1. Reprinted from Mirvish (1981) with permission of the publisher.

$$2HNO_2 \rightleftharpoons N_2O_3 + H_2O \qquad (1)$$

$$\text{Ascorbic acid } (C_6H_7O_6) + N_2O_3 \xrightarrow{k_1}$$
$$\text{dehydroascorbic acid } (C_6H_5O_6) + 2NO + H_2O \qquad (2)$$

$$\text{Ascorbate } (C_6H_6O_6^-) + N_2O_3 \xrightarrow{k_2}$$
$$\text{dehydroascorbic acid } (C_6H_5O_6) + 2NO + OH^- \qquad (3)$$

$$R_2NH + N_2O_3 \xrightarrow{k_3} R_2NNO + HNO_2 \qquad (4)$$

Since the active form of HNO_2 for nitrosamine formation is also N_2O_3 (equation 4), amines and ASC compete directly for the same nitrosating species. One mol of ASC is sufficient to reduce 2 mol of HNO_2 (i.e., 1 mol of N_2O_3), whereas 1 mol of amine reacts with 1 mol of HNO_2 (since the intermediate N_2O_3 regenerates HNO_2). According to Dahn et al. (1960), k_2 for the ascorbate reaction is $230 \times k_1$ for the ascorbic acid reaction; i.e., ascorbate reacts with N_2O_3 230 times faster than ascorbic acid. Presumably, the greater nucleophilic activity of the anion is responsible for this difference. Since the pK_a of ascorbic acid is 4.3, the ASC system is particularly effective around and above pH 4.3, where the anion concentration is high. (In fact, k_2 and k_3 were measured at pH 1.5–2.5.) Above pH 3, the ASC–nitrite reaction proceeds so rapidly that N_2O_3 formation (equation 1) becomes rate limiting. This explains why ASC is effective at pH 3 and 4, whereasureas and ammonium sulfamate (which react with nitrite most rapidly at highly acidic pHs) are relatively ineffective at the higher pH values.

The conversion of ascorbic acid and ascorbate anion into dehydroascorbic acid may proceed via the nitrite ester at the 3 position and probably involves the semiquinone (Bunton et al., 1959; Dahn et al., 1960). This is shown

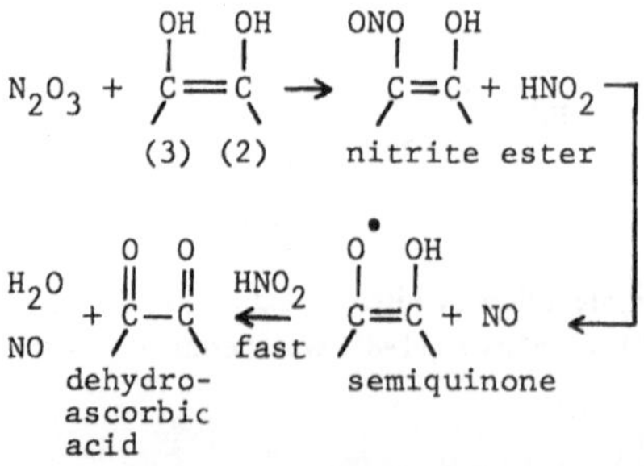

FIGURE 2. Intermediates in the reaction of nitrous anhydride (N_2O_3) with ascorbic acid. Only carbon atoms 2 and 3 are shown. Reprinted from Mirvish (1981) with permission of the publisher.

for ascorbic acid in Fig. 2. No evidence for the nitrite ester has been produced, and the reaction may proceed directly to the semiquinone.

We compared the action of ASC with that of four other inhibitors (Mirvish, 1975b). For piperazine nitrosation to give mononitrosopiperazine under given conditions (10 mM piperazine, 10 mM nitrite, 20 mM inhibitor, 10 min. reaction at pH 3), ASC, gallic acid, and sodium sulfite all blocked the reaction 100%, but cysteine and tannic acid were less effective. With 5 mM inhibitor, ASC was more effective than the other inhibitors. Similar results were obtained for the inhibition of morpholine nitrosation.

In the paper by Mirvish et al. (1972a), we proposed that readily nitrosated drugs, e.g., aminopyrine and piperazine, should be formulated with sufficient ASC to block their intragastric nitrosation by nitrite arising from food. [In fact, most nitrite in the human stomach arises from nitrite produced in the saliva by bacterial reduction of nitrate (Tannenbaum et al., 1974).] This proposal seemed particularly logical, since the pH of gastric contents after a meal is gradually lowered from 5 to 1. Accordingly, ASC might react with all the nitrite at the higher pH values, before NNO compounds could be produced. This suggestion has not been widely adopted, perhaps because the ASC dose needed to inhibit nitrosation in the human stomach remains unknown. In this connection, research is urgently needed on the ASC dose required to lower the level of the nitrite normally present in human gastric juice (Ruddell et al., 1977).

When $NaNO_2$ was added to a solution of ethylurea and ASC at pH 2.5, the main products were identified as NO and dehydroascorbate, as expected (Synnett et al., 1975). The fate of NO produced from the ASC–nitrite reaction is of interest. If the gaseous NO does not escape from the system, and excess oxygen is present, the NO can be oxidized to NO_2, which then reacts as N_2O_4 with water to give nitric and nitrous acids. Hence, this cycle (Fig. 3a) regenerates half the original nitrite (Mirvish et al., 1972a). Theoretically, if the cycle proceeds many times, twice as much ASC is needed for complete removal of nitrite than in the situation without oxygen.

If less oxygen is present, the NO_2 could react with unoxidized NO to give N_2O_3 directly. This would be hydrolyzed to regenerate 2 mol of HNO_2 (Fig. 3b). Under these conditions, ASC should not inhibit nitrosamine formation (B. Challis, personal communication). Other processes must also be considered when oxygen is present. (Further information is provided later in this section.)

Fan and Tannenbaum (1973) studied the effect of the ASC–morpholine ratio on morpholine nitrosation under aerobic conditions. When this ratio exceeded 2 : 1, nitrosomorpholine (NMOR) formation was completely

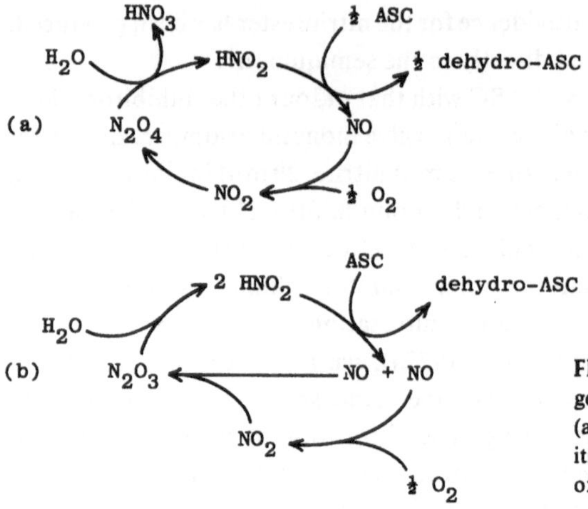

FIGURE 3. Cycles whereby oxygen could serve to regenerate half (a) or all (b) of the nitrous acid after its reduction by ASC to give nitric oxide.

blocked. When this ratio was less than 2 : 1, nitrite concentration was 40% greater when measured by the Griess reaction than when calculated from the rate of morpholine nitrosation. This suggested that ASC and nitrite reacted to form a compound determined by the Griess reagent but not available for nitrosation. No further evidence for such a compound has appeared.

Archer *et al.* (1975) studied the effect of oxygen on ASC inhibition of NMOR formation. A solution containing morpholine, nitrite, and varying amounts of ASC was reacted at pH 3–4. In the absence of air, 0.5 mol ASC/mol nitrite was needed to prevent NMOR formation, as predicted by equations 2–4. When air was bubbled into the solution via a Pasteur pipette, 1.0 mol ASC/mol nitrite was needed to prevent nitrosation. At lower ASC concentrations (but not in the absence of ASC), the nitrosation rate was increased by the presence of air. When air was bubbled in via a sparger (which produces very small bubbles), or when pure oxygen was bubbled in via a Pasteur pipette, even 1.0 mol ASC/mol nitrite did not prevent the nitrosation.

The oxidation of ASC by nitrite at pH 4 was also studied by Archer *et al.* (1975). One mole of nitrite oxidized 0.5 mol ASC under anaerobic conditions, but 1.0 mol ASC when air was bubbled in. Air alone oxidized only a small proportion of the ASC. Hence, not only does nitrite directly oxidize ASC, but it also enables oxygen to oxidize ASC. This explains why, under certain conditions, oxygen partly prevented ASC from inhibiting NMOR formation. These findings were attributed to direct oxidation by oxygen of the ASC semiquinone intermediate (Fig. 2) and perhaps to NO oxidation to NO_2, which would regenerate nitrite (Fig. 3). (The latter mechanism would be less prominent than in a closed system.)

Under conditions where ASC reacts rapidly with nitrite, amine nitrosation should not be observed until all the ASC is consumed, i.e., there should be a lag period before nitrosation begins (Archer et al., 1975). The reason is that the rapid reaction with ASC should reduce N_2O_3 to such a low level that nitrosamine formation becomes very slow. Such a lag period was observed for morpholine nitrosation in the presence of ASC and air, and an equation relating lag period to pH was found to apply (lag period increased sharply as pH rose).

Chang et al. (1979) studied the ASC–nitrite reaction by differential pulse polarography. A polarographic peak was attributed to oxyhyponitrous acid ($H_2N_2O_3$). Under some conditions, this could be the immediate product of the ASC–nitrite reaction and the precursor of NO (equations 5 and 6). Synthesized oxyhyponitrous acid reacted with N-methylaniline, diphenylamine, and iminodiacetonitrile to produce the corresponding nitrosamines. Apparently because of this reaction, ASC accelerated the nitrosation of these amines at pH 1–2. Oxyhyponitrous acid did not nitrosate simple aliphatic secondary amines, which are probably more important environmentally than the amines studied by Chang et al.

$$2HNO_2 + \text{ascorbic acid } (C_6H_7O_6) \longrightarrow$$
$$H_2N_2O_3, + \text{dehydroascorbic acid } (C_6H_5O_6) + H_2O \qquad (5)$$

$$H_2N_2O_3 \longrightarrow 2NO + H_2O \qquad (6)$$

Several studies on the nitrosation of drugs will now be discussed. Nitrosation of aminopyrine, which very readily produces DMN, was nevertheless successfully blocked by ASC (Mirvish et al., 1974). Sen and Donaldson (1974) studied the nitrosation of piperazine adipate, the usual form of piperazine used as a drug. Ascorbic acid blocked formation of the weak carcinogen mononitrosopiperazine but led to the appearance of small amounts of the strong carcinogen dinitrosopiperazine. The phenomenon depended on the presence of adipate. Nitrosation of the tertiary amine methapyrilene to give DMN and other nitrosamine derivatives was prevented by ASC (with an ASC : nitrite ratio of 2 : 1) under all conditions studied (Mergens et al., 1979). Nitrosation of various tetracyclines to give DMN was effectively inhibited by ASC (Mirvish et al., 1972a; Röper and Heyns, 1978).

Ziebarth and Scheunig (1976) compared the effect of ASC, sulfamate, and cysteine on the nitrosation of piperazine and aminopyrine. Equal concentrations by weight of the inhibitors were used, and the medium was human gastric juice. Ascorbic acid was the most effective inhibitor at all pHs examined (pH 2–5). An enhancement of nitrosation by sulfamate and cysteine was observed at pH 5–6. According to Kinawi and Schuster (1978), ephedrine nitrosation at pH 2.7–3.0 was inhibited by ASC after reaction for 60 min but was enhanced by ASC after reaction for 2–5 min.

The catalysis of nitrosation by thiocyanate and halides depends on the formation of nitrosating NOX species, e.g., NOI and NO · NCS. Since these species should also react with ASC, we would expect nitrosation by this mechanism to be inhibited by ASC. Williams (1978) measured the denitrosation of methylnitrosoaniline in the presence of thiocyanate or bromide ions and of ASC or sulfamic acid. The denitrosation rate was used to measure the efficiency of ASC and sulfamic acid as traps for NO · NCS and NOBr (which were produced by reversible reaction of the nitrosamine with NCS⁻ and Br⁻). For reaction with NOBr, ASC and sulfamic acid showed similar activities. For NO · NCS, ASC was more reactive than sulfamic acid. These reactions were carried out under more strongly acidic conditions (>0.5 N H_2SO_4) than those used by Mirvish *et al.* (1972a).

B. Use of Ascorbate in the Meat Industry

Sodium nitrite ($NaNO_2$) is added to certain meat products (e.g., frankfurters, bacon, and corned beef) to preserve the meat, especially against contamination by *Clostridium botulinum,* to improve the flavor, and to give a pink color. This color is caused by nitrosomyoglobin formed from the reaction of NO with myoglobin. Although nitrite-preserved meat products do not usually contain nitrosamines (except for the noncarcinogenic *N*-nitrosoproline), in the United States fried bacon at one time contained up to 100 ppb of the moderate carcinogen *N*-nitrosopyrrolidine (NPYR) as well as lesser amounts of the strong carcinogen DMN. This occurred when 150 ppm $NaNO_2$ were added to the bacon. The nitrosamines are produced during the frying at about 180° C.

Ascorbic acid has been included for many years in some nitrite-preserved products to improve the pink color (which it does by reducing the nitrite to NO). In practice, a solution containing both sodium nitrite and sodium ascorbate is injected into the meat. After our results were presented to a Food and Drug Administration (FDA) workshop in 1972, the meat industry and FDA became interested in adding ASC to bacon as a means of reducing NPYR formation. Laboratory studies showed that ASC inhibited NPYR formation in fried bacon and related products (Fiddler *et al.,* 1973). Sen *et al.* (1976) sprinkled antioxidant solutions on nitrite-preserved bacon just before it was fried; under these conditions, ASC was not completely and consistently effective in inhibiting NPYR formation, and propyl gallate and ascorbityl palmitate were more effective than ASC.

In a model system containing aqueous and lipid phases with reaction at 52° C, ASC alone inhibited pyrrolidine nitrosation in the aqueous phase by 43%, but did not inhibit nitrosation in the lipid phase (Pensabene *et al.,* 1976). When the system contained both ASC and ascorbityl monoesters, NPYR formation was inhibited in both phases by 40–60%. In tests on a similar two-phase system with reaction at room temperature, ASC appeared to enhance nitrosamine formation 5–25 times (Mottram and Patterson, 1977). This result may have been an artifact, since the reaction was stopped by adding alkali, and nitrogen oxides could have nitrosated amines in the lipid phase after addition of the alkali (see Section II.C). In the study by Pensabene *et al.* (1976), alkali was also added but only after several intermediate steps that may have removed much of the nitrogen oxides; also, the higher temperature would have increased HNO_2 decomposition during the reaction, so that less nitrogen oxides would be present together with the alkali.

In a protein-based model system for bacon, ASC was more efficient than cysteine or *p*-cresol as an inhibitor of pyrrolidine nitrosation (Massey *et al.,* 1978). Tanaka *et al.* (1978) compared the inhibition of nitrosamine formation by ASC and by sorbic acid (di-*trans*-2,4-hexadienoic acid), a food additive being considered as an alternative to nitrite for preserving food. In general, ASC was more effective than sorbic acid, which reacts with nitrite by addition of N_2O_3 across a C=C double bond to form the α-oxime nitrite ester. (Conceivably, this nitrite ester could itself serve as a nitrosating species.)

It is still unclear whether NPYR in fried bacon arises by decarboxylation of *N*-nitrosoproline present in the bacon before it is fried or whether pyrrolidine or some other precursor in the aqueous or lipid phase is nitrosated during frying to give NPYR. The effectiveness of ASC or other antioxidants should depend on the mechanism involved. Whatever the mechanism, since about 1975 the meat industry began to use relatively large amounts of ASC or erythorbate in bacon to reduce nitrosamine formation (erythorbate, i.e., D-ascorbate, is inactive as a vitamin but as effective as ASC in reducing nitrite). In current general practice in the United States, 120 ppm $NaNO_2$ and 500 ppm ascorbate are added to meat products. This reduces NPYR production on frying to about 10 ppb (Birdsall, 1977). A current problem is that $NaNO_2$ itself might be a weak carcinogen (Newberne, 1979), so that even a complete elimination of NPYR and DMN may not solve the regulatory questions involved in the use of nitrite-preserved meat.

C. Nitrosation in Lipids and by Nitrogen Oxides

Up to this point, we have dealt mainly with nitrosation in acidic aqueous solution, where ASC could be used to block nitrosation. Nitrosation in lipidic media cannot be inhibited by ASC because of its insolubility in these media, and in this case α-tocopherol and other lipophilic antioxidants may be more suitable agents. This approach is being studied in the case of fried bacon, where much of the NPYR may be produced in the lipid phase. In laboratory experiments, bacon was treated with 500 ppm α-tocopherol as a suspension stabilized by a surfactant in addition to the usual levels of ASC and nitrite. The amount of NPYR in the fried bacon was lowered from 10 ppb in the absence of α-tocopherol to 4–6 ppb (Walters et al., 1976; Mergens et al., 1978). Several fat- and water-soluble antioxidants that react with nitrite were added to simulated food-processing systems in the presence of emulsifiers (Gray and Dugan, 1975). Most of the test compounds, which included ASC, α-tocopherol, sodium bisulfite, various phenols, tannic acid, and cysteine, were effective inhibitors of DMN and NPYR formation from the corresponding amines.

We found that HNO_2 was partly extracted from acidic aqueous solution by organic solvents and that nitrosation of lipid-soluble amides, e.g., carbaryl, proceeded more readily in CH_2Cl_2–water mixtures than in water alone (Mirvish et al., 1978). This nitrosation was attributed to N_2O_3 produced in the organic phase from HNO_2, since reaction rate was proportional to the square of nitrite concentration (unpublished results). We also confirmed earlier observations that nitrosation by nitrogen oxides (especially N_2O_4) occurs very rapidly at 0°C in CH_2Cl_2 solution in the absence of water. For example, nitrosation of ethylurea and n-hexylurea under such conditions was almost complete in 5 sec. Nitrosation of N-butylacetamide in this system was sufficiently slow for the kinetic rate constants to be determined and, under certain conditions, proceeded 31,000 times faster than nitrosation of the same compound in water at pH 2. This finding supported the suggestion from the studies on bacon that much NNO compound formation in the environment may occur in lipidic media.

When N_2O_4 was bubbled into aqueous solutions of amines under neutral or alkaline conditions, nitrosamines and nitramines ($R_2N \cdot NO_2$) were produced (Challis and Kyrtopoulos, 1977). This occurred by direct reaction of N_2O_4 with the amines and not via hydrolysis to nitrous acid. The gases N_2O_3 and NOCL underwent similar reactions. ASC inhibits this type of nitrosation but not as effectively as phenols (B. Challis, personal communication).

Nitrosation in aqueous solution has often been stopped by making the solution alkaline in the presence of an organic solvent such as methylene chloride (CH_2Cl_2), or else the nitrosamine has been extracted with an organic solvent after the aqueous solution was made alkaline. In these cases, it has sometimes been reported that ASC or other antioxidants enhanced the nitrosation (e.g., Mirvish *et al.*, 1972a, with respect to dimethylamine nitrosation under certain conditions; Challis and Bartlett, 1975; Mottram and Patterson, 1977). A likely reason given by Dr. B. Challis (personal communication) is that the ASC–nitrite reaction produces NO which dissolves in the organic solvent and reacts there with oxygen to give NO_2. This can then nitrosate the amine, especially if nonionized amine is extracted into the solvent from the alkaline solution. Hence, the enhancement may be an artifact. In such experiments, it is convenient to stop the reaction by adding ammonium sulfamate (which converts nitrite to nitrogen) at pH 0–2. One should also perform a "zero-time" experiment to check that NNO compound is not produced when the stopping reagent is added to the solution of nitrite, amine, and ASC as soon as possible after these are mixed together.

Challis *et al.* (1978) warn that NO produced from the ASC–nitrite reaction could nitrosate amines if cupric, ferric, or iodide salts are present, since these ions catalyze amine nitrosation by NO (which does not normally occur).

III. *In Vivo* Studies

A. Acute Toxicity Experiments

This subject was reviewed by Kamm *et al.* (1975). When large single doses of dimethylamine or aminopyrine were gavaged (given by stomach tube) to rats or mice together with a large $NaNO_2$ dose, acute hepatotoxicity developed after a few days (Lijinsky and Greenblatt, 1972). This effect was detected by histological examination of the liver and by measurement of serum transaminases. With both dimethylamine and aminopyrine, the effect was attributed to intragastric formation of DMN (LD_{50} in rats, 40 mg/kg). When similar experiments were performed with aminopyrine but with ASC added to the amine solution before gavage, hepatotoxicity was completely prevented

(Kamm et al., 1973; Greenblatt, 1973). When rats received single doses of 1500 mg dimethylamine hydrochloride plus 125 mg $NaNO_2$ per kg body weight, sodium ASC doses down to 90 mg/kg completely protected the rats from necrosis (Cardesa et al., 1974). The liver was not protected from damage when ASC was injected i.p. and aminopyrine and nitrite were gavaged. Gavage of dehydroascorbate had no effect, but ascorbityl palmitate was as effective as ASC (Kamm et al., 1975).

A single intragastric dose of DMN produced acute liver necrosis in rats only when the dose reached 10 mg/kg (Cardesa et al., 1974). Hence, in the amine-plus-nitrite experiments discussed above, the absence of liver toxicity when ASC was used indicates only that DMN production did not exceed 10 mg/kg body weight. Gavage of rats with an α-tocopherol suspension in water (stabilized by an emulsifier) also completely prevented the liver toxicity caused by aminopyrine plus nitrite (Kamm et al., 1977). Like ASC, α-tocopherol reduces HNO_2 to NO.

The blocking by ASC of the hepatotoxicity of dimethylamine (1000 mg/kg) plus $NaNO_2$ (125 mg/kg) in rats was compared with that of the food stabilizers propyl gallate, butylated hydroxyanisole, butylated hydroxytoluene, and t-butylhydroquinone (Astill and Mulligan, 1977). The antioxidants (except ASC) were gavaged as solutions in corn oil. Ascorbic acid (200 mg/kg) and propyl gallate (225 mg/kg) completely protected the rats against necrosis. t-Butylhydroquinone (75 mg/kg) gave 60% protection, and butylated hydroxyanisole and butylated hydroxytoluene had no effect. Daily gavage of rats with chlordiazepoxide (Librium®) and $NaNO_2$ for 36 weeks produced liver damage attributed to *in vivo* formation of the NNO derivative; this liver damage was almost abolished when ASC was gavaged 20 min after each administration of drug plus nitrite (Preda et al., 1976). In general, acute toxicity from *in vivo* production of nitrosamines can be produced by gavage of large doses of nitrite and slowly nitrosated amines such as dimethylamine and chlordiazepoxide. In contrast, it is generally true that only amines nitrosated with moderate facility can be used successfully in carcinogenesis experiments (see next section).

B. Carcinogenicity Experiments

Sander and Bürkle (1969) were the first to induce tumors in rodents by feeding nitrite plus amines or amides. This system has since been widely studied. When pregnant rats were gavaged with ethylurea plus nitrite, hydrocephalus and nervous system tumors were induced in the offspring. Both of these effects were completely prevented when ASC was gavaged together with the ethylurea (Ivankovic et al., 1973a, 1974). This was the first demonstration that ASC inhibits carcinogenesis by nitrite plus amines or amides. In the same system, ASC did not prevent tumor induction by gavage of ethylnitrosourea (ENU). Similarly, peripheral nervous system tumorigenesis in the offspring of hamsters gavaged with ethylurea plus nitrite was prevented when the mothers also received ASC (Rustia, 1975).

In studies from our laboratories, the induction of lung adenomas in Swiss or Strain A mice was used to examine the amine/amide-plus-nitrite system. The use of lung adenomas was convenient for quantitative studies, since many adenomas per mouse were induced, and they were easy to count. Some adenomas were checked by histological examination. The amines or amides were administered in the diet and $NaNO_2$ in drinking water for 20 weeks. Since the food and water were kept at opposite ends of the cage, NNO compounds should only have been formed *in vivo*. The mice were maintained another 10 weeks and killed, and the lung adenomas counted. The method worked because most NNO compounds induce lung adenomas in these strains of mice.

Tumors were induced by treatment with nitrite plus the rapidly nitrosated compounds morpholine, piperazine, N-methylaniline, methylurea, and ethylurea, but not by nitrite plus the slowly nitrosated dimethylamine (Greenblatt et al., 1971; Mirvish et al., 1972b). Rough estimates could be made of the extent of *in vivo* nitrosation of amines, because tumor induction (number of lung adenomas/mouse minus number in control mice) was nearly proportional to the dose of nitrosamine when the nitrosamine was administered as such (this did not apply to nitrosoureas). When morpholine (6.35 g/kg food) and $NaNO_2$ (2.0 g/liter water) were administered, we estimated that 0.6% of the morpholine was nitrosated (Mirvish et al., 1975).

When precursor concentrations were varied in the piperazine-plus-nitrite system, adenoma induction was consistent with the view that nitrosation was proportional to piperazine dose and to the square of nitrite dose, in accord with the nitrosation kinetics (Greenblatt and Mirvish, 1973). When ASC was added to the food together with the amine or urea, and $NaNO_2$ was added to drinking water, induction of lung adenomas was reduced relative to the situation without ASC (Mirvish et al., 1975). Presumably, ASC competed with the amine or urea for nitrite and hence reduced the formation of NNO compounds. With 23 g ASC/kg food, lung adenoma induction by nitrite plus morpholine or piperazine was inhibited 89–91%. With 5.75 g ASC/kg food, lung tumorigenesis by morpholine plus nitrite was inhibited 72%, whereas lung tumorigenesis by piperazine plus nitrite was inhibited only 37%. This difference was attributed to the fact that morpholine is nitrosated less rapidly then piperazine, so that ASC competes more effectively with morpholine for the nitrite. Adenoma induction by methylurea plus nitrite was 98% inhibited by 11.5 g ASC/kg, and hence this system was particularly sensitive to ASC inhibition [as was the ethylurea-plus-nitrite system of Ivankovic *et al.* (1974) and Rustia (1975)]. Gallic acid (3,4,5-trihydroxybenzoic acid, a component of tannins) also strongly inhibited adenoma induction by morpholine plus nitrite.

In a contribution from the Peoples' Republic of China, gavage of rats with N-methylbenzylamine (887 mg) and $NaNO_2$ (887 mg) caused a 20% incidence of esophageal papillomas (Coordinating Group, 1974). Simultaneous gavage of a very large ascorbic acid dose (6.6 g) completely prevented the development of esophageal tumors (parenthetical numbers refer to total dose given over an unspecified period). Ascorbic acid had no effect on tumor induction by N-methyl-N-nitrosobenzylamine.

Fong and Chan (1976) treated Sprague–Dawley rats with aminopyrine plus $NaNO_2$, both given chronically in the drinking water at 1 g/liter concentrations. The water was not analyzed for the nitrosation product, DMN, although its presence was somewhat unlikely since the pH was 6.9. Some rats also received a rather low ascorbic acid dose (800 mg/kg) in the diet. The group without ASC developed a 50% incidence of tumors, chiefly lung adenomas and adenocarcinomas. The group with ASC had a 28% tumor incidence, with a similar organ distribution but with, in the lungs, a higher proportion of benign adenomas and a lower proportion of adenocarcinomas. Chang and Fong (1977) repeated the experiment as before, but with 7.0 g ASC/kg food. The group without ASC developed tumors in the liver, lungs, and kidneys; and the tumor incidence in all three organs, but especially in the liver, was reduced in the group with ASC.

We examined the effect of ASC on carcinogenesis by morpholine plus nitrite in male MRC–Wistar rats (Mirvish *et al.*, 1976). Morpholine (10 g/kg) was administered in the diet, and $NaNO_2$ (3 g/liter) in drinking water for 2 years. Some rats also received sodium ASC (23 g/kg) in the diet. The incidence of liver tumors induced by morpholine plus nitrite was reduced from 65% in the absence of ASC to 49% in the presence of ASC, and the induction period was nearly doubled from 54 to 93 weeks. Hence, *in vivo* NMOR production was probably inhibited about 50%. Unexpectedly, the group with morpholine plus nitrite plus ASC had a 54% incidence of forestomach tumors, including an 18% incidence of squamous carcinomas, whereas no forestomach tumors were observed in the morpholine-plus-nitrite group. We also tested preformed NMOR given in drinking water with and without sodium ASC given in the diet as before. The NMOR induced liver tumors (88% incidence) with a survival time of 28 weeks, and ASC had no significant effect.

The most likely interpretation of the forestomach results was that ASC served to lower the *in vivo* production of NMOR. Accordingly, liver tumors were induced more slowly by NMOR, and the rats had a longer time to develop forestomach tumors which were also induced by NMOR. A less likely hypothesis was that ASC directly enhanced development of the forestomach tumors.

In recent studies (S. S. Mirvish, R. Runge, and E. Mahboubi, unpublished data), the experiment with morpholine, nitrite, and ASC was repeated, but with a lower $NaNO_2$ level of 2 g/liter drinking water. In the rats examined thus far, those treated with morpholine plus nitrite had an 89% incidence of hepatocellular carcinoma and a 31% incidence of forestomach papillomas. In the rats treated with morpholine plus nitrite plus ASC, the liver tumor incidence was reduced to 31%, and the forestomach tumor incidence was increased to 77%. In both groups of rats, most forestomachs exhibited some degree of hyperkeratosis and acanthosis. This confirms the results of the first experiment. Since the forestomachs of both groups showed tumors and possibly premalignant lesions, the results support the hypothesis that the forestomach tumors were induced by NMOR alone.

C. Chemical Analysis of Biological Materials

Another way of discovering whether ASC inhibits *in vivo* nitrosation is to analyze biological fluids and tissues chemically for NNO compounds. This approach directly measures the effect of ASC on NNO compound formation. On the other hand, the advantages of studying carcinogenesis are that we then observe the phenomenon that we are interested in (and can detect actions of ASC other than those on NNO compound formation) and that the effect may reflect an integration over time of the exposure to NNO compounds. Only a few studies have been published in which *in vivo* formation of NNO compounds has been measured chemically, and only two of these have involved ASC.

We have already discussed the experiments of Kamm *et al.* (1975) in which ASC inhibited the acute liver toxicity induced by aminopyrine plus nitrite in rats. This paper also reported that gavage of aminopyrine (125 mg/kg) plus $NaNO_2$ (110 mg/kg) produced, 30 min later, a serum DMN level of 1.9 $\mu g/ml$. The DMN level was lowered to 0.7 $\mu g/ml$ when 18 mg/kg of sodium ASC was gavaged at the same time and to zero when 70 mg/kg of sodium ASC was gavaged.

We are presently studying methylnitrosourea (MNU) formation after administration of ^{3}H-labeled methylurea plus $NaNO_2$ mixed in a 5-g meal (Mirvish et al., 1978). MNU is determined in the stomach contents by a radiochemical procedure. When 100 mg methylurea and 4 g $NaNO_2$/kg commercial diet were administered, and the stomach contents were analyzed 3 hr later, the MNU level corresponded to 0.46% conversion from methylurea. When the food also contained 11.5 or 2.9 g sodium ASC/kg, the gastric MNU levels corresponded to 0.02 and 0.23% yields from methylurea, respectively (values were uncorrected for recovery losses). Hence, these ASC levels inhibited MNU formation by 96 and 50%, respectively. Levels of 4 g $NaNO_2$ and 11.5 g sodium ASC/kg are equimolar.

IV. Tests on Carcinogenicity and Mutagenicity of Ascorbic Acid

If ASC is to be used to inhibit the formation of NNO compounds in man, it should obviously not in itself cause cancer. Hence, tests for the carcinogenicity of ASC will now be reviewed. When AKR male and C3H female mice were fed continuously with ascorbic acid (1% in the diet), the lifespan was not altered, indicating that the spontaneous induction of leukemia (AKR mice) and mammary tumors (C3H mice) was not affected by ASC (Harman, 1962). Ascorbic acid (2.5 g/liter drinking water, given continuously) did not cause bladder tumors in Swiss mice whose bladders were implanted with cholesterol pellets and inhibited the induction of these tumors by 3-hydroxyanthranilic acid dissolved in the pellets (Pipkin et al., 1969); tumors in other organs were apparently not searched for. Lung adenomas were not induced by sodium ascorbate (23 g/kg food) fed for 20 weeks to strain A mice (Mirvish et al., 1975).

Cupric[Cu(II)] and ferric[Fe(III)] ions catalyze the oxidation by oxygen (autoxidation) of ASC (Khan and Martell, 1967). On this basis, the influence Cu(II) on ASC mutagenicity was examined by Stitch et al. (1976). Preincubated solutions of ASC (25 mM) and Cu(II)(0.025 mM) were mutagenic to S. typhimurium TA 100. ASC alone was not mutagenic. An ASC–Cu(II) mixture (about 2 and 0.02 mM, respectively) caused DNA fragmentation and repair synthesis in cultured human fibroblasts; here, too, ASC alone had no effect. Ascorbic acid caused a dose-dependent increase in sister chromatid exchanges and an inhibition of DNA synthesis in mammalian cell cultures (Galloway and Painter, 1979). The effects were partly prevented by adding catalase to the culture medium and were attributed to free radicals produced from H_2O_2, which in turn arose from ASC autoxidation. Sufficient catalase or related enzymes may be present *in vivo* to destroy any H_2O_2 produced. The autoxidation reaction is

$$ASC + O_2 \xrightarrow{\text{metal ions}} \text{dehydro-ASC} + H_2O_2 \qquad (7)$$

In conclusion, ASC does not appear to be carcinogenic in experimental animals. However, it probably would be worth retesting ASC for carcinogenicity under standard bioassay conditions, possibly with and without simultaneous feeding of Cu(II) salts.

V. Effects of Ascorbic Acid on Carcinogenicity and Mutagenicity of N-Nitroso Compounds

As already mentioned, ASC did not affect carcinogenesis in the rat by ENU given transplacentally (Ivankovic *et al.*, 1973b), by NMOR (Mirvish *et al.*, 1976), or by methylnitrosobenzylamine (Coordinating Group, 1974). We tested the effect of ASC, given chronically in the diet, on lung adenoma induction by mononitrosopiperazine and NMOR administered to mice in the drinking water (Mirvish *et al.*, 1975). We reported that ASC produced a small (15 to 59%) increase in adenoma yield. This could have been caused by a greater intake of nitrosamine-containing drinking water in the group with ASC, although such an increase was not observed in the few measurements made of water consumption.

We subsequently tested the effect of ASC given in the diet on lung tumorigenesis in Strain A mice by DMN, given as two i.p. injections (Table 2). In this case, the nitrosamine dose could not be affected by the ASC. We also examined the effect of gallic acid given in the diet at a level equimolar to that of ASC. The group with ASC showed a decrease in DMN tumorigenesis, whereas gallic acid had no effect. Similar results were obtained when ASC was administered from 1 week before to 1 week after the DMN injections, or from 1 week before the first DMN injection for 20 weeks. These experiments showed large standard deviations and should be repeated.

Edgar (1974) suggested that ASC might inhibit nitrosamine carcinogenesis. This suggestion was based on a preliminary report by Kamm *et al.* (1973), later withdrawn (Kamm *et al.*, 1975), that ASC partly prevented the liver dam-

TABLE 2. Effect of Ascorbic Acid on Lung Tumorigenesis by
Dimethylnitrosamine in Male Strain A Mice[a,d]

Additional treatment	Treatment period (age in weeks)	Effective number of mice	Lung adenomas/mouse Mean ± S.D.	p
None	—	33	8.2 ± 8.1	Ref.[b]
Na ASC	10–13	40	4.0 ± 3.3	<0.005
Na ASC	10–30	35	5.4 ± 3.4	<0.05
Gallic acid	10–13	42	8.5 ± 3.4	N.S.[c]
Gallic acid	10–30	36	9.4 ± 9.6	N.S.[c]

[a] All groups received two i.p. injections of DMN in aqueous solution given at ages of 11 and 12 weeks. Dimethylnitrosamine dose was 5 mg/kg body weight per injection. A commercial powdered rodent diet was used with Na ASC or gallic acid (21.8 g/kg) added to the diet as in Mirvish et al. (1975).
[b] Reference group.
[c] Not significant.
[d] Reprinted from Mirvish (1981) with permission of the publisher.

age produced by a single dose of DMN. Greenblatt (1973) and Cardesa et al. (1974) also found that ASC did not alter DMN toxicity. Hence, we thought it unlikely that ASC would affect carcinogenesis directly (Mirvish and Shubik, 1974).

Edgar's suggestion was based on his review of evidence that ASC shows nucleophilic properties. Hence, ASC might react directly with the alkylating species (carbonium ions) that are believed to be produced during the metabolic activation of nitrosamines. On this basis, Guttenplan (1977) tested the effect of ASC on mutagenesis by NNO compounds, using *Salmonella typhimurium* TA-1530. The bacteria were incubated directly in a solution containing ASC and the NNO compound. Ascorbic acid inhibited mutagenesis by 1-methyl-3-nitro-1-nitrosoguanidine (MNNG) in the absence of liver microsomes.

In a more detailed study, Guttenplan (1978) showed that ASC inhibited MNNG mutagenicity in *S. typhimurium* because it reacted chemically with this compound (on the basis that mutagenicity paralleled MNNG concentration after it had reacted with ASC). Cupric [Cu(II)] and ferric [Fe(III)] ions, which catalyze ASC autoxidation (Khan and Martell, 1967), were tested as catalysts. Both Cu(II) and, less effectively, Fe(III) accelerated the ASC–MNNG reaction (as measured chemically), suggesting that this reaction involves ASC oxidation (see also Galloway and Painter, 1979). Ascorbic acid did not affect mutagenesis by MNU or spontaneous MNU decomposition in the presence or absence of Cu(II). An unidentified direct-acting mutagen produced by the nitrosation of spermidine was destroyed by ASC (Kokatnur et al., 1978).

Ascorbic acid also inhibited the microsome-mediated mutagenicity of DMN, and this inhibition was enhanced by Cu(II) (Guttenplan, 1977). The effective levels of ASC and Cu(II) were higher than those for the experiments with MNNG. It was suggested that ASC reduced an active metabolite of DMN or that a DMN metabolite alkylated ASC. The ASC levels in these experiments were 2–6 mM, lower than those used to demonstrate the mutagenicity of ASC–Cu(II) mixtures (Stich *et al.*, 1976) and not far above ASC levels that can occur in human tissues. The inhibition of DMN carcinogenesis by ASC (Table 2) could be explained by Guttenplan's results.

Lo and Stich (1978) used the induction of DNA repair in cultured human fibroblasts and related effects as means to monitor methylguanidine nitrosation and to show that ASC and other reducing agents inhibited this nitrosation. The main product detected was probably the highly mutagenic, but only moderately carcinogenic, methylnitrosocyanamide. The final product of methylguanidine nitrosation is the moderately mutagenic but highly carcinogenic MNU (Mirvish, 1971). Hence, a bioassay based on mutagenesis can give misleading results if carcinogenesis is the main subject of interest. The same bioassay was used to demonstrate that ASC inhibited the microsome-mediated DNA damage caused by DMN.

VI. Ascorbic Acid and Carcinogenesis in Man

Gastric cancer in man could be caused by nitrosoureas or other nitrosamides produced intragastrically from amides in food and nitrite derived from food or saliva (Mirvish, 1971, 1977; Haenszel and Correa, 1975; Cuello *et al.*, 1976; Weisburger, 1979). If this hypothesis is correct, ASC could play a significant role in inhibiting *in vivo* formation of the nitrosamides. The evidence for this hypothesis is beyond the scope of this review. However, it is relevant that there is a negative association between gastric cancer incidence and the consumption of fresh fruit (e.g., citrus) and vegetables (e.g., lettuce) that contain ASC. This association has been observed in Holland (Meinsma, 1964) and Colombia (Cuello *et al.*, 1976) as well as in the United States, Japan, Scandinavia, and England (reviewed by Haenszel and Correa, 1975). These observations suggest that ASC reduces the incidence of gastric cancer by inhibiting nitrosamide formation in the food and/or *in vivo*. Other naturally occurring compounds that react with nitrite, such as tannins, could also play a role here. The incidence of gastric cancer is falling progressively in the United States and some other countries. In addition to other factors discussed by Weisburger (1979), the increased consumption of fresh and frozen fruits and vegetables could play a role here.

If we accept the view that nitrosamides may be involved in the etiology of gastric cancer, then we should strongly recommend that people in areas at high risk for gastric cancer (e.g., Japan and Colombia) adopt appropriate changes in their diet including a greater intake of fresh fruit and vegetables or of ASC (Weisburger, 1977).

A contributing factor to the high incidence of nasopharyngeal cancer in southern China may be the high consumption of salted fish coupled with an ASC deficiency in early life (Ho, 1978). This association suggests that *in vivo* formation of an NNO compound was inhibited by ASC. Feeding of salted fish from Hong Kong induced nasal cavity tumors in rats.

Esophageal cancer is especially common in parts of Iran, South Africa, and China (Day, 1975). Nitrosamines are likely etiologic agents, since certain of these compounds (e.g., unsymmetric dialkylnitrosamines) are the most common carcinogens for the rodent esophagus. If nitrosamines are involved, and especially if they are formed *in vivo*, then exposure to ASC should be negatively correlated with the disease. This may be true at least in Iran, where the occurrence of esophageal cancer was correlated with deficiencies in vitamins A and C and in riboflavin (Hormozdiari *et al.*, 1975).

With respect to colorectal cancer, human feces contain nitrite and nitrate that probably arise by bacterial degradation of proteins (Tannenbaum *et al.*, 1978) and a direct-acting mutagen that may be related to a nitrosamide (Varghese *et al.*, 1978; Bruce *et al.*, 1979). The mutagen concentration was reduced by lowering the fat and increasing the fiber content of the diet and by feeding ASC or α-tocopherol. The ASC dose was 4 g/day given daily for several days. Since an increased fat and decreased fiber content in the diet is associated with a high incidence of colorectal cancer, the findings suggested that the mutagen is an etiologic agent. The rationale for using ASC and α-tocopherol was that they would remove nitrite from the intestinal contents and hence inhibit formation of the mutagen.

VII. Summary and Conclusions

In acidic aqueous solution, ASC inhibits the formation of nitrosamines and nitrosoureas from nitrite and the corresponding amines or ureas because it reduces nitrite to nitric oxide. Ascorbate anion is more reactive than ascorbic acid. Hence, ASC is more effective than most other reducing agents at relatively high pHs of 3–5 where the ASC anion is predominant. In the presence of oxygen, higher levels of ASC are needed to inhibit nitrosamine formation; the mechanism probably involves a direct reaction of oxygen with

ASC semiquinone and oxidation of nitric oxide to give, eventually, nitrite. Certain nitrogen oxides readily produce NNO compounds in lipidic media and lipid–water mixtures; in this case, ASC is ineffective as an inhibitor (although α-tocopherol and other lipidic antioxidants could be used). This phenomenon can cause an artifactual enhancement by ASC of aqueous nitrosation if the correct experimental conditions are not chosen.

We have suggested that ASC be administered with readily nitrosated drugs to inhibit *in vivo* conversion to carcinogenic NNO compounds, but the experimental basis for the suggestion has not been tested in man. In the food industry, ASC is widely used to inhibit NPYR formation during the frying of bacon; the mechanism for this inhibition remains unclear.

In vivo, ASC reduced or abolished the acute toxicity caused by gavage of nitrite plus dimethylamine or aminopyrine. Ascorbic acid also inhibited tumor induction by simultaneous administration of nitrite plus amines or alkylureas in rats, mice, and hamsters. These effects were attributed to nitrite reduction as in the chemical experiments. In other experiments, ASC lowered the amount of NNO compounds produced *in vivo* and determined by chemical analysis.

Ascorbic acid is apparently not carcinogenic in itself but was mutagenic in the presence of cupric and ferric ions; in this case, hydrogen peroxide produced by ASC autoxidation was probably the active agent. Ascorbic acid appeared to inhibit the induction of lung adenomas in mice by DMN; it also inhibited the microsome-mediated mutagenicity of DMN, especially in the presence of cupric ions. Ascorbic acid reacts chemically with MNNG and a spermidine nitrosation product and, hence, inhibited their direct-acting mutagenicity.

Gastric cancer in man may be caused by nitrosoureas or other nitrosamides produced in the stomach. This hypothesis is supported by the negative association between gastric cancer incidence and the consumption of ASC-containing fresh fruits and vegetables. The high incidence of nasopharyngeal and esophageal cancer in certain areas may be caused in part by nitrosamines and may be correlated with a deficiency in ASC. Human feces contain a mutagen that may be a nitrosamide. Conditions thought to cause an increased incidence of colon cancer also increased the level of this mutagen, suggesting an etiologic relationship, and oral administration of ASC reduced the mutagen level.

The following practical conclusions can be drawn.

1. Ascorbic acid is an efficient inhibitor of acidic aqueous nitrosation, especially at relatively high pHs.

2. The conditions under which ASC inhibits intragastric nitrosation in man should be established so that ASC can be evaluated as an inhibitor of drug nitrosation *in vivo*.
3. Use of ASC in the meat industry is reducing human exposure to nitrosamines in fried bacon.
4. An increased intake of ASC-containing fruits and vegetables or of ASC should be encouraged in areas of high gastric cancer.
5. The connection between ASC and the level of fecal mutagens should be further explored.

ACKNOWLEDGMENTS. I thank Dr. B. Challis (New England Institute of Life Sciences, Waltham, Mass.) for his useful criticisms. Drs. K. Karlowski, O. Bulay, R. Runge, and D. Birt collaborated with me in recent work reviewed here. J. S. Sams, S. R. Arnold, K. Devish, F. Goldenberg, and D. Delimont provided technical assistance in this work. Writing of this review and work performed in this laboratory were supported by grant PO1 CA 25100 and contract NO1 CP33278 from the National Cancer Institute, and by grant BC-39G from the American Cancer Society.

References

Archer, M. D., Tannenbaum, S. R., Fan, T. Y., and Weisman, M., 1975, Reaction of nitrite with ascorbate and its relation to nitrosamine formation, *J. Natl. Cancer Inst.* **54**:1203.
Astill, B. D., and Mulligan, L. T., 1977, Phenolic antioxidants and the inhibition of hepatotoxicity from *N*-dimethylnitrosamine formed *in situ* in the rat stomach, *Food Cosmet. Toxicol.* **15**:167.
Birdsall, J. J., 1977, *N*-Nitrosopyrrolidine in bacon obtained from 10 commercial bacon production plants, in: *Proceedings of the 2nd International Symposium on Nitrite in Meat Products, Central Agricultural Publication Documentation* (B. J. Linbergen, and B. Krol, eds.), pp. 211–213, Pudoc Press, Wageningen, Netherlands.
Bruce, W. R., Varghese, A. J., Wang, S., and Dion, P., 1979, The endogenous production of nitroso compounds in the colon and cancer at that site, in: *Naturally Occurring Carcinogens — Mutagens and Modulators of Carcinogenesis* (E. C. Miller, J. A. Miller, I. Hirono, T. Sugimura, and S. Takayama, eds.), pp. 221–228, University Park Press, Baltimore.
Bunton, C. A., Dahn, H., and Loewe, L., 1959, Oxidation of ascorbic acid and similar substances by nitrous acid, *Nature* **183**:163.
Cameron, E., Pauling, L., and Leibovitz, B., 1979, Ascorbic acid and cancer: A review, *Cancer Res.* **39**:663.
Cardesa, A., Mirvish, S. S., Haven, G. T., and Shubik, P., 1974, Inhibitory effect of ascorbic acid on the acute toxicity of dimethylamine plus nitrite in the rat, *Proc. Soc. Exp. Biol. Med.* **145**:124.
Challis, B. C., and Bartlett, C. D., 1975, Possible cocarcinogenic effects of coffee constituents, *Nature* **254**:532.

Challis, B. C., and Kyrtopoulos, S. A., 1977, Rapid formation of carcinogenic *N*-nitrosamines in aqueous alkaline solutions, *Br. J. Cancer* **35**:693.
Challis, B. C., Edwards, A., Hunma, R. R., Kyrtopoulos, S. A., and Outram, J. R., 1978, Rapid formation of *N*-nitrosamines from nitrogen oxides under neutral and alkaline conditions, in: *Environmental Aspects of N-Nitroso Compounds* (E. A. Walker, M. Castegnaro, L. Griciute, and E. R. Lyle, eds.), pp. 127–142, International Agency for Research on Cancer, Lyon.
Chan, W. C., and Fong, Y. Y., 1977, Ascorbic acid prevents liver tumor production by aminopyrine and nitrite in the rat, *Int. J. Cancer* **20**:268.
Chang, S. F., Harrington, G. W., Rothstein, M., Shergalis, W. A., Swern, D., and Vohra, S. K., 1979, Accelerating effect of ascorbic acid on *N*-nitrosamine formation and nitrosation by oxyhyponitrite, *Cancer Res.* **39**:3871.
Coordinating Group for Research on the Etiology of Esophageal Cancer of North China, 1974, *The Epidemiology of Esophageal Cancer in North China and Preliminary Results in the Investigation of its Etiological Factors,* National Academy of Medical Sciences, Peking.
Cuello, C., Correa, P., Haenszel, W., Gordillo, G., Brown, C., Archer, M., and Tannenbaum, S., 1976, Gastric cancer in Colombia. I. Cancer risk and suspect environmental agents, *J. Natl. Cancer Inst.* **57**:1015.
Dahn, H., Loewe, L., and Bunton, C. A., 1960, Über die Oxydation von Ascorbinsäure durch salpetrige Säure. Teil VI: Übersicht und Diskussion der Ergebnisse, *Helv. Chim. Acta* **43**:320.
Day, N. E., 1975, Some aspects of the epidemiology of esophageal cancer, *Cancer Res.* **35**:3304.
Edgar, J. A., 1974, Ascorbic acid and biological alkylating agents, *Nature* **248**:136.
Fan, T. Y., and Tannenbaum, S. R., 1973, Natural inhibitors of nitrosation reactions: The concept of available nitrite, *J. Food Sci.* **38**:1067.
Fiddler, W., Pensabene, J. W., Piotrowski, E. G., Doerr, R. C., and Wasserman, A. E., 1973, Use of sodium ascorbate or erythorbate to inhibit formation of *N*-nitrosodimethylamine in frankfurters, *J. Food Sci.* **38**:1084.
Fong, Y. Y., and Chan, W. C., 1976, The effect of ascorbate on amine–nitrite carcinogenicity, in: *Environmental N-Nitroso Compounds: Analysis and Formation* (E. A. Walker, P. Bogovski, and L. Griciute, eds.), pp. 461–464, International Agency for Research on Cancer, Lyon.
Galloway, S. M., and Painter, R. B., 1979, Vitamin C is positive in the DNA synthesis inhibition and sister–chromatid exchange tests, *Mutat. Res.* **60**:321.
Gray, J. I., and Dugan, L. R., 1975, Inhibition of *N*-nitrosamine formation in model food systems, *J. Food Sci.* **40**:981.
Greenblatt, M., 1973, Ascorbic acid blocking of aminopyrine nitrosation in NZO/B1 mice, *J. Natl. Cancer Inst.* **50**:1055.
Greenblatt, M., and Mirvish, S. S., 1973, Dose–response studies with concurrent administration of piperazine and sodium nitrite to strain A mice, *J. Natl. Cancer Inst.* **50**:119.
Greenblatt, M., Mirvish, S. S., and So, B. T., 1971, Nitrosamine studies: Induction of lung adenomas by concurrent administration of sodium nitrite and secondary amines in Swiss mice, *J. Natl. Cancer Inst.* **46**:1029.
Guttenplan, J. B., 1977, Inhibition by L-ascorbate of bacterial mutagenesis induced by two *N*-nitroso compounds, *Nature* **268**:368.
Guttenplan, J. B., 1978, Mechanisms of inhibition by ascorbate of microbial mutagenesis induced by *N*-nitroso compounds, *Cancer Res.* **38**:2018.
Haenszel, W., and Correa, P., 1975, Developments in the epidemiology of stomach cancer over the past decade, *Cancer Res.* **35**:3452.
Harman, D., 1962, Role of free radicals in mutation, cancer, aging and the maintenance of life, *Radiat. Res.* **16**:753.

Ho, J. H. C., 1978, An epidemiologic and clinical study of nasopharyngeal carcinoma, *Int. J. Radiat. Oncol. Biol. Biophys.* **4**:183.

Hormozdiari, H., Day, N. E., Aramesh, B., and Mahboubi, E., 1975, Dietary factors and esophageal cancer in the Caspian littoral of Iran, *Cancer Res.* **35**:3493.

Ivankovic, S., Preussmann, R., Schmähl, D., and Zeller, J., 1973a, Verhütung von Nitrosamid-bedingtem Hydrocephalus durch Ascorbinsäure nach praenataler Gabe von Äthylharnstoff und Nitrit an Ratten, *Z. Krebsforsch.* **79**:145.

Ivankovic, S., Zeller, W. J., Schmähl, D., and Preussmann, R., 1973b, Verhinderung der pranatal carcinogenen Wirkung von Äthylharnstoff und Nitrit durch Ascorbinsäure, *Naturwissenschaften* **60**:525.

Ivankovic, S., Preussmann, R., Schmähl, D., and Zeller, J. W., 1974, Prevention by ascorbic acid of *in vivo* formation of *N*-nitroso compounds, in: *N-Nitroso Compounds in the Environment* (P. Bogovski and E. A. Walker, eds.), pp. 101–102, International Agency for Research on Cancer, Lyon.

Kamm, J. J., Dashman, T., Conney, A. H., and Burns, J. J., 1973, Protective effects of ascorbic acid on hepatotoxicity caused by sodium nitrite plus aminopyrine, *Proc. Natl. Acad. Sci. USA* **70**:747.

Kamm, J. J., Dashman, T., Conney, A. H., and Burns, J. J., 1975, Effect of ascorbic acid on amine–nitrite toxicity, *Ann. N.Y. Acad. Sci.,* **258**:169.

Kamm, J. J., Dashman, T., Newmark, H., and Mergens, W. J., 1977, Inhibition of amine–nitrite hepatotoxicity by alpha-tocopherol, *Toxicol. Appl. Pharmacol.* **41**:575.

Khan, M. M. T., and Martell, A. E., 1967, Metal ion and metal chelate catalyzed oxidation of ascorbic acid by molecular oxygen. I. Cupric and ferric ion catalyzed oxidation, *J. Am. Chem. Soc.* **89**:4176.

Kinawi, A., and Schuster, T., 1978, Reaktionskinetische Untersuchengen zur Entstehung von *N*-Nitrosoephedrin *in vitro* and *in vivo, Arzneim. Forsch.* **28**:219.

Kokatnur, M. G., Murray, M. L., and Correa, P., 1978, Mutagenic properties of nitrosated spermidine, *Proc. Soc. Exp. Biol. Med.* **158**:85.

Lijinsky, W., and Greenblatt, M., 1972, Carcinogen dimethylnitrosamine produced *in vivo* from nitrite and aminopyrine, *Nature* [*New Biol.*] **236**:177.

Lijinsky, W., Conrad, E., and Bogart, R.V.D., 1972, Formation of carcinogenic nitrosamines by interaction of drugs with nitrite, in: *N-Nitroso Compounds—Analysis and Formation* (P. Bogovski, R. Preussmann, and E. A. Walker, eds.), pp. 130–133, International Agency for Research on Cancer, Lyon.

Lo, L. W., and Stich, H. F., 1978, The use of short-term tests to measure the preventive action of reducing agents on formation and activation of carcinogenic nitroso compounds, *Mutat. Res.* **57**:57.

Massey, R. C., Crews, C., Davies, R., and McWeeny, D. J., 1978, A study of the competitive nitrosations of pyrrolidine, ascorbic acid, cysteine and *p*-cresol in a protein-based model system, *J. Sci. Food Agric.* **29**:815.

Meinsma, L., 1964, Voeding en kanker, *Voeding* **25**:357.

Mergens, W. J., Kamm, J. J., Newmark, H. L., Fiddler, W., and Pensabene, J., 1978, Alpha-tocopherol: Use in preventing nitrosamine formation, in: *Environmental Aspects of N-Nitroso Compounds* (E. A. Walker, M. Castegnaro, L. Griciute, and R. E. Lyle, eds.), pp. 199–212, International Agency for Research on Cancer, Lyon.

Mergens, W. J., Vane, F. M., Tannebaum, S. R., Green, L., and Skipper, P. L., 1979, *In vitro* nitrosation of methapyrilene, *J. Pharm. Sci.* **68**:827.

Mirvish, S. S., 1971, Kinetics of nitrosamide formation from alkylureas, *N*-alkylurethans and alkylguanidines: Possible implications for the etiology of human gastric cancer, *J. Natl. Cancer Inst.* **46**:1183.

Mirvish, S. S., 1975a, Blocking the formation of N-nitroso compounds with ascorbic acid in vitro and in vivo, Ann. N.Y. Acad. Sci. **258**:175.
Mirvish, S. S., 1975b, Formation of N-nitroso compounds: Chemistry, kinetics, and in vivo occurrence, Toxicol. Appl. Pharmacol **31**:325.
Mirvish, S. S., 1977, N-Nitroso compounds: Their chemical and in vivo formation and possible importance as environmental carcinogens. J. Toxicol. Environ. Health **2**:1267.
Mirvish, S., 1981, in: Cancer: Achievements, Challenges and Prospects for the 1980's (J. H. Burchenal and H. F. Oettgen, eds.), pp. 557–587, Grune & Stratton, New York.
Mirvish, S. S., and Shubik, P., 1974, Ascorbic acid and nitrosamines, Nature **250**:684.
Mirvish, S. S., Wallcave, L., Eagen, M., and Shubik, P., 1972a, Ascorbate–nitrite reaction: Possible means of blocking the formation of carcinogenic N-nitroso compounds, Science **177**:65.
Mirvish, S. S., Greenblatt, M., and Kommineni, V. R. C., 1972b, Nitrosamide formation in vivo: Induction of lung adenomas in Swiss mice by concurrent feeding of nitrite and methylurea or ethylurea, J. Natl. Cancer Inst. **48**:1311.
Mirvish, S. S., Gold, B., Eagen, M., and Arnold, S., 1974, Kinetics of the nitrosation of aminopyrine to give dimethylnitrosamine, Z. Krebsforsch. **82**:259.
Mirvish, S. S., Cardesa, A., Wallcave, L., and Shubik, P., 1975, Induction of mouse lung adenomas by amines and ureas plus nitrite and by N-nitroso compounds: Effect of nitrite dose and of ascorbate, gallate, thiocyanate, and caffeine, J. Natl. Cancer Inst. **55**:633.
Mirvish, S. S., Pelfrene, A., Garcia, H., and Shubik, P., 1976, Effect of sodium ascorbate on tumor induction in rats treated with morpholine and sodium nitrite, and with nitrosomorpholine, Cancer Lett. **2**:101.
Mirvish, S. S., Karlowski, K., Sams, J., and Arnold, S. D., 1978, Studies related to nitrosamide formation: Nitrosation in solvent : water and solvent systems, nitrosomethylurea formation in the rat stomach, and analysis of a fish product for ureas, in: Environmental Aspects of N-Nitroso Compounds (E. A. Walker, M. Castegnaro, L. Griciute, and R. E. Lyle, eds.), pp. 161–174, International Agency for Research on Cancer, Lyon.
Mottram, D. S., and Patterson, R. L. S., 1977, The effect of ascorbate reductants on N-nitrosamine formation in a model system resembling bacon fat, J. Sci. Food Agric. **28**:352.
Newberne, P. M., 1979, Nitrite promotes lymphoma incidence in rats, Science **204**:1079.
Pensabene, J. W., Fiddler, W., Feinberg, J., and Wasserman, A. E., 1976, Evaluation of ascorbyl monoesters for the inhibition of nitrosopyrrolidine formation in a model system, J. Food Sci. **41**:199.
Pipkin, G. E., Schlegel, J. U., Nishimura, R., and Shultz, G. N., 1969, Inhibitory effect of L-ascorbate on tumor formation in urinary bladders implanted with 3-hydroxyanthranilic acid, Proc. Soc. Exp. Biol. Med. **131**:522.
Preda, N., Popa, L., and Galea, V., 1976, N-Nitroso compound formation by chlordiazepoxide and nitrite interaction in vitro and in vivo: Protective action of ascorbic acid, in: Environmental N-Nitroso Compounds: Analysis and Formation (E. A. Walker, P. Bogovski, and L. Griciute, eds.), pp. 301–304, International Agency for Research on Cancer, Lyon.
Ridd, J. H., 1961, Nitrosation, diazotisation, and deamination, Q. Rev. Chem. Soc. **15**:418.
Röper, H., and Heyns, K., 1978, Possible nitrosodimethylamine formation in comparative in vitro nitrosation experiments with six different tetracycline antibiotics, in: Environmental Aspects of N-Nitroso Compounds (E. A. Walker, M. Castegnaro, L. Griciute, and R. E. Lyle, eds.), pp. 219–237, International Agency for Research on Cancer, Lyon.
Ruddell, W. S., Blendis, L. M., and Walters, C. L., 1977, Nitrite and thiocyanate in the fasting and secreting stomach and in saliva, Gut **18**:73.
Rustia, M., 1975, Inhibitory effect of sodium ascorbate on ethylurea and sodium nitrite carcinogenesis and negative findings in progeny after intestinal inoculation of precursors into pregnant hamsters, J. Natl. Cancer Inst. **55**:1389.

Sander, J., and Bürkle, G., 1969, Induktion maligner Tumoren bei Ratten durch gleichzeitige Verfuttenrung von Nitrit und sekindaren Aminen, *Z. Krebsforsch.* **73**:54.

Sen. N. P., and Donaldson, B., 1974, The effect of ascorbic acid and glutathione on the formation of nitrosopiperazines from piperazine adipate and nitrite, in: *N-Nitroso Compounds: Analysis and Formation* (P. Bogovski, E. A. Walker, and W. Davis, eds.), pp. 103–106, International Agency for Research on Cancer, Lyon.

Sen, N. P., Donaldson, B., Seaman, S., Iyengar, J. R., and Miles, W. F., 1976, Inhibition of nitrosamine formation in fried bacon by propyl gallate and L-ascorbyl palmitate, *J. Agric. Food. Chem.* **24**:397.

Stich, H. F., Karim, J., Koropatnick, J., and Lo, L., 1976, Mutagenic action of ascorbic acid, *Nature* **260**:722.

Synnett, J. A., Unger, I., and Strunz, G., 1975, On the reactions of $NaNO_2$ with ethyl urea in the presence and absence of ascorbic acid, *Naturwissenschaften* **62**:138.

Tanaka, K., Chung, K. C., Hayatsu, H., and Kada, T., 1978, Inhibition of nitrosamine formation *in vitro* by sorbic acid, *Food Cosmet. Toxicol.* **16**:209.

Tannenbaum, S. R., Sinskey, A. J., Weisman, M., and Bishop, W., 1974, Nitrite in human saliva: Its possible relationship to nitrosamine formation, *J. Natl. Cancer Inst.* **53**:19.

Tannenbaum, S. R., Fett, D., Young, V. R., Land, P. D., and Bruce, W. R., 1978, Nitrite and nitrate are formed by endogenous synthesis in the human intestine, *Science* **200**:1487.

Varghese, A. J., Land, P. C., Furrer, R., and Bruce, W. R., 1978, Non-volatile *N*-nitroso compounds in human feces, in: *Environmental Aspects of N-Nitroso Compounds* (E. A. Walker, M. Castegnaro, L. Griciute, and R. W. Lyle, eds.), pp. 257–264, International Agency for Research on Cancer, Lyon.

Walters, C. L., Edwards, M. W., Elsey, T. S., and Martin, M., 1976, The effect of antioxidants on the production of volatile nitrosamines during the frying of bacon, *Z. Lebensm. Unters. Forsch.* **162**:377.

Weisburger, J. H., 1977, Vitamin C and prevention of nitrosamine formation, *Lancet* **2**:607.

Weisburger, J. H., 1979, Mechanism of action of diet as a carcinogen, *Cancer* **43**:1987.

Williams, D. L. H., 1978, Comparison of the efficiencies of ascorbic acid and sulphamic acid as nitrite traps, *Food. Cosmet. Toxicol.* **16**:365.

Ziebarth, D., and Scheunig, G., 1976, Effects of some inhibitors on the nitrosation of drugs in human gastric juice, in: *Environmental N-Nitroso Compounds: Analysis and Formation* (E. A. Walker, P. Bogovski, and L. Griciute, eds.), pp. 279–290, International Agency for Research on Cancer, Lyon.

5

α-Tocopherol (Vitamin E) and Its Relationship to Tumor Induction and Development

HAROLD L. NEWMARK and
WILLIAM J. MERGENS

I. Introduction

In recent years, emphasis on the role of the chemical and biological environment in carcinogenesis has emerged. Some have suggested that the majority of all human cancers may be environmentally related (Higginson, 1976). Such developments have, in part, their origins in the recognition that geographical differences in cancer patterns exist in the world, and they are certainly related to variations in environment (Clemmesen, 1965; Doll *et al.*, 1970; Segi *et al.*, 1969). In general, it has also been observed that as migrant groups leave their previous environment and adopt a new one, their propensity toward specific cancers also shifts to the prevailing risk of the new country or even local area. Further weight has been added to this idea through the identification in the human environment of numerous carcinogenic substances such as polynuclear aromatic hydrocarbons, nitrosamines, nitrosamides, and aflatoxins. The presence of many of these entities in our environment and food supplies or from *in vivo* formation leaves little doubt about potential exposure to man.

HAROLD L. NEWMARK and WILLIAM J. MERGENS • Hoffman-LaRoche, Inc., Nutley, New Jersey 07110.

A. Mechanisms of Tumor Induction/Inhibition

By no means have all the carcinogenic agents or causative factors (initiators or promoters) in our environment been identified. However, much has been accomplished in understanding tumor induction. Only a few chemical carcinogens are direct acting; most require metabolic activation. One major generalization that has been determined (J. A. Miller, 1970, 1979; J. A. Miller and Miller, 1969; E C. Miller and Miller, 1971, 1972) is that the ultimate chemical carcinogenic form is an alkylating agent (or more generally, an electrophile).

An alkylating agent, once formed within the cell, can chemically attack a variety of available substances in the cell with a wide range of damaging effects. These effects probably are not tumorigenic unless the alkylation attack occurs on the cellular DNA, resulting in the development of aberrant heretible information. A reasonable hypothesis for tumorigenesis is that if the rate of cellular DNA alterations induced by alkylation, radiation, etc. exceeds the cellular rate of repair of these alterations (e.g., by excision), then a tumor can be induced. Although the interaction of ultimate carcinogens with DNA is the most likely cause of chemical carcinogenesis, the possibility of the importance of the interaction of ultimate carcinogens with other targets within the cell (i.e., protein, RNA) should be further explored.

A corollary of the electrophile concept is that all efforts should be made to reduce the "load" of potential alkylating agents. At present, there seems to be little quantitative information, except in some unusual, mostly industrial hazard situations, concerning the major sources of intracellular alkylating (i.e., carcinogenic) substances in man. Early results from the study of human stools by Bruce (personal communication, 1978) suggest that the mutagens found in feces, apparently formed in the lower GI tract, behave in similar fashion to N-nitroso compounds. These may be a major source of carcinogens in man. Attention is thus focused on means of reducing or deflecting the potential formation of intracellular alkylating agents.

Figure 1 outlines the formation of an alkylating agent as the last occurrence prior to the initiation of a carcinogenic event. It should be observed that inhibition of tumor formation can be approached at a number of different steps in the proposed pathway. Chemoprophylaxis can range from prevention of formation of a carcinogen, through alteration of the metabolism of the agent through decreased enzymatic activation or increased enzymatic detoxification, all the way to scavenging of the alkylating agent, per se.

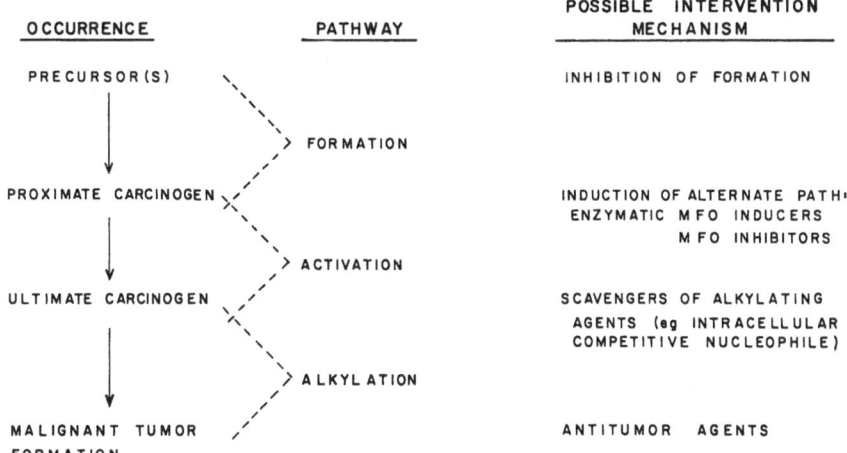

FIGURE 1. Carcinogenesis scheme.

II. Vitamin E as an Antitumor Agent

The effectiveness of vitamin E as an anticarcinogenic dietary supplement is less well documented than similar application and investigations dealing with other chemical agents (Berenblum, 1929; Crabtree, 1941; Wattenberg, 1971, 1977, 1978a,b; Falk, 1971), hormonal action (Houssay et al., 1951; Shay et al., 1960; Meisels, 1966; Belman and Troll, 1972; Kledzik et al., 1974; Hamilton et al., 1975), other vitamins (Saffiotti et al., 1967; Sporn et al., 1977), and caloric restriction (White, 1961; A. Tannenbaum and Silverstone, 1953). Vitamin E has, however, been used for several studies on the prevention of tumor formation.

A. Ultraviolet Light-Induced Carcinogenesis

Ultraviolet light (UVL) is known to produce cancer (Roffo, 1933) in hairless mice. In two subsequent studies, Black and Chan (1975) found that a dietary antioxidant mixture consisting of 2% (w/w) of additives 1.2% ascorbic acid, 0.5% butylated hydroxyanisole (BHT), 0.2% dl-α-tocopherol, and 0.1% reduced glutathione was effective in reducing the number and severity of direct UVL-induced squamous cell carcinomas in skin of hairless mice. Chan and Black (1977) also found reduced frequency of premalignant lesions and their subsequent development into tumors in mice whose dorsal median was painted with 3-methylcholanthrene followed by weekly applications of 0.5% croton oil for 15 weeks.

The influence of vitamin E (5 mg/100 g body weight i.m.) on the effect of local X-ray irradiation of two intramuscularly transplanted tumors in the rat was studied by Kagerud *et al.* (1978a,b). A significantly enhanced toxic effect of irradiation on the tumor was found. This is in contrast to the tumor-protecting effect previously reported with large doses of tocopherol (Sakamoto and Sakka, 1973). The latter study employed 100 mg/100 g body weight given intraperitoneally 0.5 hr before irradiation, whereas Kagerud noted that the most pronounced effect of tocopherol was observed when the vitamin was administered in a single dose of 5 mg/100 g body weight 7 days before irradiation. Plasma, muscle, and tumor levels of tocopherol were examined. Maximum concentrations were found 1 day, 3 days, and 3–14 days after administration, respectively.

B. Polynuclear Aromatic Hydrocarbons

In an early report, Severi (1935) indicated that vitamin E diminished resistance to the general toxic action of coal tar and promoted the appearance of neoformations but hindered their malignant evolution in male white mice. In female mice, vitamin E was found to increase resistance to toxicity, had no influence on latency, somewhat promoted neoformation, and had an uncertain effect on malignant evolution. In the author's interpretation, the results were rendered equivocal because of the small number of animals remaining in the study at its conclusion as a result of high mortality.

In 1939, Carruthers investigated the effect of dietary vitamin E obtained from refined crude cottonseed oil on the incidence and metastasis of tumors induced by 3-methylcholanthrene. The administration of vitamin E concentrate had no significant effect on the carcinogenic effect of 3-methylcholanthrene dissolved in lard or spermaceti and injected subcutaneously. The etiology of tumors induced by 3-methylcholanthrene was considered questionable by the author, however, because approximately 30% of the animals developed epidermoid carcinomas. Most other investigators have reported sarcomas from administration of 3-methylcholanthrene. Jaffe (1946) reported a 50% reduction in the incidence of sarcomas arising from the intraperitoneal injection of 3-methylcholanthrene when mice were supplemented with wheat germ oil, although no explanation of the mechanism of the protective effect was given. A concomitant marked reduction in the toxicity of 3-methylcholanthrene was observed in the supplemented mice.

Haber and Wissler (1962), using C57 leaden strain female mice receiving 30–100 times the normal dietary intake of α-tocopherol and injected subcutaneously with 100 μg/ml of 3-methylcholanthrene in mineral oil, reported that only about half as many sarcomas appeared in the group on the vitamin-E-enriched diet than in the nonsupplemented controls. An additional experiment on black male C57 mice also showed a 50% reduction in sarcoma incidence in the mice administered 7 mg/g of vitamin E. Tocopherol has been observed to delay the development of tumors caused by other hydrocarbons such as benzo[a]pyrene and coal tars (Severi, 1935; Karrer and Demole, 1938; Cameron and Meltzer, 1937), although the results have not always been consistent (Jaffe, 1946; Haddow, 1937).

Swick and Baumann (1951) reported that in rats, hepatomas induced by 3'-methyl-4-dimethylaminoazobenzene (3'-MeDAB) accumulated dietary α-tocopherol more rapidly than did adjacent liver tissue. In depletion experiments, hepatomas held tocopherol more tenaciously than normal tissue. The Jensen sarcoma, the Walker carcinoma, and the Flexner–Jobling carcinoma also absorbed tocopherol more rapidly than liver or muscle. Dietary vitamin E decreased the incidence of hepatomas when large amounts (5% corn oil plus 1 mg/g α-tocopherol in the feed) of tocopherol were fed after the administration of 3'-MeDAB. The vitamin increased tumor incidence slightly when fed between two periods of dye feeding, whereas variations in vitamin E intake made during the time the carcinogen was fed had little effect on final tumor incidence. Harr et al. (1972) found that the combination of selenite supplementation of vitamin E-adequate, low-selenium diets substantially decreased the effect of cancer induction by N-2-fluorenylacetamide (FAA). Bonmassar et al. (1968) injected mice subcutaneously with benzo[a]pyrene dissolved in ethyl oleate (100 μg/day for 20 days) and found that α-tocopherol (30 μg/day) administered simultaneously with the carcinogen for 20 days shortens the time of appearance of the tumors, but most tumors in the vitamin E-treated animals disappeared a few weeks later, and consequently the mortality was largely reduced.

Many polynuclear aromatic hydrocarbons exert their carcinogenic action by metabolism to an arene oxide, hydration to a dihydro diol, and additional oxidation to a diol–epoxide. A study by Shamberger (1966) used the initiator 7,12-dimethylbenz[a]anthracene (DMBA) in combination with croton oil in the mouse model. The roles of several antioxidant compounds were evaluated in preventing tumor growth. The addition of 0.0005% sodium selenide to the croton oil resulted in a 90% decrease in the number of tumors. The authors also found that the incorporation of 0.25% dl-α-tocopheryl acetate resulted in a 62% suppression in tumor response over a 16-week period.

Using this same carcinogen (DMBA), Lee and Chen (1979) recently reported an enhancement of tumorigenesis in rats by vitamin E deficiency. The results indicate that rats suffering from vitamin E deficiency at the time of DMBA exposure (i.v.) are more susceptible to the development of mammary tumors. Isolated liver microsomes from rats treated *in vivo* with the liver carcinogen 2-aminofluorene (AF) have a tendency toward a reduced incorporation of amino acids into protein. Hultin and Arrhenius (1964) reported this inhibitory effect to be dependent on the level of vitamin E and to be more pronounced when the animals were maintained on diets low in vitamin E. When liver slices are incubated with dimethylnitrosamine, dimethylaminophenylazoquinoline, or 2-aminofluorene (Arrhenius and Hultin, 1961; Hultin *et al.*, 1960), the activity of the slices in incorporating labeled amino acids into protein is progressively diminished. This effect is mainly because of a decreased incorporation activity of the microsomes (Skaae and Nafstad, 1978). More recently, for the carcinogen dimethylnitrosamine (DMN), Skaare and Nafstad (1978) suggested, and Dashman and Kamm (1979) have demonstrated that the administration of relatively high doses of vitamin E (55 mg/kg per day, i.m.) to rats for 3 days results in a significant decrease in acute hepatotoxicity of DMN. The decrease in toxicity is apparently associated with a decrease in hepatic metabolism of DMN. Since the metabolism of DMN is mediated by the liver microsomal mixed-function oxidase (MFO), these latter authors have suggested that DMN demethylase and ethylmorphine demethylase activities and cytochrome P-450 activities were decreased in animals pretreated with 45–100 mg/kg of vitamin E administered i.m.

III. Nitroso Compounds

A class of carcinogenic compounds that has received considerable attention by researchers since the late 1960s consists of the *N*-nitroso compounds (i.e., nitrosamines and nitrosamides). This class of compounds has been shown to include members with remarkable carcinogenic properties. There are many who suggest that because of their potency and the fact that they have been found in many foods and elsewhere in our environment, the *N*-nitroso compounds could represent a major source of human cancer, at least in the gastrointestinal system.

The use of vitamin E as an inhibitory agent in investigational studies is finding increased application. This is interesting because the role of vitamin E is as yet incompletely understood. Much work is directly related to the prevention of nitrosamine formation by vitamin E, whereas other studies suggest that other mechanisms outlined in Fig. 1, such as the retardation of oxidative activation, may also provide possible interpretations of the role of this vitamin. The remainder of this chapter will attempt to summarize studies involving vitamin E and its relation to other agents in blocking N-nitroso compound formation. In this blocking function, vitamin E may play a major role in reduction or prevention of induction of carcinogenesis.

A. Carcinogenicity

Since 1956, when dimethylnitrosamine (DMN) was first demonstrated to be a potent primary carcinogen in rats (Magee and Barnes, 1956), N-nitroso compounds have been receiving increased attention as potential major sources of cancer. The environmental precursors of nitrosamines are ubiquitous, so it is not surprising that small quantities of nitrosamines have been found in the air (Fine *et al.*, 1976), water (Cohen and Bachman, 1978), and food supplies (Eisenbrand *et al.*, 1978; Gough *et al.*, 1977, 1978a; Sen *et al.*, 1978), as well as being formed *de novo in vivo* (Rounbehler *et al.*, 1977; Fine *et al.*, 1977; S. Tannenbaum, 1979).

The chief N-nitroso compounds are the nitrosamines and the nitrosamides. A brief tabulation of their chief properties as carcinogens is found in Table 1.

TABLE 1. Carcinogenic Properties of N-Nitroso Compounds

General
80% found to be carcinogenic
Tend to be organ specific
Often potent at very low doses
Nitrosamines
Stable compounds
Highly soluble and permeable
Require metabolic activation
Nitrosamides
Unstable in water and alkali
Do not require metabolic activation
Contact carcinogens as well as organ specific

B. Mutagenicity

Carcinogenic N-nitroso compounds are also generally mutagenic, although the correlation of carcinogenicity and mutagenicity is not perfect. Nitrosamines require microsomal or host-mediated metabolism to become mutagenic, whereas the carcinogenic nitrosamides do not require metabolism for mutagenesis, i.e., they are direct-acting mutagens.

C. Mechanism of Activation

1. Nitrosamines

The mechanism of activation of nitrosamines has been postulated by Druckrey et al. (1969), Dutton and Heath (1956), and Magee (1956). In this scheme, intracellular oxidative enzymes combined with molecular rearrangement yield an alkyl carbonium ion that can act as a powerful alkylating agent on nucleophiles, including the DNA in the cell. The variation in substitution of the N-nitroso group of the nitrosamines by different alkyl, aryl, and heterocyclic groups produces the tissue or organ specificity of the cancer induced (Wishnok et al., 1978). It also modifies the rate and type of activation (Lijinsky and Taylor, 1978) of the alkylating agent that would be the ultimate carcinogen.

2. Nitrosamides

Nitrosamides generally do not seem to require metabolic activation for carcinogenesis. At least, no oxidative enzymatic reactions are required, only simpler and less energy-requiring chemical transformations to form an alkylating agent that would be the active ultimate carcinogen. This same property correlates with the generally far weaker chemical stability of nitrosamides as compared to nitrosamines. An application of these differential stability properties is that analytical procedures have been successfully developed for finding low levels (parts per billion) of nitrosamines, at least volatile ones. The nitrosamines are generally stable in a variety of extraction, purification, and sample preparation schemes. On the other hand, reliable methods for low levels of nitrosamides have not yet appeared. Variation in alkyl, aryl, or heterocycle substitution of the nitrosamides can sufficiently modify the properties of the molecule (distribution coefficient, tissue binding, etc.) to achieve organ specificity as a carcinogen when these compounds are administered systemically. However, nitrosamides also possess the capacity for local tumorigenesis if applied locally, either experimentally or through *in vivo* generation in a particular area such as the lower GI tract.

The current hypothesis of chemical changes of a nitrosamide to the ultimate carcinogenic alkylating agent is as follows:

$$R-N(NO)-C(=O)-NH_2 \longrightarrow R-N\equiv N^+$$
$$\downarrow + H_2O$$
$$HO-C(=O)-NH_2 + R-N=NOH$$
$$\downarrow$$
$$CO_2 + NH_3$$

D. Implications for Carcinogenesis

Thus, N-nitroso compounds are powerful procarcinogens that are converted to reactive metabolites that alkylate. These alkylations should probably be considered as additive to nucleic acid alteration from other sources, e.g., polycyclic hydrocarbons, radiation, viruses, etc. The total carcinogenic load is therefore the sum or additive effect of all of the factors that alter the somatic cellular DNA during the lifetime of the organism. However, at least some tissues have a repair mechanism for "splicing out" alkylated nucleic acid bases produced by a nitrosamine (Arfellini *et al.*, 1978; Craddock and Henderson, 1977; Pegg and Hui, 1978). For example, the liver is the prime site of carcinogenesis by dimethylnitrosamine (DMN) regardless of the route of administration if it is given chronically in low or moderate doses, but the liver also has a high capacity for repair of this alkylation. However, if DMN is given in single high doses, some crosses the blood–brain barrier, producing alkylated sites in brain DNA. This damage is very long lasting, suggesting that the brain has little repair capacity for alkylation produced by DMN.

Although these data are from animal experiments, they should be considered in relation to human carcinogenesis, since human blood levels of DMN have been reported in the range from 0.1–1.5 ppb (Lakritz *et al.*, 1980), and it has also been found in urine and feces of normal humans (Wang et al., 1978). Thus, DMN appears to be formed *in vivo* at an appreciable rate, perhaps as high as 70 to 700 μg per day in humans (S. Tannenbaum et al., 1978). If this amount is considered in proportion to the food intake of humans, about 500 g on a dry basis, it would be equivalent to 0.14–1.4 ppm of the food. In rats, DMN has been shown to be definitely carcinogenic at 5 ppm and barely so at 2 ppm in their feed (Terracini et al., 1967). Even considering the risks and errors inherent in extrapolating such animal data to man, the possibility that *in vivo* formation of a known potent carcinogen may be within an order of magnitude of carcinogenesis based on animal data is striking. It focuses attention on means to control, reduce, or eliminate carcinogenesis from this possible source.

Cancer induction by N-nitroso compounds may depend on the balance in a tissue between the rate of DNA alteration by alkylation of activated N-nitroso moieties and the rate of cellular repair of the DNA damage. Discussion of research into means of stimulating cellular DNA repair or of increasing resistance to DNA alkylation by activated proximal carcinogens is beyond the scope of this chapter. However, to reduce the "load potential" of sources of DNA alteration, attention must also be focused on means to reduce the input of N-nitroso compounds to the organism from the environment and to reduce the formation of N-nitroso compounds *in vivo*. Recent reports indicate that both ascorbic acid (vitamin C) and α-tocopherol (vitamin E) are useful tools with which to accomplish both goals (Kamm et al., 1973; Mirvish et al., 1972; Mergens et al., 1980).

IV. Formation of N-Nitroso Compounds

A. General Principles

In order to understand how to control carcinogenesis caused by N-nitroso compounds, it is necessary to consider their chemical properties and methods of formation. A factor of prime importance in this regard is that the N-nitroso compounds, once formed, do not easily or readily revert back to precursors.

The nitrosamines are generally very stable compounds in neutral, alkaline, and weakly acidic solutions. They are uncharged, very soluble, and can readily diffuse through many media and "barriers" including rubber gloves (Gough et al., 1978b; Sansone and Tenari, 1978; Walker et al., 1978). N-Nitroso compounds can be decomposed by heating in strong acid or by exposure to ultraviolet light. Their comparatively good stability has permitted development of reliable methods for the ready isolation of nitrosamines in complex analytical schemes (Fan et al., 1978).

Nitrosamides, however, are generally far less stable, and this has complicated development of reliable analytical methods for measuring their presence in low levels in tissues, foods, etc. However, the reactions caused by their instability do not result in their reversion back to precursors but to reactive intermediates leading to alkylating agents. Thus, in the case of both nitrosamines and nitrosamides, once formed, there is a risk of carcinogenesis by their conversion to an alkylating agent *in vivo*.

It is therefore interesting to determine if (1) formation of these N-nitroso compounds can be prevented or blocked and (2) whether the terminal active alkylating agent can be prevented from attacking the cellular DNA. In fact, a large body of reports has appeared in recent years on the successful use of blocking agents including ascorbic acid (vitamin C) and α-tocopherol (vitamin E) to prevent N-nitroso compound formation (Mirvish et al., 1972, 1975, 1976; Mirvish, 1975a; Greenblatt, 1973; Kamm et al., 1973, 1974, 1977; Fong and Chan, 1976; Kinawi et al., 1977; Preda et al., 1976; Cardesa et al., 1974; Kawabata et al., 1974; Ivankovic et al., 1974; Archer et al., 1975; Fan and Tannenbaum, 1974; Sen and Donaldson, 1974; Sen et al., 1974, 1976; Gray and Dugan, 1975; Ziebarth and Scheunig, 1976; Mergens et al., 1978). Only a few reports have appeared, however, suggesting methods of blunting the alkylation effects of N-nitroso compounds once formed (Edgar, 1974; Guttenplan, 1977).

In classical organic chemistry, nitrosamines were considered only as the reaction products of secondary amines with an acidified solution of a nitrite salt or ester. Today, it is recognized that nitrosamines can be produced from primary, secondary, and tertiary amines, and nitrosamides from secondary amides. Douglass et al. (1978) have published a good review of nitrosamine formation. For the purposes of this writing, it will suffice to say that amine and amide precursors for nitrosation reactions to form N-nitroso compounds are indeed ubiquitous in our food supply, environment, and particularly *in vivo*. These precursors of nitrosamines and nitrosamides compose a large part of our living organic world. Therefore, to study means of blocking N-nitroso compound formation, it is necessary to look at the nature of the nitrosating agents and the chemistry of formation of N-nitroso compounds.

B. Aqueous Systems

In aqueous solution, the optimum condition for nitrosation (Mirvish, 1975b) is usually found to be about pH 3–4 and reflects the mutual optimization of two conditions, (1) the formation of the nitrosating intermediate N_2O_3 and (2) the concentration of the more reactive unprotonated form of the amine which is governed by the following equations:

$$NO_2^- + H^+ \longrightarrow HONO$$
$$2HONO \rightleftharpoons N_2O_3 + H_2O$$
$$R_2NH + H^+ \longrightarrow R_2NH_2^+$$
$$R_2NH + N_2O_3 \longrightarrow R_2NNO + HONO$$

This suggests then that amines with pK_a in the range of 4–6 will be more rapidly nitrosated than those with pK_a values in the range of 9–11. This has been borne out in practice many times. Amines such as N-methylaniline (4.84),* piperazine (5.9, 9.8), and aminopyrine (5.04) are much more rapidly nitrosated than piperdine (11.2), dimethylamine (10.72), and pyrrolidine (11.27).

In alkaline aqueous solution, on the other hand, one would expect that nitrosations would not occur at all because of the absence of an active nitrosating intermediate. Thus, one convenient way of stopping nitrosation reactions in aqueous media is to alkalize the reaction mixture. However, Challis et al. (1978) have shown that N-nitrosamines and N-nitramines are readily formed in aqueous solution between pH 7 and 14 when the nitrosation agents are the gases N_2O_3 and N_2O_4. Interestingly, amines not only compete effectively with the expected OH^- hydrolysis reaction, but the nucleophilic reactivity of various amines becomes virtually independent of pK_a value. In this case, the alkaline pH of the aqueous solvent exhibits a "leveling" effect on dissolved amines in that all the amines are unprotonated and become equivalent in reactivity. Challis et al. (1978) noted that under their experimental conditions 2×10^{-3} M amine competed effectively with 55.5 M H_2O and 0.1 M OH^- for the nitrosating agent and suggested that possibly more reactive isomers of N_2O_3 and N_2O_4 are generated by the gaseous NO and NO_2 components. Here, N-nitrosamines result from reaction of the unsymmetrical tautomer (ON—NO_3), whereas the symmetrical tautomer (O_2N—NO_2) produces an N-nitramine possibly via a four-center transition state. The results for N_2O_3 may be explained similarly in terms of the corresponding

---

*Number in parentheses refers to pK_a of the amine.

ON—NO$_2$ ⇌ ON—ONO tautomers. This conclusion has a precedent (Steel et al., 1952) in the case of N$_2$O$_4$ but not for N$_2$O$_3$.

Tautomers of N$_2$O$_3$ and N$_2$O$_4$

	Symmetrical	Unsymmetrical
Dinitrogen trioxide	O=N—O—N=O	O=N—N(=O)$_2$
Dinitrogen tetroxide	O$_2$N—NO$_2$	O$_2$N—O—NO

In moderately acidic aqueous nitrite solution, the nitrosating agent is essentially nitrous acid anhydride, N$_2$O$_3$, formed from nitrous acid, HONO (pK_a = 3.14 at 25°C), which is in turn formed from acidification of nitrite ions. Stronger acidification can yield a very reactive nitrosating agent, H$_2$ONO$^+$. Of even greater interest in nitrosation *in vivo* is the catalytic effect of certain anions that form more reactive nitrosating agents (Boyland et al., 1971; Boyland and Walker, 1974; Fan and Tannenbaum, 1973; Schweinsberg, 1974). Thiocyanate is the most active such catalyst, followed by halides in the order I$^-$, Br$^-$, Cl$^-$. This effect is often strong at low pH.

C. Nonaqueous Systems

In nonaqueous (nonpolar) solvent systems, nitrosation also proceeds. Once the conditions are set for a nitrosating agent and susceptible amine to enter a lipid nonpolar phase, the reaction is generally extremely rapid. Free amines readily dissolve in aprotic lipid solvent systems as the unprotonated base, yielding a high proportion (if not all) of the more reactive free base form of the molecule for nitrosation. The active intermediates of the nitrosating agents N$_2$O$_3$ or even NO$_2$ are gases with appreciable solubility in lipid nonpolar solvent systems. This is in marked contrast to the poor lipid solubility of nitrite ion NO$_2^-$. The existence of a nitrosating agent in aprotic solvents has been known for a long time and was recently demonstrated by Mirvish et al., (1978) who recorded the UV spectra of "dried HNO$_2$" in methylene chloride. The chemistry of these reactions can be summarized as follows (Lovejoy and Vosper, 1968):

$$2R_2NH + N_2O_3 \longrightarrow R_2NH_2^+NO_2^- + R_2NNO$$
nitrite salt   nitrosamine

$$2R_2NH + N_2O_4 \longrightarrow R_2NH_2^+NO_3^- + R_2NNO$$
nitrate salt   nitrosamine

The formation of nitrosamines in aprotic solvents has applicability to many practical lipophilic systems including foods (particularly bacon), cigarette smoke, cosmetics, and some drugs. But the very rapid kinetics of nitrosation reactions in lipid solution indicates that the lipid phase of emulsions or analogous multiphase systems can act as "catalyst" to facilitate nitrosation reactions that may be far slower in purely aqueous media (Okun and Archer, 1977; Kim et al., 1980; Mergens et al., 1980). This is apparently true in some cosmetic emulsion systems and may have important applicability to nitrosation reactions in vivo, particularly in the GI tract. In these multiphase systems, the pH of the aqueous phase may be poor for nitrosation in aqueous media (e.g., neutral or alkaline pH) because of the very small concentration of HONO or N_2O_3 that can exist at these pH ranges. However, the small amount of N_2O_3 readily enters the lipid where the nitrosation reaction is very rapid. The nitrosation reaction is almost completely unidirectional towards the formation of N-nitroso compounds. The net result is that the presence of the lipid in such an emulsion brings together low concentrations of free base (which increases in the lipid as the pH goes up towards alkalinity) and nitrosating agent (N_2O_3) which react rapidly and probably completely to form N-nitroso compounds. In physiological lipids, especially in the GI tract, the free hydroxyl groups of substances such as monoglycerides, some phosphatides, cholesterol, bile acids, and salts, etc. may contribute by functioning as transnitrosating agents.

D. Transnitrosation

Many organic nitro compounds and nitroso compounds can act as effective sources of nitrosation of susceptible amines and amides. For example, Bronopol™ (2-nitro-2-bromo-1,3-propanediol) was formerly used extensively as an antimicrobial preservative in cosmetics until it was found to react readily with diethanolamine to form nitrosodiethanolamine (Douglass et al., 1978). This has lead to the hypothesis that the potential carcinogenicity of nitro compounds may be because of their capacity as nitrosation sources in vivo. If the model is valid, ascorbic acid or tocopherol could serve to reduce the carcinogenicity. In a limited trial based on this concept, the mutagenicity of 5-nitroisopropylimidazole was reduced significantly, but was not completely eliminated, by the presence of either ascorbic acid or α-tocopherol in the test system (Newmark and Mergens, 1981). In protocols for carcinogenicity testing of nitro compounds, it may be useful to compensate the higher test doses of the administered compound with ascorbic acid and tocopherol to insure that the nitrosation-blocking capacity native to the natural feed is not overwhelmed.

Phenolic compounds are particularly important in transnitrosation and may even function as nitrosation catalysts, as discussed in Section V.B.2.

V. Blocking N-Nitroso Compound Formation

A. Principles

The work *in vitro* of Mirvish *et al.* (1972) on the prevention of dimethylnitrosamine formation from oxytetracycline and nitrite paved the way for a new approach in blocking nitrosamine formation using ascorbic acid. Independent *in vivo* studies by Kamm *et al.* (1973) showed that the simultaneous feeding of ascorbic acid could prevent amine–nitrite-induced hepatotoxicity in rats from aminopyrine and sodium nitrite. Ascorbic acid was also demonstrated to prevent carcinogenesis induced by feeding aminopyrine and sodium nitrite to animals (Greenblatt, 1973).

These protective effects are currently believed to be caused by the ability of ascorbic acid or α-tocopherol to compete with susceptible amines (such as aminopyrine or oxytetracycline) for the available nitrite ion (i.e., nitrosating species). This premise is based on the work of Dahn *et al.* (1960) who studied the anaerobic oxidation of ascorbic acid by nitrous acid (HONO). These workers reported that the initial attack by the nitrosating species is on the 3-hydroxy group of ascorbic acid, forming the nitrite ester which subsequently decomposes to yield the semiquinone. Further reaction of the semiquinone with an additional mole of nitrosating species completes the oxidation of ascorbate to dehydroascorbic acid.

Archer *et al.* (1975) suggested that between pH 1.5 and 5.0, the anaerobic nitrosation of secondary amines in the presence of ascorbic acid involves two competitive second-order reactions as follows:

$$\text{Amine} + \text{N}_2\text{O}_3 \xrightarrow{k_1} \text{Nitrosamine} + \text{NO}_2^- + \text{H}^+ \qquad (1)$$

$$\text{Ascorbate} + N_2O_3 \xrightarrow{k_2} \text{dehydroascorbic acid} + 2NO + 2H_2O \quad (2)$$

If $k_2 \gg k_1$, then ascorbate will successfully compete with amine for available nitrite. The above reaction scheme also suggests that any reducing agent capable of rapidly destroying nitrite could be a potential protective agent against nitrosamine formation.

In one approach to preventing nitrosamine formation by the use of blocking (or scavenging) agents, a model system was developed to evaluate the ability of reducing agents to destroy nitrite ion, relative to that of ascorbic acid. The results of several of these experiments are shown in Figs. 2 and 3. The particular reaction conditions for these studies were simulated gastric fluid (USP XIX) at pH 3 and pH 5, respectively, at 37° C. The water-insoluble compounds were dispersed using a weight ratio of 6:1 polysorbate 20: antioxidant. Several results are of particular interest in this aqueous system. Caffeic and ferulic acids were found to be very reactive agents in this system. These two antioxidant compounds are basically cinnamic acids with ad-

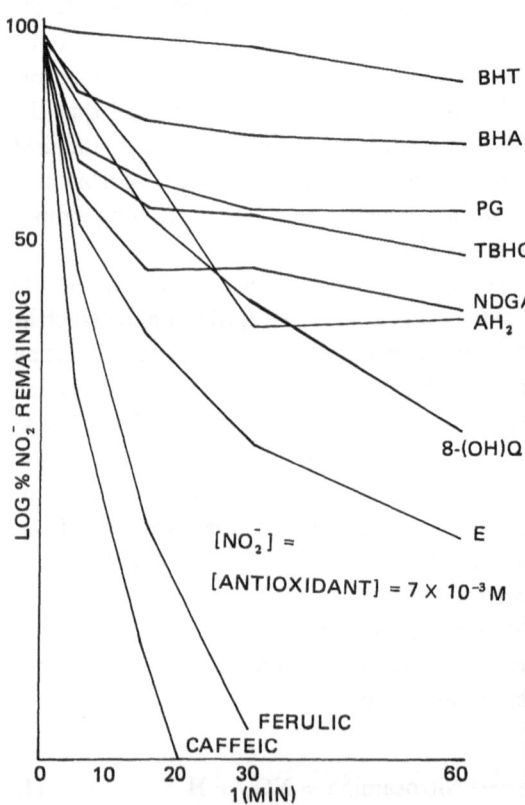

FIGURE 2. Nitrite consumption by antioxidant compounds at pH 3, 37° C, in simulated USP gastric fluid. $[NO_2^-] = [\text{antioxidant}] = 7 \times 10^{-3}$ M. Water-insoluble compounds were dispersed in the aqueous phase using a 6:1 weight ratio of polyoxyethylene(zo)sorbitan monolaurate to antioxidant. NO_2^- determinations performed by Greiss reaction. Key: BHT, butylated hydroxytoluene; BHA, butylated hydroxyanisole; PG, propyl gallate; TBHQ, tertiary butylhydroquinone; NDGA, nordihydroguariatic acid; AH_2, ascorbic acid; (8-OH)Q, 8-hydroxyquinoline; E, dl-α-tocopherol; ferulic, ferulic acid; caffeic, caffeic acid.

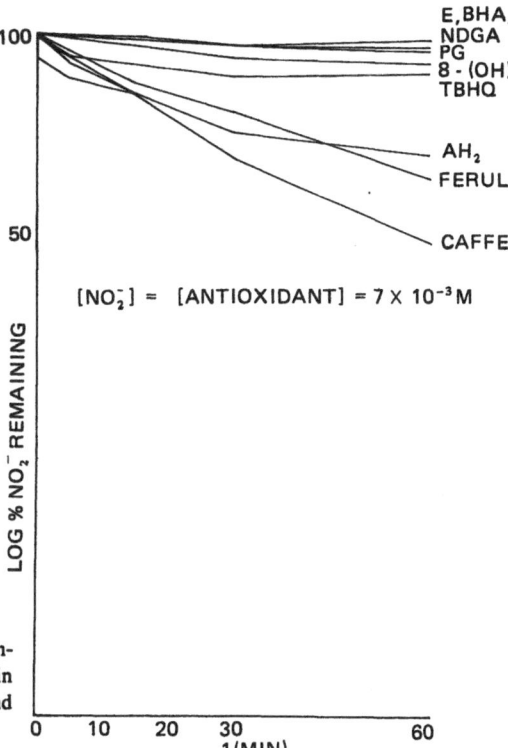

FIGURE 3. Nitrite consumption by antioxidant compounds at pH 5, 37°C, in simulated USP gastric fluid. Key and conditions are the same as in Fig. 2.

ditional phenolic hydroxyl groups and appear to react very vigorously with nitrite. They are present in the free state only in small quantities in foods of vegetable origin but constitute a significant portion, in polymeric form, of the lignin fibers that hold woody plant cells together. Aside from these two agents, α-tocopherol (vitamin E) was found to be most effective at the acid pHs, whereas ascorbic acid was found to most rapidly destroy nitrite ion at pH 5.

Included in the data are a number of substances used as antioxidants in foods, particularly to prevent oxidative rancidity in fats. These include propyl gallate (PG), butylated hydroxytoluene (BHT), butylated hydroxyanisole (BHA), tertiary butyl hydroquinone (TBHQ), as well as α-tocopherol. There is a lack of correlation between general antioxidant efficacy and nitrite-blocking reactivity. Indeed, it appears almost the reverse, with BHA and BHT, usually considered the best lipid antioxidants, being very poor as nitrite blockers. These data *in vitro* correlate well with the report of Astill and Mulligan (1977) showing similar results *in vivo* of the effect of a variety of antioxidants in blocking the liver toxicity of orally administered dimethylamine and sodium nitrite. The nitrite-blocking reaction is basically a chemical reduction, with a definite and often irreversible oxidative change in the blocking agent. Antioxidants in lipid systems often function by scavenging free radicals and transferring the energy without destruction of the antioxidant (Cort, 1974). This represents a sharp difference between the mechanism of "antioxidants" as such and nitrosamine formation-blocking agents. Some compounds can be both, but not necessarily.

The reaction of nitrite with tocopherol in aqueous dispersion slows down considerably when the pH is raised from 3 to 5. The reactivity of ascorbate, on the other hand, does not vary to such a great degree. If one considers the differences in the method of dispersion of these two components in the aqueous gastric fluid, several conclusions can be drawn. Ascorbate is directly soluble in water. Dahn et al. (1960) have pointed out that the more reactive form of ascorbic acid in reacting with a nitrosating intermediate is the anionic form. This would indicate that in these simulated gastric fluid experiments involving the ascorbic acid reduction, both the generation of the nitrosating intermediate and the more reactive form of ascorbic acid are pH dependent. The more acidic conditions favor the formation of the nitrosating intermediate and the less reactive form of ascorbic acid. As the pH becomes more neutral, less nitrosating intermediate is being formed, but at the same time the more reactive anionic form of ascorbic acid is being generated. Hence, it appears that, in aqueous media, ascorbic acid is a more efficient reactant at neutral to slightly acidic solutions.

α-Tocopherol is more reactive than ascorbic acid at pH 3 but considerably less reactive at pH 5. One explanation for this behavior is that in this system the tocopherol exists in a lipid micelle and, therefore, in this range a change in pH would have little effect on the state of protonation of the tocopherol. However, lower pH increases the formation of the lipophilic nitrosating agent N_2O_3 ($2NO_2^- + 2H^+ \longrightarrow HONO \longrightarrow N_2O_3 + H_2O$) which can readily enter the lipid micelle phase and rapidly react with the tocopherol. It is often forgotten that the nonionized "gaseous" substances such as NO, N_2O_3, NO_2, etc. are far more soluble in nonpolar (lipophilic) solvents than in polar (hydrophilic) solvents. Thus, in the presence of the lipid micelle offers a source of "concentration" of nitrosating species by extraction into this lipophilic phase. Tocopherol, if present under these conditions, can be particularly effective in reacting with the nitrosating agent since both are "concentrated" in the lipid micellar phase. This is important for reactivity in the nonaqueous phase or in acidic conditions in aqueous dispersions. This is not the case, however, as was previously pointed out, for ascorbic acid which is primarily active only in the aqueous phase. The α-tocopherol experiment essentially reflects the effect of pH on the formation of the lipophilic form of the nitrosating intermediate. One important observation is the apparent strong ability of α-tocopherol to react with a nitrosating intermediate in an aprotic solvent, in this case the emulsion micelle (Mergens *et al.*, 1978).

From these initial experiments it becomes apparent that nitrosamine formation could take place in any number of different conditions. More importantly, the prevention of nitrosamine formation by the use of blocking agents requires an understanding of the phase in which nitrosamine formation was taking place.

B. Blocking Agents

Most agents effective in blocking N-nitroso formation are reducing agents capable of transforming the nitrosating species to nitric oxide (NO) or oxides of nitrogen of lower oxidation state. In the process, the reducing agent is itself oxidized and thus consumed. In addition to the excess of blocking agent needed for effective competition against the nitrosation reaction on a competitive kinetic basis, it is usually necessary to have an excess blocking agent to prevent reoxidation of the NO to NO_2 or N_2O_3 which would regenerate the nitrosating capacity. This oxidation is catalyzed by trace metals and depends on the presence of oxygen. In most systems, such as food, *in vivo* reactions, etc., this reoxidation potential poses no serious hazard. However, thin film exposures such as a cosmetic applied to the skin pose serious problems when exposed to atmospheres containing nitrogen oxides, such as urban polluted air or particularly smoke-filled rooms.

A large variety of reducing agents can function as blocking agents of N-nitroso compound formation.

1. Sulfur Compounds

Sulfur compounds function essentially in aqueous media (Gray and Dugan, 1975; Hisatune, 1961; Jones, 1973). These include sodium bisulfite, ammonium sulfamate, sulfamic acid, cysteine, glutathione, and mercaptans in general.

2. Phenols

Phenols, particularly diphenols, may block nitrosation by reduction of the nitrosating agent to NO, and in so doing, they are oxidized to form a quinone. Nitrosating inhibition *in vivo* and/or *in vitro* has been shown for gallic acid, propyl gallate, tannic acid, vanillin, hydroquinone, and thymol. However, unsubstituted carbons on the aromatic ring can also be C-nitrosated to form an aromatic nitroso compound. Although this also ostensibly removes the nitrosating agent, the nitrosophenol formed can itself nitrosate a susceptible amine.

Walker *et al.* (1979) have shown that phenols catalyze nitrosation reactions to form N-nitroso compounds, apparently by the formation of a nitrosophenol intermediate that then acts as a transnitrosater of a susceptible amine (or amide). Thus, a phenolic compound, to be useful as a blocking agent against nitrosation, should ideally be molecularly structured to be readily oxidized, e.g., to a quinone and thus act as a reducing agent and should also be completely substituted on the aromatic ring to prevent C-nitrosation from occurring.

3. α-Tocopherol (Vitamin E)

α-Tocopherol, the chief form of vitamin E, is a natural substance with just these chemical properties. In addition, the chemical moiety has a side chain of three isoprenoid units that apparently functions to aid in absorption into the organism and particularly into tissue cells. The strongly lipophilic nature of the tocopherols leads to their concentration in the hydrophobic portions or subcellular components of the cells. In these locations, α-tocopherol normally performs its major function as lipid antioxidant, both by scavenging lipophilic free radicals and by reducing potent (and often toxic) cellular lipid-oxidizing agents. There are other tocopherols and tocotrienols (tocopherols with unsaturated side chains) in foods of plant origin. Although these are very important in the plant kingdom as lipid antioxidants, they have far less importance in mammals, primarily because of poor absorption and retention in the organism. The structure of the α-, β-, γ-, and ϵ-tocopherols are shown in Fig. 4.

From the viewpoint of blocking of nitrosation reactions, these structures are very interesting. Although all of the tocopherols can act as reducing phenols to form quinones in reducing a nitrosating agent to NO, only the α-tocopherol, being completely substituted on the aromatic ring, can completely avoid forming a C-nitroso derivative that can potentially transnitrosate or even catalyze a nitrosation reaction of a nitrosatable amine or amide (Quaife, 1948). Kamm *et al.* (1977) and Mergens *et al.* (1978) have shown that α-tocopherol is a very effective blocking agent against nitrosation

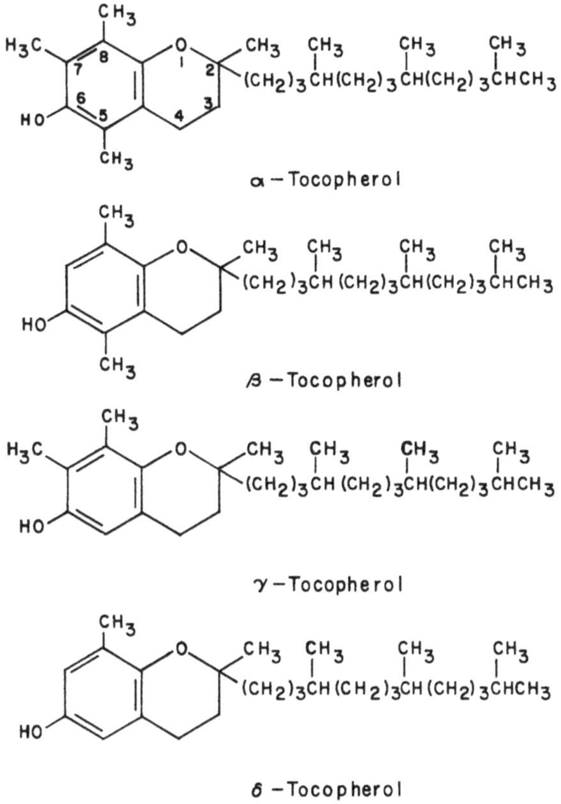

FIGURE 4. Chemical structure of some tocopherols.

reactions, whereas γ-tocopherol is somewhat less effective both *in vitro* and *in vivo*. This superiority of α-tocopherol over γ-tocopherol as a nitrosation inhibitor is in marked contrast to the superiority of the γ- over the α-tocopherol as an *in vitro* or food-type antioxidant. The difference in mechanism apparently depends on the availability of substitution positions on the aromatic ring of the γ-tocopherol in blocking nitrosation reactions as compared with the mechanisms of lipid oxidation blocking.

In reaction with a nitrosating agent, α-tocopherol is converted (oxidized) to α-tocoquinone (Kamm *et al.*, 1977), an irreversible reaction that also is the first step in the normal metabolism of α-tocopherol (Csallany *et al.*, 1962; Weber and Wiss, 1964) and yields the first reaction product formed by losses of tocopherol in foods through oxidation in processing and storage (Bauernfeind, 1977). Thus, tocoquinone is a normal constituent in foods as well as a metabolite of α-tocopherol.

The "vitamin E" of commerce is a loose term that includes several different chemical moieties (American Pharmaceutical Assocation) including the d-α-tocopherol, dl-α-tocopherol, and their acetic and succinic esters. α-Tocopherol has three asymmetric centers at positions 2, 4', and 8'. The chief distinctions are as follows:

1. The assymetric center at position 2, where the side chain joins the chromane ring, is in the optically active d position in the "natural" form of the vitamin. The racemic dl form produced by total synthesis is composed of an equal mixture of the d form and the l form at position 2, the latter having only about one-half the biological activity of the vitamin of the d form. The biological activity is determined by biological tests that are at least partly dependent on relative efficiency of absorption and retention into the organism and cellular components (Draper, 1970), so that the d form is considered to have 1.36 times the activity of the synthetic dl form. On this basis, the relative biological activities of the α-tocopherols have been assigned in terms of units, not milligrams, of activity. However, in terms of nitrosation-blocking ability, both the d and dl forms have equal capacity. Thus, they can be considered equivalent on weight basis rather than on a unit of biological activity. The assymetry at positions 4' and 8' appear to have little effect on biological activity.

2. Most commercially available vitamin E is in the form of esters, particularly acetate and hemisuccinate. The esters do not naturally appear in foods but were developed as means of stabilizing the isolated "natural" d form as well as the synthetic dl form from oxidation of the phenol group during processing and storage, particularly in pharmaceutical dosage forms such as tablets and capsules. These esters per se are inactive as antioxidants of N-nitroso-blocking agents. On ingestion, they are slowly and often incompletely hydrolyzed in the GI tract by the pancreatic lipases with the aid of bile as an emulsifier. The acetate may be partly absorbed unhydrolyzed and is only very slowly hydrolyzed on parenteral administration (Newmark et al., 1975). Unfortunately, some studies of vitamin E in cancer research (such as the effect on reduction of carcinogenesis by experimental agents) have used α-tocopherol acetate with little or no attention paid to the rate, site, or extent of hydrolysis to the active free phenolic form. It would be far more prudent to utilize the natural form, the free unesterified phenolic α-tocopherol, d (natural) or dl (synthetic), in all such studies in the future. This may be especially true of studies *in vivo* seeking activity of α-tocopherol in the upper portion of the GI tract (stomach, duodenum, etc.) where little or no free active tocopherol can be expected to be formed when tocopheryl acetate or succinate is administered.

TABLE 2. Absorption of dl-α-Tocopherol in Man

Oral dose (mg)	Percent absorbed (24 hr)
10	96.9 ± 13.0
30	87.3 ± 13.5
50	72.6 ± 11.6
100	81.5 ± 6.1
500	67.6 ± 19.4
1500	70.3 ± 27.9
2000	55.2 ± 28.8

3. Both d- and dl-α-tocopherols are oils, essentially insoluble in water and miscible with edible fats and oils. In foods, tocopherols are naturally present in the dispersions of lipid in the food; they in turn produce fine dispersions in the GI tract on digestion, along with the lipids (triglycerides, phosphatides, etc.) with which they are associated. For use of α-tocopherol experimentally for *in vivo* studies, various systems are available (both mechanical and physiochemical using surfactants) to prepare aqueous dispersions of the oleaginous tocopherol in order to achieve effective interfacial area for interaction with substances such as nitrosating agents in the aqueous phase (Pensabene *et al.*, 1978).

4. α-Tocopherol is not completely absorbed from the GI tract. Absorption efficiency decreases as the administered dose increases, as indicated in studies in man by Schmandke *et al.* (1967) and illustrated in Table 2.

In unpublished work with W. R. Bruce (personal communication) we have confirmed that individuals taking 400 mg dl-α-tocopherol per day in a form that forms a fine emulsion on ingestion eliminate about one-third of the dose in the feces. The actual level was in the range of 500–1000 ppm of dl-α-tocopherol in the feces which compares favorably with the 500 ppm level found effective in blocking nitrosamine formation during the frying of bacon. Thus, the administration of free α-tocopherol in a form that yields a fine emulsion on ingestion can supply an effective nitrosation inhibitor for the entire GI tract, at least in the lipophilic phase.

4. Other Blocking Agents

There are apparently other blocking agents in natural foods. In at least a few animal feed pellets made from natural ingredients, the nitrite reaction capacity was found to be appreciably greater than the combined content of ascorbic acid and free tocopherol (W. J. Mergens, unpublished data, 1978).

We have found that caffeic and ferulic acids react vigorously with nitrite but have not determined whether the products of the reaction can transnitrosate to a susceptible amine. Lignin fibers in plant foods partly represent polymers of these compounds that also appear to react with nitrite. It has also been suggested that the reductones present in foods may function as effective blockers of nitrosamine formation (A. E. Wasserman, personal communication, 1979).

C. Integration of Blocking Systems

In Fig. 5, an attempt is made to summarize our current concepts of nitrosation reactions in aqueous solution, gas state, and nonpolar solvents (i.e., lipids), with the expected exchanges of nitrosating sources among the three phases. The ordinate at the left denotes the oxidation state of the nitrogen in the various oxides, ions, etc. in the highly interreactive system. Only oxides or ions containing nitrogen in the +3 or +4 state can nitrosate. Oxidation to the +5 state (nitrate) removes the capacity to nitrosate, as does reduction to the +2 state (Nitric oxide, NO) or to the +1 state (nitrous oxide). Ascorbic acid in aqueous solution and α-tocopherol in lipid or nonpolar solvents or the lipid or micellar phase of an emulsion both act by reducing the nitrosating agent to NO. This also suggests that in multiphase systems such as actually exist in tissues *in vivo*, in the contents of the GI tract, in many foods such as bacon, etc., both ascorbic acid and tocopherol should be used in combination to block nitrosation, in order to be more effective. For example, since the active nitrosating intermediate N_2O_3 can rapidly move in and out of lipid and aqueous phases, blocking (i.e., reducing) agents should ideally be present in both.

Ascorbic acid is normally an excellent reducing agent and oxygen scavenger in aqueous systems. However, it can also act as a prooxidant and/or a source of free radicals. For example, in nonenzymatic reactions with aqueous oxygen in the presence of trace metals, particularly cupric or ferric ions, it produces hydrogen peroxide:

$$\text{Ascorbic acid} + O_2 \xrightarrow{\text{Metal ions}} \text{dehydroascorbic acid} + H_2O_2$$

The peroxide can attack the unsaturated double bonds of fatty acids, etc., generating free radicals from the lipid peroxide systems. α-Tocopherol, as an antioxidant, partly acts as a free radical scavenger (Cort, 1974). Enzy-

α-Tocopherol and Tumor Induction and Development

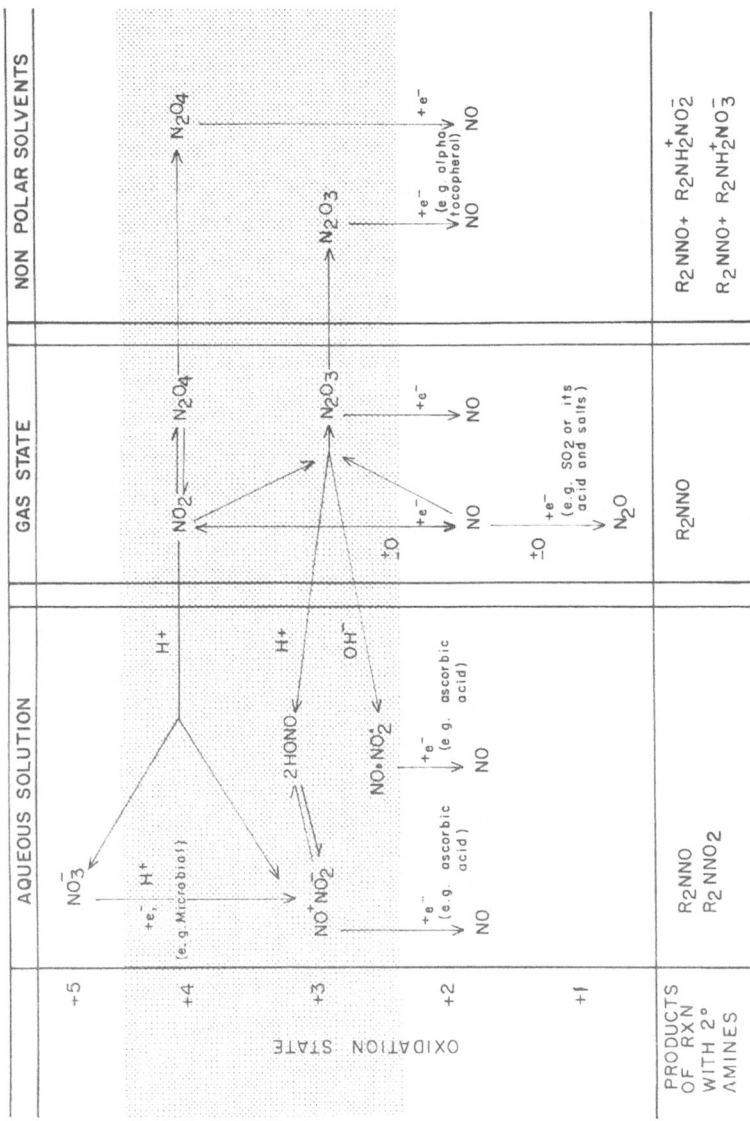

FIGURE 5. Some possible dismutations and transformations of the oxides of nitrogen. Shaded area designates oxidation states of nitrogen capable of nitrosating an amine. See text for explanation.

matically, however, ascorbic acid is oxidized normally without peroxide formation.

$$\text{Ascorbic acid} + O_2 \xrightarrow{\text{polyphenol oxidase}} \text{dehydroascorbic} + H_2O$$

In biological systems, α-tocopherol (vitamin E) probably acts to quench the nonenzymatic side reactions of ascorbic acid with trace metals by free radical scavenging. In many of the reactions involved in nitrosation, a free radical mechanism has been postulated. The free radical-scavenging properties of α-tocopherol would seem to complement the aqueous reducing properties of ascorbic acid by preventing the propagation of free radical mediated reactions.

Thus, the active form of vitamins C and E (ascorbic acid and free α-tocopherol) can be seen to act as a complementary pair of agents in blocking nitrosation reactions by two mechanisms:

1. Acting simultaneously as nitrosating agent reductants in both aqueous (vitamin C) and lipid or micellar phases (vitamin E).
2. Acting as a complementary pair of agents to block free radical propagation, as well as chemical reduction of nitrosating agents.

Some data in bacon studies (Fiddler *et al.*, 1974), cigarette smoke (Mergens *et al.*, 1978), and *in vivo* (Bruce, 1979) indicate the utility of the approach of using the combination of ascorbic acid and α-tocopherol.

VI. α-Tocopherol Applications

Free α-tocopherol has been demonstrated to be a useful practical inhibitor of formation of the tumorigenic *N*-nitroso compounds (Kamm *et al.*, 1977; Mergens *et al.*, 1978). Some specific applications are reviewed below.

A. Bacon

In the United States, pork bellies are processed into bacon with an aqueous solution input by pumping to achieve 120 ppm sodium nitrite and 550 ppm sodium ascorbate. This system serves to protect the bacon from the growth of toxin from *Cl. botulinum* without forming nitrosamines during storage. When the bacon is fried during preparation for eating, the water is lost by vaporization, generating the readily lipid-mobile N_2O_3 nitrosating agent from the residual nitrite in the bacon. This readily produces nitrosamines in the fat phase, particularly nitrosopyrrolidine. The source of the pyrrolidine is proline which is a major constituent of the collagen fibers in the fat layer. The presence of α-tocopherol in the range of 250–500 ppm in the bacon at the time of frying has been demonstrated to be effective in reducing nitrosamines in the bacon (Fiddler et al., 1978). The presence of tocopherol also markedly (e.g., two- to fourfold) reduces the nitrosamine in the vapors formed during bacon frying (W. J. Mergens, unpublished data, 1979).

B. Other Foods

Extensive surveys have been made to determine if significant quantities of nitrosamines are present in foods. Although low levels have been found in many foods other than bacon, the total quantities appear to contribute only a small amount to the daily diet, at least in the few countries where estimates have been made. In Great Britain, the dietary intake of preformed nitrosamines has been estimated at 0.5 μg/day Gough et al., 1978a), and about 0.6 μg/day in West Germany (Eisenbrand et al., 1978). The major sources of these dietary nitrosamines include (1) application of nitrosating agents for preservation, including sodium nitrite in processed meats or smoked fish, etc., which supplies nitrogen oxides to the foods, and (2) microbiological conversion of nitrogenous components of foods, particularly nitrates, to nitrites. Food preservation techniques dependent on formation of nitrites have evolved in many cultures throughout the world over millenia. The carcinogenic risks engendered have only recently come into focus, as have potential tools for reducing these risks.

1. Fish

Marquardt et al. (1977) have shown that nitroso compounds produced by smoking fish or treating it with nitrite are mutagenic and have suggested that this may be related to the higher incidence of gastric cancer in Japan. The fish lipids, usually highly unsaturated, contain variable amounts of tocopherol, depending on the dietary intake of the fish and decreasing variably with the storage and processing technologies applied after the fish is caught. The ascorbic acid content of fish is very low. Therefore, we suggest that the variable production of N-nitroso compounds produced on smoking or nitrite treatment of fish may be inversely related to the residual tocopherol levels in the fish lipids. Treatment of fish with added tocopherol prior to smoking or nitrite treatment, may be an effective way to add to the natural levels of nitrosamine-blocking agents in the fish tissues.

2. Fermented Foods

In any food product where the processing includes a microbiological fermentation, there is a good likelihood that nitrite will be produced from a nitrogenous component. Thus, variable but low levels of nitrosamines have been found in some cheese products (Sen *et al.*, 1978). Quite possibly, the variability of the nitrosamines found is inversely related to the tocopherol level in the milk used to make the cheese, since no appreciable ascorbic acid or other blocking agents are present in milk. Beer, both in the United States and West Germany, was found (Fazio *et al.*, 1980; Spiegelhalder *et al.*, 1980) to have appreciable levels of nitrosamines, but this can be corrected, apparently, by changes in technology to reduce the nitrogen oxides of direct flame malt drying from producing nitrosamines in the malt. In China, "pickling" of vegetables for storage may be associated with esophageal and nasopharyngeal cancer in humans and farm animals (Kaplan and Tsuchitani, 1978; Newmark and Mergens, 1981). It has been suggested that the application of α-tocopherol itself, or mixing the vegetables in the pickling process with high-tocopherol-containing cereal foods such as wheat germ may prevent formation of carcinogenic N-nitroso compounds.

C. Rectal and Colonic Carcinogenesis

The growth of microorganisms is frequently associated with production of nitrite. Substrates can include a wide variety of physiologically available nitrogen sources, including ammonia, urea, nitrate, etc. Thus, the microbiological growth in the small and large intestine appears to be a major source of nitrite availability in man (S. Tannenbaum *et al.*, 1978). This production of nitrosating agent capacity is assumed to be the source of fecal mutagens found in at least some individuals (Varghese *et al.*, 1978). These fecal mutagens have been reduced by the use of ascorbic acid and α-tocopherol in a few carefully controlled humans as follows (W. R. Bruce, personal communication 1978):

Ascorbic acid	4 g/day	50% reduction
dl-α-Tocopherol	400 mg/day	60–70% reduction
dl-α-Tocopherol plus ascorbic acid	400 mg/day 400 mg/day	75–90% reduction

De Cosse et al. (1975), in a pilot study, have indicated a reduction of rectal polyps in a few familial polyposis patients on an intake of 3 g/day of ascorbic acid, using a slow-release form aimed at releasing at least some of the blocking agent in the lower portions of the intestinal tract.

D. Lung Cancer

Nitrogen oxides in the atmosphere are a regular feature of urban life. Levels of 1 ppm are common in cities, and some, like Los Angeles, occasionally reach 2.5 ppm (Wayne, 1962). Cigarette smoke, while varying with the type of tobacco, manufacturer, filter, etc., delivers 2–3 mg of nitrogen oxides per day to a pack-a-day smoker in the main-stream smoke (Bokhoven and Niessen, 1961; W. J. Mergens and H. L. Newmark, unpublished data, 1974). Side-stream smoke may contain ten times as much (Brunnemann and Hoffmann, 1978). Nitrogen oxides, usually a mixture of several but predominantly NO and NO_2 in this mixture, can act as powerful nitrosating agents by the following equilibration:

$$NO + NO_2 \rightleftharpoons N_2O_3$$

Inhalation tests have demonstrated that inhaled NO_2 is largely absent in expired air, suggesting that it is rapidly absorbed or consumed in reactions in the lung (Bokhoven and Niessen, 1961). If an individual breathes 1.5 liters per breath, 12 breaths per minute (normal resting breathing for an adult), in an atmosphere of 1 ppm of NO_2, over 1 mmol is absorbed per day. Depending on the amount of NO absorbed simultaneously, a nitrosation capacity equivalent to 70–140 mg of sodium nitrite can be taken directly into the lungs each day.

This quantity of nitrogen oxides impinging on the lung tissue would be expected to be highly reactive. It is no surprise that several reports have appeared indicating that cigarette smokers have a significantly lower ascorbic acid serum level than do nonsmokers (Pelletier, 1968). This could result from the reaction of ascorbic acid with nitrogen oxides of the cigarette smoke coming into the mouth and lung.

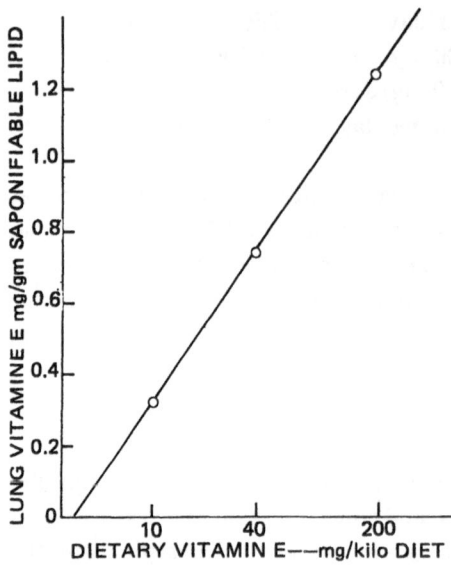

FIGURE 6. Relationship of dietary tocopherol to tocopherol levels in lung lipid. Male Sprague-Dawley rats were fed an E-low purified diet containing 8% "stripped" safflower oil from weaning to 15 weeks of age. The above groups were fed the same diet with varying levels of dl-α-tocopheryl acetate.

The ascorbic levels in lung tissue can be altered by high daily intakes, but only by a comparatively small factor. However, in a rat study, the tocopherol level (mg tocopherol/g lipid) in lung tissue increased directly as the logarithm of the daily intake (L. Machlin, unpublished data, 1974) (see Fig. 6). This is in agreement with the elevation of tocopherol in other tissues as a function of daily intake previously reported (Yang and Desai, 1977). It thus appears possible to build up lung tissue resistance to nitrosation attack from inhalation of nitrogen oxides. Studies in rats have demonstrated the beneficial effect of dietary vitamin E supplementation in protecting lung tissue damage from short exposure to controlled atmospheres containing low levels of NO_2 (Thomas et al., 1967; Dowell et al., 1971; Menzel, 1979; Menzel et al., 1972; Ramirez and Dowell, 1971).

E. Bladder Cancer

Infections in the bladder have been associated with the detection of N-nitroso compounds in the urine (Hicks et al., 1978; Radmonski et al., 1977). The microorganisms are believed to be the source of the nitrite or other nitrosating agent, synthesizing it from urea or other nitrogenous compounds in normal urine held in the bladder. For these nitrosamines formed *in situ*, high oral intakes of ascorbic acid could be very useful. The ascorbic acid would have the double effect of blocking nitrosation reactions and lowering the pH of the urine to aid in clearing the infection. Tocopherol does not normally appear in urine.

Nitrosamines have been reported in the urine of normal men and women without bladder infections (Kakizoe et al., 1979). It is believed that these N-nitroso compounds may originate in the lower GI tract. If this is so, then the combined use of ascorbic acid and free tocopherol would be the most useful combination agent to suppress urinary N-nitroso compounds, since Bruce (1979) has demonstrated this combination to be the most effective in reducing fecal mutagens from the same source.

F. N-Nitroso Compounds in Blood

Dimethylnitrosamine has been measured in blood and seems to range from 0.1 to 1.5 ppb in normal men and women (Lakritz et al., 1980; Fine et al., 1977). This compound probably originates in the lower GI tract and may be representative of other N-nitroso compounds originating there but inducing tumors elsewhere because of their organ specificity. If so, then a significant reduction of nitrosation in the GI tract would be desirable by daily intake of ascorbic acid and free α-tocopherol in the dose range shown by Dion et al. (1980) to produce major suppression of fecal mutagens.

In a single unconfirmed human observation, it was reported that a high intake of ascorbic acid did indeed lower the blood level of dimethylnitrosamine (D. H. Fine, personal communication, 1978).

G. Gastric Cancer

Although the incidence of gastric cancer has declined markedly during the past 20 years in the United States, it remains very common in countries such as Japan, Iceland, Chile, and Colombia (Weisburger et al., 1977). The incidence is particularly high in certain specific areas of Colombia (Cuello et al., 1976) and in the town of Worksop in England (Hill et al., 1973), both apparently related to a very high level of nitrates in the drinking water and local soils. The relative lack of refrigeration for food storage in these areas permits microbiological production of nitrite from the high nitrogenous content of locally grown crops. This intake of nitrite has been suggested by Correa et al. (1975) to be a cause of cellular damage to the gastric lining, leading to a hypertrophic gastritis associated with decreased acid production. This achlorhydria permits microbiological fermentation to occur in the stomach itself. The high dietary nitrate intake, coupled with microbiological conversion of nitrate to nitrite, probably leads to significant formation of N-nitroso compounds. Prolongation of this set of conditions has been suggested as the mechanism of gastric carcinogenesis in these areas.

In limited studies of patients with chronic gastric achlorhydria from other disease states such as pernicious anemia and chronic atrophic gastritis, increase of gastric pH, particularly above pH 5, has been associated with: (1) very large increase in microbiological growth; (2) qualitative resemblance of gastric flora to microorganisms of the lower GI tract; (3) increase in nitrite content; and (4) increase of mutagenic activity, all in samples of gastric contents (Bartholemew et al., 1980; Walker et al., 1980).

An analogous condition could also occur on long-term administration of drugs (e.g., cimetidine) that inhibit secretion of gastric acid, allowing microbiological fermentation conditions to be produced in the stomach (Bartholemew et al., 1980).

In both conditions described above, the formation of carcinogenic N-nitroso compounds could be prevented by the administration of blocking agents in or with the food at each meal. For this purpose, the combination of ascorbic acid with α-tocopherol would appear to be a safe complimentary pair of agents to function simultaneously in both aqueous and lipid phases of the food. Although many fresh foods contain appreciable amounts of these substances, it would appear to be prudent to use the mixture or combination routinely as supplementation for the purpose of blocking N-nitroso formation. This could be applied to populations living in high-risk areas such as those with high nitrates in soil and water, and also to patients on a regimen of drugs that suppress gastric secretion.

VII. Ascorbic Acid and Tocopherol Effect on Preformed Nitrosamines

There are only a few documented suggestions, and even less data, that administration of ascorbic acid or α-tocopherol could alter the toxicity or carcinogenicity of N-nitroso compounds once present in tissues. Kamm et al. (1974) found that the administration of sodium ascorbate had no consistent effect on hepatotoxicity induced by the administration of nitrosodimethylamine to rats. However, Dashman and Kamm (1979) reported that the administration of high doses of α-tocopherol (55 mg/kg per day) parenterally to rats resulted in a significant decrease in acute hepatotoxicity of dimethylnitrosamine. These authors showed that these high doses of α-tocopherol inhibited microsomal mixed-function oxidase enzymes, thus decreasing the hepatotoxicity of the nitrosamine by inhibiting its rate of metabolism to the proximal toxic agent. A similar report from Skaare and Nafstad (1978) reported that α-tocopheryl acetate administered either orally (0.02% of diet) or parenterally (200 mg/kg) reduced hepatotoxicity induced by dimethylnitrosamine in rats. Selenium, which is biochemically related to some of the functions of α-tocopherol *in vivo*, had no protective action. The lipid antioxidant ethoxyquin (EMQ), which has vitamin E-like activity in some biological systems, also failed to protect rats against dimethylnitrosamine hepatotoxicity. On the contrary, EMQ increased the severity of acute hepatic necrosis induced by dimethylnitrosamine (Skaare *et al.*, 1977). More work is needed to determine if α-tocopherol administration can prevent toxicity or carcinogenicity from exposure to preformed *N*-nitroso compounds. Presumably, high doses will be needed to retard metabolic activation by oxidative enzymes. To be effective, these high doses should be administered in a form with high biological availability, such as the aqueous injectable form used by Dashman and Kamm (1979).

VIII. Summary

The *N*-nitroso compounds are a potential source of carcinogenesis in humans.

Although *N*-nitroso compounds appear to be ubiquitous in our environment, being present in low levels in foods, cosmetics, drugs, atmosphere, etc., a far larger source seems to be endogenous formation *in vivo*.

N-Nitroso compounds, once formed, are converted *in vivo* to reactive electrophilic ultimate carcinogens. Therefore, the most practical method of eliminating carcinogenesis by nitrosamines is to prevent their formation by diverting potential nitrosating agents to nonnitrosating substances (e.g., nitric oxide) by the use of appropriate blocking agents.

α-Tocopherol is an effective blocking agent against *N*-nitroso compound formation, particularly in the lipid phase. Its activity as a blocking agent against nitrosamine formation does not directly relate to its antioxidant activity. It should probably be used in conjunction with ascorbic acid because of the mutually complementary actions of the two vitamins in blocking nitrosamine formation in both aqueous and lipid media. As safe nutrient ingredients in many food systems as well as being available from commercial synthesis, the combination of vitamins C and E, properly formulated for optimum biological effect, represent very useful compounds for the nutritional inhibition of formation of tumorigenic *N*-nitroso compounds.

ACKNOWLEDGMENTS. The authors are deeply appreciative to Dr. Alan Conney for his aid and encouragement in the preparation of this chapter.

References

American Pharmaceutical Association, 1975, Vitamin E, in: The National Formulary XIV, pp. 758–768, American Pharmaceutical Association, Washington.

Archer, M. C., Tannenbaum, S. R., Fan, T.-Y., and Weisman, M., 1975, Reaction of nitrite with ascorbate and its relation to nitrosamine formation, *J. Natl. Cancer Inst.* 54(5):1203.

Arfellini, G., Grilli, S., and Prodi, G., 1978, In vivo DNA repair after N-methyl-N-nitrosourea administration to rats of different ages, *Z. Krebsforsch. Klin. Onkol.* 91:157.

Arrhenius, E., and Hultin, T., 1961, The effect of 2-aminofluorene and related aromatic amines on the protein and ribonucleic acid metabolism of liver slices, *Exp. Cell Res.* 22:476.

Astill, B. D., and Mulligan, L. T., 1977, Phenolic antioxidants and the inhibition of hepatotoxicity from N-dimethylnitrosamine formed *in situ* in the rat stomach, *Food Cosmet. Toxicol.* 15:167.

Bartholomew, B. A., Hill, M. J., Hudson, M. J., Ruddell, W. S. J., and Walters, C. L., 1980, Gastric bacteria, nitrate, nitrite and nitrosamines in patients with pernicious anemia and in patients treated with cimetidine, in: *N-Nitroso Compounds: Analysis, Formation and Occurrence* (E. A. Walker, M. Griciute, M. Castegnaro, and M. Borzsonyi, eds.), pp. 595–606, International Agency for Research on Cancer, Lyon.

Bauernfeind, J. C., 1977, The tocopherol content of food and influencing factors, *CRC Crit. Rev. Food Sci. Nutr.* 8(4):337.

Belman, S., and Troll, W., 1972, The inhibition of croton oil-promoted mouse skin tumorigenesis by steroid hormones, *Cancer Res.* 32:450.

Berenblum, I., 1929, The modifying influence of dichloro-ethyl sulphide on the induction of tumors in mice by tar, *J. Pathol. Bacteriol.* 32:425.

Black, H. S., and Chan, J. T., 1975, Suppression of ultraviolet light-induced tumor formation by dietary antioxidants, *J. Invest. Dermatol.* 65:412.

Bokhoven, C., and Niessen, H. J., 1961, Amounts of oxides of nitrogen and carbon monoxide in cigarette smoke, with and without inhalation, *Nature* 192:458.

Bonmassar, E., Dallavalle, R., and Giuliani, G., 1968, Influsso della vitimina E e del gallato di propile sulla cancerogenesi da benzopirene nel topo, *Arch. Ital. Patol. Clin. Tumori* 11:245.

Boyland, E., and Walker, S. A., 1974, Thiocyanate catalysis of nitrosamine formation and some dietary implications, in: *N-Nitroso Compounds in the Environment* (P. Bogovski and E. A. Walker, eds.), pp. 132–136, International Agency for Research on Cancer, Lyon.

Boyland, E., Nice, E., and Williams, K., 1971, The catalysis of nitrosation by thiocyanate from saliva, *Food Cosmet. Toxicol.* 9:639.

Bruce, W. R., Varghese, A. J., Wang, S., and Dion, P., 1979, The endogenous production of nitroso compounds in the colon and cancer at that site, in *Naturally Occurring Carcinogens—Mutagens and Modulators of Carcinogenesis, Proceedings of the 9th International Symposium of The Princess Takamatsu Cancer Research Fund, Tokyo, 1979* (E. C. Miller, J. A. Miller, I. Hirono, T. Sugimura, and S. Takayama, eds.), pp. 221–228, University Park Press, Baltimore.

Brunnemann, K. D., and Hoffman, D., 1978, Chemical studies on tobacco smoke. LIX. Analysis of volatile nitrosamines in tobacco smoke and polluted indoor environments, in: *Environmental Aspects of N-Nitroso Compounds* (E. A. Walker, M. Castegnaro, L. Griciute, and R. E. Lyle, eds.), pp. 343–356, International Agency for Research on Cancer, Lyon.

Cameron, A. T., and Meltzer, S., 1937, The effects of certain diets on the production of tar carcinoma in mice, *Am. J. Cancer* 30:56.

Cardesa, A., Mirvish, S. S., Haven, G. T., and Shubik, P., 1974, Inhibitory effect of ascorbic acid on the acute toxicity of dimethylamine plus nitrite in the rate, *Proc. Soc. Exp. Biol. Med.* **145**:124.

Carruthers, C., 1939, Vitamin E and experimental tumors, *Am. J. Cancer* **35**:546.

Challis, B. C., Edwards, A., Hunma, R. R., Kryptopolous, S. A., and Outram, J. R., 1978, Rapid formation of N-nitrosamines from nitrogen oxides under neutral and alkaline conditions, in: *Environmental Aspects of N-Nitroso Compounds* (E. A. Walker, M. Castegnaro, L. Griciute, and R. E. Lyle, eds.), pp. 127–142, International Agency for Research on Cancer, Lyon.

Chan, J. T., and Black, H. S., 1977, The mitigating effect of dietary antioxidants on chemically induced carcinogenesis, *Experientia* **34**:110.

Clemmesen, J., 1965, *Statistical Studies in the Aetiology of Malignant Neoplasams I. Review and Results*, Munksgaard, Copenhagen.

Cohen, J. B., and Bachman, J. D., 1978, Measurement of environmental nitrosamines, in: *Environmental Aspects of N-Nitroso Compounds* (E. A. Walker, M. Castegnaro, L. Griciute, and R. E. Lyle, eds.), pp. 357–372, International Agency for Research on Cancer, Lyon.

Correa, P., Haenszel, W., Cuello, C., Tannenbaum, S. R., and Archer, M., 1975, A model for gastric cancer epidemiology, *Lancet* **2**:58.

Cort, W. M., 1974, Antioxidant activity of tocopherols, ascorbyl palmitate, and ascorbic acid and their mode of action, *J. Am. Oil Chem. Soc.* **51**(7):321.

Crabtree, H. G., 1941, Retardation of the rate of tumor induction by hydrolyzing chlor compounds, *Cancer Res.* **1**:39.

Craddock, U. M., and Henderson, A. R., 1977, De novo replication and repair replication of DNA during diethylnitrosamine-induced carcinogenesis, *Cancer Lett.* **3**:277.

Csallany, A. S., Draper, H. H., and Shah, S. N., 1962, Conversion of d-α-tocopherol-C^{14} to tocopheryl-p-quinone in vivo, *Arch. Biochem. Biophys.* **98**:142.

Cuello, C. Correa, P., Haenszel, W., Gordillo, G., Brown, C., Archer, M. C., and Tannenbaum, S. R., 1976, Gastric cancer in Colombia I. Cancer risk and suspect agents, *J. Natl. Cancer Inst.* **57**:1015.

Dahn, H., Loewe, L., and Buntor, C. A., 1960, Uber die Oxydation von Ascorbinsauer durch salpetrige Saure, Tiel VI: Ubersicht und Diskussion der Ergebnisse, *Helv. Chim. Acta.* **43**:320.

Dashman, T., and Kamm, J. J., 1979, Effects of high doses of vitamin E on dimethylnitrosamine hepatotoxicity and drug metabolism in the rat, *Biochem. Pharmacol.* **28**:1485.

De Cosse, J. J., Adams, M. B., Kuzma, J. F., LoGerfo, P., and Condon, R. E., 1975, Effect of ascorbic acid on rectal polyps of patients with familial polyposis, *Surgery* **78**:608.

Dion, P. W., Bright-See, E. B., Furrer, R., Eng, V. W. S., and Bruce, W. R., 1980, The effects of dietary fat, ascorbic acid and alpha-tocopherol on fecal mutagens, in: *Proceedings of AACR*, in press.

Doll, R., Muir, C., and Waterhouse, J. A. H., eds., 1970, *Cancer Incidence in five Continents. A Technical Report*, Vol. II, Springer-Verlag, Berlin, Heidelberg, New York.

Douglass, M. L., Kabacoff, B. L., Anderson, G. A., and Cheng, M. C., 1978, The chemistry of nitrosamine formation, inhibition and destruction, *J. Soc. Cosmet. Chem.* **29**:581.

Dowell, A. R., Kilburn, K. H., and Pratt, P. C., 1971, Short-term exposure to nitrogen dioxide, *Arch. Intern. Med.* **128**:74.

Draper, H. H., 1970, The tocopherols, in: *International Encyclopedia of Food and Nutrition*, Vol. 9, Fat-Soluble Vitamins (R. A. Morton, ed.), pp. 333–393, Pergamon Press, Elmsford, N. Y.

Druckrey, H., Preussman, R., and Ivankovic, S., 1969, N-Nitroso compounds in organotropic and transplacental carcinogenesis, *Ann. N. Y. Acad. Sci.* **163**:676.

Dutton, A. H., and Heath, D. F., 1956, Demethylation of dimethylnitrosamine in rats and mice, *Nature* **178**:644.

Edgar, J. A., 1974, Ascorbic acid and biological alkylating agents, *Nature* **248**:136.

Eisenbrand, G., Spiegelhalder, B., Janzowski, C., Kann, J., and Preussmann, R., 1978, Volatile and non-volatile *N*-nitroso compounds in foods and other environmental media, in: *Environmental Aspects of N-Nitroso Compounds* (E. A. Walker, M. Castegnaro, L. Griciute, and R. E. Lyle, eds.), pp. 311–324, International Agency for Research on Cancer, Lyon.

Falk, H. L., 1971, Anticarcinogenesis—an alternative, *Prog. Exp. Tumor Res.* **14**:105.

Fan, S. T., Krull, I. S., Ross, R. D., Wolff, M. H., and Fine, D. H., 1978, Comprehensive analytical procedures for the determination of volatile and non-volatile, polar and non-polar *N*-nitroso compounds, in: *Environmental Aspects of N-Nitroso Compounds* (E. A. Walker, M. Castegnaro, L. Griciute, and R. E. Lyle, eds.), pp. 3–17, International Agency for Research on Cancer, Lyon.

Fan, T. Y., and Tannenbaum, S. R., 1973, Factors influencing the rate of formation of nitrosomorpholine from morpholine and nitrite: Acceleration by thiocyanate and other anions, *J. Agric. Food Chem.* **21**:237.

Fan, T. Y., and Tannenbaum, S. R., 1974, Natural inhibitors of nitrosation reactions, concept of available nitrite, *J. Food Sci.* **38**:1067.

Fazio, T., Havery, D. C., and Howard, J. W., 1980, Determination of volatile *N*-nitrosamines in foodstuffs. I. A new clean-up technique for confirmation by GLC-MS. II. A continued survey of foods and beverages, in: *N-Nitroso Compounds: Analysis, Formation and Occurrence* (E. A. Walker, M. Griciute, M. Castegnaro, and M. Borzsonyi, eds.), pp. 419–431, International Agency for Research on Cancer, Lyon.

Fiddler, W., Pensabene, J. W., and Wasserman, A. E., 1974, The role of lean and adipose tissue on the formation of nitrosopyrrolidine in fried bacon, *J. Food Sci.* **39**:1070.

Fiddler, W., Pensabene, J. A., Piotrowski, E. G., Phillips, J. G., Keating, J., Mergens, W. J., and Newmark, H. L., 1978, Inhibition of formation of volatile nitrosamines in fried bacon by the use of cure-solubilized alpha-tocopherol, *J. Agr. Food Chem.* **26**:653.

Fine, D. H., Rounbehler, D. P., Belcher, N. M., and Epstein, S. S., 1976, *N*-Nitroso compounds: Detection in ambient air, *Science* **192**:1328.

Fine, D. H., Ross, D., Rounbehler, D., Silvergleid, A., and Song, L., 1977, Formation *in vivo* of volatile *N*-nitrosamines in man after ingestion of cooked bacon and spinach, *Nature* **263**:753.

Fong, Y. Y., and Chan, W. C., 1976, Effect of ascorbate on amine–nitrite carcinogenicity, in: *Environmental N-Nitroso Compounds: Analysis and Formation* (E. A. Walker, P. Bogovski, and L. Griciute, eds.), pp. 461–464, International Agency for Research on Cancer, Lyon.

Gough, T. A., Webb, K. S., and Eaton, R. F., 1977, Simple chemiluminescent detector for the screening of foodstuffs for the presence of volatile nitrosamines, *J. Chromatogr.* **137**:293.

Gough, T. A., Webb, K. S., and Coleman, R. F., 1978a, Estimate of the volatile nitrosamine content of UK food, *Nature* **272**:161.

Gough, T. A., Webb, K. S., and McPhail, M. F., 1978b, Diffusion of nitrosamines through gloves, in: *Environmental Aspects of N-Nitroso Compounds* (E. A. Walker, M. Castegnaro, L. Griciute, and R. E. Lyle, eds.), pp. 531–534, International Agency for Research on Cancer, Lyon.

Gray, J. I., and Dugan, L. R., Jr., 1975, Inhibition of *N*-nitrosamine formation in model food systems, *J. Food Sci.* **40**:981.

Greenblatt, M., 1973, Ascorbic acid blocking of aminopyrine nitrosation in MZO/Bl mice, *J. Natl. Cancer Inst.* **50**:1055.

Guttenplan, J. B., 1977, Inhibition by L-ascorbate of bacterial mutagenesis induced by two *N*-nitroso compounds, *Nature* **268**:368.

Haber, S., and Wissler, R., 1962, Effect of vitamin E on carcinogenicity of methylcholanthrene, *Proc. Soc. Exp. Biol. Med.* **111**:774.

Haddow, A., 1937, The influence of wheat germ oil in the diet on the induction of tumors in mice, *Am. J. Cancer* **29**:363.

Hamilton, J. M., Flaks, A., Saluja, P. G., and Maguire, S., 1975, Hormonally induced renal neoplasia in the male syrian hamster and the inhibitory effect of 2-bromo-α-ergocryptine methanesulfonate, *J. Natl. Cancer Inst.* **54**:1385.

Harr, J. R., Exon, J. H., Whanger, P. D., and Weswig, P. H., 1972, Effects of dietary selenium on N-2-fluorenyl-acetamide (FAA)-induced cancer in vitamin E supplemented, selenium depleted rats, *Clin. Toxicol.* **5**(2):187.

Hicks, R. M., Gough, T. A., and Walters, C. L., 1978, Demonstration of the presence of nitrosamines in human urine: Preliminary observations on a possible etiology for bladder cancer in association with chronic urinary tract infection, in: *Environmental Aspects of N-nitroso Compounds* (E. A. Walker, M. Castegnaro, L., Griciute, and R. E. Lyle, eds.), pp. 465–475, International Agency for Research on Cancer, Lyon.

Higginson, J., 1976, A hazardous society? Individual versus community responsibility in cancer prevention, *Am. J. Public Health* **66**:359.

Hill, M. J., Hawksworth, G. M., and Tattersall, G., 1973, Bacteria, nitrosamines and stomach cancer, *Br. J. Cancer* **28**:572.

Hisatune, I. C., 1961, Thermodynamic properties of some oxides of nitrogen, *J. Phys. Chem.* **65**:2249.

Houssay, A., Higgins, G. M., and Bennett, W. A., 1951, The influence exerted by desoxycorticosterone acetate upon the production of adrenal tumors in gonadectomized mice, *Cancer Res.* **11**:297.

Hultin, T., and Arrhenius, E., 1964, Effects of carcinogenic amines on amino acid incorporation by liver systems. III. Inhibition by aminofluorene treatment and its dependence on vitamin E, *Cancer Res.* **25**:124.

Hultin, T., Arrhenius, E., Lon, H., and Magee, P. N., 1960, Toxic liver injury. Inhibition by dimethylnitrosamine of incorporation of labeled amino acids into proteins of rat liver preparations *in vitro*, *Biochem. J.* **76**:109.

Ivankovic, S., Preussmann, R., Schmahl, D., and Zeller, J. W., 1974, Prevention by ascorbic acid of *in vivo* formation of N-nitroso compounds, in: *N-Nitroso Compounds in the Environment* (P. Bogovski and E. A. Walker, eds.), pp. 101–102, International Agency for Research on Cancer, Lyon.

Jaffe, N., 1946, The influence of wheat germ oil on the production of tumors in rats by methylcholanthrene, *Exp. Med. Surg.* **4**:278.

Jones, K., 1973, The chemistry of nitrogen, in: *Comprehensive Inorganic Chemistry*, Vol. 2 (J. C. Bailar, Jr., H. J. Emeleus, R. Nyholm, and R. F. Trotman-Dickenson, eds.), pp. 372–374, Pergamon Press, New York.

Kagerud, A., Holm, G., Larsson, H., and Peterson, H. I., 1978a, Tocopherol and local X-ray irradiation of two transplantable rat tumors, *Cancer Lett.* **5**:123.

Kagerud, A., Klintenberg, C., Lund, N., and Peterson, H. I., 1978b, Influence of tocopherol on tumor cell oxygenation, *Cancer Lett.* **5**:185.

Kakizoe, T., Wang, T. T., Eng, V. W. S., Furrer, R., Dion, P., and Bruce, W. R., 1979, Volatile N-nitrosamines in the urine of normal donors and of bladder cancer patients, *Cancer Res.* **39**:829.

Kamm, J. J., Dashman, T., Conney, A. H., and Burns, J. J., 1973, Protective effect of ascorbic acid on hepatotoxicity caused by nitrite plus aminopyrine, *Proc. Natl. Acad. Sci. USA* **70**:747.

Kamm, J. J., Dashman, T., Conney, A. H., and Burns, J. J., 1974, The effect of ascorbate on amine-nitrite hepatotoxicity, in: *N-Nitroso Compounds in the Environment* (P. Bogovski and E. A. Walker, eds.), pp. 200–204, International Agency for Research on Cancer, Lyon.

Kamm, J. J., Dashman, T., Newmark, H. L., and Mergens, W. J., 1977, Inhibition of amine-nitrite hepatotoxicity by α-tocopherol, *Toxicol. Appl. Pharmacol.* **41**(3):575.

Kaplan, H. S., and Tsuchitani, P. J., eds., 1978, *Cancer In China*, Alan R. Liss, Inc., New York.

Karrer, P., and Demole, V., 1938, Synthesis and biological titration of vitamin E, *Schweiz. Med. Wochenschr.* **33**:954.

Kawabata, T., Shazuki, H., and Ishibashi, T., 1974, N-Nitroso compounds in food. VIII. Effect of ascorbic acid on the formation of N-nitrosodimethylamine *in vitro*, *Nippon Suisan Gakkaishi* **40**:1251.

Kim, Y. -K., Tannenbaum, S. R., and Wishnok, J. S., 1980, Nitrosation of dialkylamines in the presence of bile acid conjugates, in: *N-Nitroso Compounds: Analysis, Formation and Occurrence* (E. A. Walker, M. Griciute, M. Castegnaro, and M. Borzsonyi, eds.), pp. 207–214, International Agency for Research on Cancer, Lyon.

Kinawi, V. A., Doring, D., and Witte, I., 1977, Reaktionkinetische Untersuchungen zur Entstehung von 7-Chlor-2-N-nitrosomethylamino-3-phenyl-^{3}H-1,4-benzodiazepin-4-oxid, *Arzneim. Forsch.* **27**:747.

Kledzik, G. S., Brandley, C. J., and Meites, J., 1974, Reduction of carcinogen-induced mammary cancer incidence in rats by early treatment with hormones or drugs, *Cancer Res.* **17**:317.

Lakritz, L., Simenhoff, M. L., Dunn, S. R., and Fiddler, W., 1980, N-Nitrosodimethylamine in human blood, *Food Cosmet. Toxicol.* **18**:77.

Lee, C., and Chen, C., 1979, Enhancement of mammary tumorigenesis in rats by vitamin E deficiency, *Proc. AACR ASCO* **20**:132.

Lijinsky, W., and Taylor, H. W., 1978, Relative carcinogenic effectiveness of derivatives of nitrosodiethylamine in rats, *Cancer Res.* **28**:2391.

Lovejoy, D. L., and Vosper, A. J., 1968, Dinitrogen trioxide VI. Reactions of dinitrogen trioxide with primary and secondary amines, *J. Chem. Soc.* [*A*] **10**:2325.

Magee, P. N., 1956, Toxic liver injury; the metabolism of dimethylnitrosamine, *Biochem. J.* **64**:676.

Magee, P. N., and Barnes, J. M., 1956, The production of malignant primary hepatic tumors in the rat by feeding dimethylnitrosamine, *Br. J. Cancer* **10**:114.

Marquardt, H., Rufino, F., and Weisburger, J. H., 1977, Mutagenic activity of nitrite treated foods: Human stomach cancer may be related to dietary factors, *Science* **196**:1000.

Meisels, A., 1966, Effect of sex hormones on the carcinogenic action of dimethyl-benzanthracene on the uterus of intact and castrated mice, *Cancer Res.* **26**:757.

Menzel, D. B., 1979, Nutritional needs in environmental intoxication: Vitamin E and air pollution, an example, *Environ. Health Perspect.* **29**:105.

Menzel, D. B., Roehm, J. N., and Lee, S. D., 1972, Vitamin E: The biological and environmental antioxidant, *J. Agric. Food Chem.* **20**(3):481.

Mergens, W. J., Kamm, J. J., Newmark, H. L., Fiddler, W., and Pensabene, J., 1978, Alpha-tocopherol: Uses in preventing nitrosamine formation, in: *Environmental Aspects of N-Nitroso Compounds* (E. A. Walker, M. Castegnaro, L. Griciute, and R. E. Lyle, eds.), pp. 199–212, International Agency for Research on Cancer, Lyon.

Mergens, W. J., Chau, J., and Newmark, H. L., 1980, The influence of ascorbic acid and *dl*-alpha-tocopherol on the formation of nitrosamines in an *in vitro* gastrointestinal model system, in: *N-Nitroso Compounds: Analysis, Formation and Occurrence* (E. A. Walker, M. Griciute, M. Castegnaro, and M. Borzsonyi, eds.), pp. 259–267, International Agency for Research on Cancer, Lyon.

Miller, E. C., and Miller, J. A., 1971, The mutagenicity of chemical carcinogens: Correlations, problems, and interpretations, in: *Chemical Mutagens—Principles and Methods for Their Detection*, Vol. 1 (A. Hollaender, ed.), pp. 83–119, Plenum Press, New York.

Miller, E. C., and Miller, J. A., 1972, Environment and cancer, in: *24th Annual Symposium on Fundamental Cancer Research*, p. 5, Williams & Wilkins, Baltimore.

Miller, J. A., 1970, Carcinogenesis by chemicals: An overview, G.H.A. Clowes Memorial Lecture, *Cancer Res.* **30**:559.

Miller, J. A., 1979, Concluding remarks on chemicals and chemical carcinogenesis, in: *Carcinogens: Identification and Mechanisms of Action* (A. C. Griffin and C. R. Shaw, eds.), pp. 455–469, Raven Press, New York.

Miller, J. A., and Miller, E. C., 1969, Physicochemical mechanisms of carcinogenesis, in: *The Jerusalem Symposia on Quantum Chemistry and Biochemistry*, Vol. I (E. D. Bergman and B. Pullman, eds.), p. 237, The Israel Academy of Sciences and Humanities, Jerusalem.

Mirvish, S. S., 1975a, Blocking the formation of N-nitroso compounds with ascorbic acid *in vitro* and *in vivo*, *Ann. N.Y. Acad. Sci.* **258**:175.

Mirvish, S. S., 1975b, Formation of N-nitroso compounds: Chemistry kinetics and *in vivo* occurrence, *Toxicol. Appl. Pharmacol.* **31**:325.

Mirvish, S. S., Wallcave, L., Eagen, M., and Shubik, P., 1972, Ascorbate–nitrite reaction: Possible means of blocking the formation of carcinogenic N-nitroso compounds, *Science* **177**:65.

Mirvish, S. S., Cardesa, A., Wallcave, L., and Shubik, P., 1975, Induction of mouse lung adenomas by amines or ureas plus nitrite and by N-nitroso compounds: Effect of ascorbate, gallic acid, thiocyanate and caffeine, *J. Natl. Cancer Inst.* **55**:633.

Mirvish, S. S., Pelfrene, A. F., Garcia, H., and Shubik, P., 1976, Effect of sodium ascorbate on tumor induction in rats treated with morpholine and sodium nitrite, and with nitrosomorpholine, *Cancer Lett.* **2**:101.

Mirvish, S. S., Karlowski, K., Sams, J. P., and Arnold, S. D., 1978, Studies related to nitrosamide formation: Nitrosation in solvent: water and solvent systems, nitrosomethylurea formation in the rat stomach and analysis of a fish product for ureas, in: *Environmental Aspects of N-Nitroso Compounds* (E. A. Walker, M. Castegnaro, L. Griciute, and R. E. Lyle, eds.), pp. 161–174, International Agency for Research on Cancer, Lyon.

Newmark, H. L., and Mergens, W. J., 1981, Applications of ascorbic acid and tocopherol as inhibitors of nitrosamine formation and oxidation in foods, in: *Criteria of Food Acceptance* (J. Solms and R. L. Hall, eds.), pp. 379–390, Forster Verlag AG/Forster Publishing Ltd., Zurich.

Newmark, H. L., Pool, W., Bauernfeind, J. C., and DeRitter, E., 1975, Biopharmaceutic factors in parenteral administration of vitamin E, *J. Pharm. Sci.* **64**(4):655.

Okun, J. D., and Archer, M. C., 1977, Kinetics of nitrosamine formation in the presence of micelle-forming surfactants, *J. Natl. Cancer Inst.* **58**(2):409.

Pegg, A., and Hui, G., 1978, Removal of methylated purines from rat liver DNA after administration of dimethylnitrosamine, *Cancer Res.* **38**:2011.

Pelletier, O., 1968, Smoking and vitamin C levels in humans, *Am. J. Chem. Nutr.* **21**:1259.

Pensabene, J. W., Fiddler, W., Mergens, W. J., and Wasserman, A. E., 1978, Effect of alpha-tocopherol formulations on the inhibition of nitrosopyrrolidine formation in model food systems, *J. Food Sci.* **43**:801.

Preda, N., Popa, L., Galea, V., and Simo, G., 1976, N-Nitroso compound formation by chlordiazepoxide and nitrite interaction *in vitro* and *in vivo*: Protective action of ascorbic acid, in: *Environmental N-Nitroso Compounds: Analysis and Formation* (E. A. Walker, P. Bogovski, and L. Griciute, eds.), pp. 301–304, International Agency for Research on Cancer, Lyon.

Quaife, M. L., 1948, Nitrosotocopherols, their use in the chemical assay of the individual tocopherols in a mixture of the α, β, γ and δ forms, *J. Biol. Chem.* **175**:605.

Radmonski, J. L., Greenwald, P., Hearn, W. L., Block, N., and Woods, F. M. 1977, Nitrosamine formation in bladder infections and its role in the etiology of bladder cancer, *J. Urol.* **120:**48.

Ramirez, J. R., and Dowell, A. R., 1971, Silo-fillers disease: Nitrogen dioxide-induced lung injury. Long term follow up and review of the literature, *Ann. Intern. Med.* **74:**569.

Roffo, A. H., 1933, Heliotropism of cholesterol in relation to skin cancer, *Am. J. Cancer* **17:**42.

Rounbehler, D. P., Ross, R., Fine, D. H., Iqbal, Z. M., and Epstein, S. S., 1977, Quantitation of dimethylnitrosamine in the whole mouse after biosynthesis *in vivo* from trace levels of precursors, *Science* **197:**917.

Saffiotti, U., Montesano, R., Sellakumar, A. R., and Borg, S. A., 1967, Experimental cancer of the lung. Inhibition by vitamin A of the induction of tracheobronchial squamous, metaplasia and squamous cell tumors, *Cancer* **20:**857.

Sakamoto, K., and Sakka, M., 1973, Reduced effect of irradiation on normal and malignant cells irradiated *in vivo* in mice pretreated with vitamin E, *Br. J. Radiol.* **46:**538.

Sansone, E. B., and Tenari, Y. B., 1978, The permeability of laboratory gloves to selected nitrosamines, in: *Environmental Aspects of N-Nitroso Compounds* (E. A. Walker, M. Castegnaro, L. Griciute, and R. E. Lyle, eds.), pp. 517–529, International Agency for Research on Cancer, Lyon.

Schmandke, H., Sima, C., and Maune, R., 1967, Die Absorbierung uber α-Tocopherol bei Menschen, *Int. Z. Vitaminforsch.* **39:**296.

Schweinsberg, F., 1974, Catalysis of nitrosamine synthesis, in: *N-Nitroso Compounds in the Environment* (P. Bogovski and E. A. Walker, eds.), pp. 80–85, International Agency for Research on Cancer, Lyon.

Segi, M., Kurihara, M., and Matsuyama, T., 1969, *Cancer Mortality for Selected Sites in 24 Countries, No. 5 (A64-65),* Dept. of Public Health, Tokakii University School of Medicine, Sendai.

Sen, N. P., and Donaldson, B., 1974, The effect of ascorbic acid and glutathione on the formation of nitrosopiperazines from piperazine adipate and nitrite, in: *N-Nitroso Compounds in the Environment* (P. Bogovski and E. A. Walker, eds.), pp. 103–106, International Agency for Research on Cancer, Lyon.

Sen, N. P., Donaldson, B., Charbonneau, C., and Miles, W. F., 1974, Effect of additives on the formation of nitrosamines in meat curing mixtures containing spices and nitrites, *J. Agric. Food Chem.* **22:**1125.

Sen, N. P., Donaldson, B., Seaman, S., Iyengar, J. R., and Miles, W. F., 1976, Inhibition of nitrosamine formation in fried bacon by propyl gallate and L-ascorbyl palmitate, *J. Agric. Food Chem.* **24:**397.

Sen, N. P., Donaldson, B. A., Seaman, S., Iyengar, J. R., and Miles, W. F., 1978, Recent studies in Canada on the analysis and occurrence of volatile and non-volatile N-nitroso compounds in foods, in: *Environmental Aspects of N-Nitroso Compounds* (E. A. Walker, M. Castegnaro, L. Griciute, and R. E. Lyle, eds.), pp. 373–393, International Agency for Research on Cancer, Lyon.

Severi, R., 1935, Influenza di una dieta a vario contenuto in vitamina E sullo suiluppo dei tumori da catrame nel topo, *Pathologica* **27:**524.

Shamberger, R. J., 1966, Protection against carcinogenesis by antioxidants, *Experientia* **22:**116.

Shay, H., Harris, C., and Gruenstein, M., 1960, Further studies in prevention of experimentally induced breast cancer in the rat. Some endocrine aspects, *Acta Union Int. Contre Cancer* **16(1):**225.

Skaare, J. U., and Nafstad, I., 1978, Interaction of vitamin E and selenium with the hepatotoxic agent dimethylnitrosamine, *Acta Pharmacol. Toxicol.* **43:**119.

Skaare, J. U., Nafstad, I., and Dahle, H. K., 1977, Enhanced hepatotoxicity of dimethylnitrosamine by pretreatment of rats with the antioxidant ethoxyquin, *Toxicol. Appl. Pharmacol.* **42:**19.

Spiegelhalder, B., Eisenbrand, G., and Preussmann, R., 1980, Occurrence of volatile nitrosamines in food: A survey of the West German market, in: *N-Nitroso Compounds: Analysis, Formation and Occurrence* (E. A. Walker, M. Griciute, M. Castegnaro, and M. Borzsonyi, eds.), pp. 467–477, International Agency for Research on Cancer, Lyon.

Sporn, M. B., Squire, R. A., Brown, C. C., Smith, J. M., Wenk, M. L., and Springer, S., 1977, 13-*Cis* retinoic acid: Inhibition of bladder carcinogenesis in the rat, *Science* **195**:487.

Swick, R. W., and Bauman, C. A., 1951, Tocopherol in tumor tissues and effects of tocopherol on the development of liver tumors, *Cancer Res.* **11**(12):948.

Tannenbaum, A., and Silverstone, H., 1953, Nutrition in relation to cancer, *Adv. Cancer Res.* **1**:451.

Tannenbaum, S. R., 1979, Endogenous formation of nitrite and *N*-nitroso compounds, in: *Naturally Occurring Carcinogens—Mutagens and Modulators of Carcinogenesis, Proceedings of the 9th International Symposium of The Princess Takamatsu Cancer Research Fund, Tokyo, 1979,* (E. C. Miller, J. A. Miller, I. Hirono, T. Sugimura, and S. Takayama, eds.), pp. 211–220, University Park Press, Baltimore.

Tannenbaum, S. R., Fett, D., Young, V. R., Land, P. D., and Bruce, W. R., 1978, Nitrite and nitrate are formed by endogenous synthesis in the human intestine, *Science* **200**:1487.

Terracini, B., Magee, P. N., and Barnes, J. M., 1967, Hepatic pathology in rats on low dietary levels of dimethylnitrosamine, *Br. J. Cancer* **21**:559.

Thomas, H. V., Mueller, P. K., and Lyman, R. L., 1967, Lipoperoxidation of lung lipids in rats exposed to nitrogen dioxide, *Science* **159**:532.

USP XIX, 1975, Simulated gastric fluid, p. 765, United States Pharmacopeial Convention, Inc., Rockville, Md.

Varghese, A. J., Land, P. C., Furrer, R., and Bruce, W. R., 1978, Non-volatile *N*-nitroso compounds in human feces, in: *Environmental Aspects of N-Nitroso Compounds* (E. A. Walker, M. Castegnaro, L. Griciute, and R. E. Lyle, eds.), pp. 257–264, International Agency for Cancer Research, Lyon.

Walker, E. A., Castegnaro, M., Garren, L., and Pignatelli, B., 1978, Limitations to the protective effect of rubber gloves for handling nitrosamines, in: *Environmental Aspects of N-Nitroso Compounds* (E. A. Walker, M. Castegnaro, L. Griciute, and R. E. Lyle, eds.), pp. 535–543, International Agency for Research on Cancer, Lyon.

Walker, E. A., Pignatelli, B., and Castegnaro, M., 1979, Catalytic effect of *p*-nitrosophenol on the nitrosation of diethylamine, *J. Agric. Food Chem.* **27**(2):393.

Walker, E. A., Castegnaro, M., Pignatelli, B., and Munoz, N., 1980, *N*-nitrosamines in gastric juice and atrophic gastritis. A pilot study, in: *N-Nitroso Compounds: Analysis, Formation and Occurrence* (E. A. Walker, M. Griciute, M. Castegnaro, and M. Brozsonyi, eds.), pp. 633–641, International Agency for Research on Cancer, Lyon.

Wang, T., Kakizoe, T., Dion, P., Furrer, R., Vargese, A. J., and Bruce, W. R., 1978, Volatile nitrosamines in normal human feces, *Nature* **276**:280.

Wattenberg, L., 1971, The role of the portal of entry in inhibition of tumorigenesis, *Prog. Exp. Tumor Res.* **14**:89.

Wattenberg, L. W., 1977, Inhibition of carcinogenic effects of polycyclic hydrocarbons by benzylisothiocyanate and related compounds, *J. Natl. Cancer Inst.* **58**:395.

Wattenberg, L., 1978a, Inhibitors of chemical carcinogenesis, *Adv. Cancer Res.* **26**:197.

Wattenberg, L. W., 1978b, Guest editorial: Inhibition of chemical carcinogenesis, *J. Natl. Cancer Inst.* **60**:11.

Wayne, L. G., 1962, *The Chemistry of Urban Atmospheres, Technical Progress Report Vol. III,* Los Angeles County Air Pollution Control District, December 1962.

Weber, F., and Wiss, O., 1964, Synergism of *d* and *l*-α-tocopherol during absorption, *Biochem. Biophys. Res. Commun.* **14**:186.

Weisburger, J. H., Cohen, L. A., and Wynder, E. L., 1977, On the etiology and metabolic epidemiology of the main human cancers, in: *Origins of Human Cancer* (H. H. Hiatt, J. D. Watson, and J. A. Winsten, eds.), pp. 567–602, Cold Spring Harbor Laboratory, Cold Spring Harbor, New York.

White, F. R., 1961, The relationship between underfeeding and tumor formation, transplantation, and growth in rats and mice, *Cancer Res.* **21**:281.

Wishnok, J. S., Archer, M. C., Edelman, A. S., and Rand, W. M., 1978, Nitrosamine carcinogenicity: A quantitative Hansch–Taft structure–activity relationship, *Chem. Biol. Interact.* **20**:43.

Yang, N. Y. J., and Desai, I. D., 1977, Effect of high levels of dietary vitamin E on liver and plasma lipids and fat-soluble vitamins in rats, *J. Nutr.* **107**:1418.

Ziebarth, D., and Scheunig, G., 1976, Effect of some inhibitors on the nitrosation of drugs in human gastric juice, in: *Environmental N-Nitroso Compounds: Analysis and Formation* (E. A. Walker, P. Bogovski, and L. Griciute, eds.), pp. 279–290, International Agency for Research on Cancer, Lyon.

6

Trace Elements and Metals as Anticarcinogens

MARYCE M. JACOBS and A. CLARK GRIFFIN

I. Introduction

The inhibition of tumor induction and development by trace elements and metals has only recently become a major area of exploration in the research community. Although thousands of publications report trace element and metal modifications of enzymes and other subcellular components, on only few occasions has the relevance of these observations to the carcinogenic process been evaluated. Interest in these modifying factors has been somewhat blunted because of their sometimes mercurial ability to either augment or inhibit the carcinogenic process. As environmentalists and epidemiologists have associated modifiers with increased and reduced cancer rates and as nutritionists have labeled certain heretofore unrecognized trace elements and metals "nutrients," the cancer researcher has turned his attention to specific events in the multistage origin of tumors that are potential targets for modification.

In this chapter, we shall present an annotated discussion of the anticarcinogenic, antimutagenic, anticlastogenic, and other inhibitory properties of trace elements and metals. The majority of reports cite the effect of a single modifier in animal, bacterial, and *in vitro* test systems. The detoxification of one element by another and the net contribution to an antitumorigenic effect

---

MARYCE M. JACOBS • Eppley Institute for Research in Cancer, University of Nebraska Medical Center, Omaha, Nebraska 68105. A. CLARK GRIFFIN • Department of Biochemistry, The University of Texas System Cancer Center, M. D. Anderson Hospital and Tumor Institute, Houston, Texas 77030.

will be briefly described. In animal test systems, the carcinogen, animal species, relative dose levels of carcinogen and modifier, diet, route of administration, and/or spontaneous tumor profile will be provided. The ability of a trace element or metal to augment or inhibit a chemically induced or spontaneous tumor incidence is often closely associated with one or more of the above parameters in the animal test system.

Many trace elements and metals inhibit carcinogenesis in animal systems. Continued investigation of their effects in bacterial, cell culture, and other *in vitro* systems have aided in elucidating the mechanism(s) by which the elements act as anticarcinogens. *Selenium* (Se) inhibits chemically induced tumors in rats and spontaneous tumors in mice. *In vitro* studies showed Se to inhibit mutagens of *Salmonella*, to prevent chemically induced chromosome breakage, and to inhibit selected enzymes required for activation of some chemical carcinogens. Zinc, which is essential for normal proliferative processes, also inhibits carcinogenesis. In contrast, a zinc deficiency rather than a supplement inhibited Walker 256 carcinoma in rats, Lewis lung tumor, and several mouse leukemias. Supplemental copper inhibits a variety of chemically induced tumors in rats and potentiates the anticarcinogenic action of some alkylating agents. Platinum has been used clinically in the treatment of cancers. Compounds of this element have the ability to stop cell division. Although in small amounts iodine prevents goiter, in larger amounts it prevents tumor growth. Arsenic decreases the incidence of adenomas and carcinomas of the lung in mice. Germanium-fed rats have significant reductions in tumors of liver, lung, mammary, and adrenals. Magnesium also has antitumor properties.

In addition to antineoplastic effects of a single element on nonmetal carcinogens, trace elements can also inhibit metal carcinogens. Selenium and zinc inhibit cadmium carcinogenesis, and manganese inhibits nickel carcinogenesis. Although the focus of this chapter will be on trace elements as inhibitors of carcinogenesis, consideration will also be given to the inhibitory effects of trace elements and metals in *in vitro* test systems and of metal–metal detoxification.

II. Selenium

A. Clinical

Both inorganic and organic forms of selenium have exhibited a protective role against the origin of malignant disease. An increased incidence of colon, rectum, breast, and other cancers in humans in geographic regions where Se is deficient has been demonstrated in the United States (Jansson et al., 1975, 1976; Shamberger and Willis, 1971) and on a global scale (Schrauzer, 1976; Jansson et al., 1977). The reduced breast cancer incidence in Asian populations as compared with the United States may reflect the combined protection of two to four times higher Se and approximately 2 times lower polyunsaturated fatty acid (PUFA) contents of Asian diets (Wilson and Petrakis, 1976). Since Schwartz and Foltz (1957) recognized Se as an essential nutrient and active component of factor 3, Se has been shown to prevent lipid peroxidation (Hoekstra, 1975) through its role as a component of the selenoenzyme glutathione peroxidase (Flohe et al., 1973). The low PUFA and high Se in the diets as well as the presence of glutathione peroxidase in mammary tissue collectively contribute to the reduced breast cancer incidence in the Asian population.

In addition to the epidemiological link between low Se and high cancer incidence, several clinical trials have reinforced this association. Lower blood Se levels and glutathione peroxidase activity have been observed in patients with gastrointestinal and other cancers (Broghamer et al., 1976; McConnell et al., 1975; Shamberger et al., 1973; Robinson et al., 1979). In areas of the United States where there is a high (0.06–0.1 ppm) Se content in forage crops, there are significantly lower cancer death rates from neoplasms of the tongue, esophagus, stomach, intestine, rectum, liver, pancreas, larynx, lungs, and bladder in men and women (Shamberger et al., 1976). Deaths from Hodgkin's disease and lymphoma were also reduced in geographic areas high in Se.

The therapeutic attributes of organic Se were noted in one report in which oral administration of selenium cystine significantly lowered the total leukocyte count in patients with acute and chronic leukemia (Weisberger and Suhrland, 1955). Another clinical application of selenium-containing compounds has been the use of ^{75}Se-labeled methionine in tumor diagnosis. Pancreatic, liver, and parathyroid tissues actively concentrate the radiopharmaceutical, allowing for external organ scanning (Shapiro, 1973). The imaging of the pancreas with [^{75}Se]selenomethionine, however, has had low reliability. Recent studies in dogs and mice attribute this in part to growth hormone (Atkins and Som, 1979). In the presence of growth hormone, pancreatic uptake of ^{75}Se is depressed with concurrent depression in the pancreas-to-liver concentration ratio. The use of [^{75}Se]adenosyl selenomethionine as a radiopharmaceutical for diagnostic scanning of the prostate is being examined experimentally in rats and may have future clinical application (Eakins, 1979).

B. Animal

The spontaneous tumor incidence and the incidence of chemically induced tumors have been inhibited by inorganic and organic forms of Se in selected mouse, rat, and other animal strains. Selenium supplements decreased the incidence of spontaneous mammary tumors in C_3H mice (Schrauzer and Ishmael, 1974), of intestinal adenocarcinomas in sheep (Wedderburn, 1972), and colon (Jacobs *et al.*, 1977a) and liver (Clayton and Baumann, 1949; Griffin and Jacobs, 1977; Harr *et al.*, 1973) tumors in rats.

Schrauzer and colleagues (Schrauzer and Ishmael, 1974; Schrauzer *et al.*, 1978a,b) have demonstrated that additions of 0.1 to 2 ppm Se as selenite to the drinking water of inbred female C_3H/St mice enormously reduced the spontaneous mammary tumor incidence. The untreated control incidence of 82% was reduced to 10% by addition of 2 ppm Se in the form of SeO_2 to the drinking water for 15 months (Schrauzer and Ishmael, 1974). In comparison, the addition of 2 ppm arsenite to the drinking water increased the age of onset, growth rate, and incidence of multiple tumors. Combination of Se with As diminished the deleterious effects of As (Schrauzer *et al.*, 1978b).

Jacobs (1977) and Jacobs *et al.* (1977a) reported that 4 ppm Se supplements as sodium selenite to the drinking water reduced the colon tumor incidence in 1,2-dimethylhydrazine (DMH)-treated rats from 87% to 40%. Supplemental Se decreased the total number of colon tumors induced by DMH more than threefold and by methylazoxymethanol (MAM) almost twofold. In their studies, adult male Sprague–Dawley rats received 20 weekly subcutaneous injections of 20 mg/kg body weight of either DMH or MAM. The decreased tumorigenicity of DMH may reflect Se inhibition of the oxidative activation of DMH through azomethane and azoxymethane to form MAM. The lowered tumorigenicity of MAM may be because of Se inhibition of alcohol or aldehyde dehydrogenase metabolism of MAM or of Se inhibition of nonenzymatic reactions of MAM (Zedeck *et al.*, 1979). Alternatively, metabolites of the sodium selenite supplement formed *in vivo* may directly interact with either of the colon carcinogens or with DMH metabolites, giving rise to the reduced tumorigenicity. Comprehensive reviews of the biochemical events subject to possible Se intervention and the metabolic aspects of Se action have been published elsewhere (Diplock, 1976; Jansson and Jacobs, 1976).

The comparative effects of Se and antioxidants of DMH induction of colon tumors in male Sprague–Dawley rats have been presented in detail (Jacobs and Griffin, 1979). Supplements of 4 ppm Se as Na_2SeO_3 to the drinking water, 1.2% ascorbic acid (V_C) to the diet, or 0.5% butylated hydroxytoluene (BHT) to the diet of DMH-treated rats reduced the colon tumor incidence of DMH controls from 64% to 31% (Se), 38% (V_C), and 43% (BHT). The colon tumor incidence in DMH-treated rats receiving a combination of Se plus V_C increased to 83%, whereas the combination of Se plus BHT decreased the colon tumor incidence to 55%.

A variety of hepatocarcinogens has been inhibited by Se in animal models. Clayton and Baumann (1949) reported a reducer liver tumor incidence in rats fed alternating diets containing either supplemental Se or the azo dye 3′-methyl-4-dimethylaminoazobenzene (3′MeDAB). In these studies, albino rats were maintained on semisynthetic diets and were given 0.064% 3′MeDAB for 2 weeks. Subsequently, the animals were placed on dye-free diet supplemented with 5 ppm Se as sodium selenite. Finally, the rats were provided a Se-free but dye-containing diet for an additional 4 weeks. The liver tumor incidence was reduced approximately 50% as compared to control animals receiving basal diet during the intermediate period. This study is one of the early reports of an inhibition of Se on tumor development.

More recently, Griffin and Jacobs (1977) submitted male Sprague–Dawley rats simultaneously to supplemental Se and to azo dye in the diet to obtain a reduction in hepatic tumors. The 3′MeDAB (0.05%) was incorporated into the diet for 8 weeks and then removed. During carcinogen administration and for an additional 4 weeks prior to sacrifice, the rats were maintained on 6 ppm Se supplements. The Se was provided as either sodium selenite in the drinking water or as an organic form in yeast (*Saccharomyces cerevesiae*) containing 118 μg Se/g yeast. The inorganic Se reduced the tumor incidence from 92% to 46%, and the organic Se reduced the incidence from 92% to 64%.

In another male Sprague–Dawley rat model Grant *et al.* (1977) noted a protective effect of dietary sodium selenite on lesions induced by aflatoxin B1. Animals were provided 25 μg aflatoxin B_1 per os 5 days a week for 4 weeks and Se (0.03–5 ppm) in the diet. After 17 months, a low (20%) incidence of hepatocarcinomas was observed in 1-ppm-Se-treated rats. Changes in dietary Se gave rise to variations in glutathione peroxidase activities and tissue Se levels. The authors observed that dietary Se and repeated aflatoxin B_1 interact to form large bizarre renal tubule cells.

Shamberger (1970) has reported that Se decreased tumor induction in animals' skin painted with 7,12-dimethylbenzanthracene (DMBA). The utility of this carcinogen in deciphering the multistage origin of tumors has long been recognized. One of the authors M. M. Jacobs is conducting an exhaustive study on the effects of Se provided by different routes of administration on DMBA-painted mice. Perhaps the data (unpublished) will aid in our understanding of the tumorigenic process.

The hepatocarcinogen 2-acetylaminofluorene (AAF) undergoes metabolic activation through N-hydroxy-AAF to several proposed metabolites including N-hydroxy-aminofluorene. Adult male Sprague–Dawley rats were provided 0.03% AAF in the diet for 14 weeks followed by AAF-free diet. The basal diet was Purina Laboratory Chow®. Simultaneous administration of a 4-ppm Se supplement (Na_2SeO_3) in the drinking water reduced the hepatic tumor incidence 50% (Marshall et al., 1979). In further studies, our laboratory has reported that Se inhibited AAF activation with apparent specificity for hydroxylation of certain positions of the AAF molecule (Marshall et al., 1978, 1979). The N-hydroxylase activity was reduced with a corresponding reduction in the anticipated N-OH-AAF metabolite and an increase in the ring-hydroxylated intermediate, 3-OH-AAF. The antitumorigenic effect of Se may very well reflect the reduction in the formation of the highly carcinogenic metabolite, N-OH-AAF, and the production of the noncarcinogenic metabolite, 3-OH-AAF.

In earlier studies by Harr et al. (1973), Se reduced the number of tumors in rats given AAF. The group of rats receiving 0.03% AAF in the diet and 4 ppm Se (Na_2SeO_3) in the drinking water for 14 weeks had a final tumor incidence of 4/14 rats. The control group receiving dietary AAF and no additional Se had a tumor incidence of 9/13 rats. Harr et al. (1973) also reported hepatic toxicity, neoplasia, and tumor induction at extrahepatic sites including mammary gland. It is important to distinguish their experimental model from that in the above studies. Harr et al. (1973) employed young female OSU–Brown rats fed a low Se ration supplemented with 60 ppm vitamin E. To this formula diet 0.015% AAF added. Either 0-, 0.1-, 0.5-, or 2.5-ppm Se supplements were provided in the drinking water. Differences in Se-to-carcinogen ratios, rat strains, age, and basal diets each contribute to different effects of Se. Harr et al. (1973) proposed that the selenite was either preventing carcinogenesis or modifying the rate of induction.

C. Bacterial

Both the mutagenicity and the antimutagenicity of Se compounds in bacterial systems have been demonstrated. Noda et al. (1979) have reported the weak mutagenicity of selenate (SeO_4^{2-}) selenite (SeO_3^{2-}) in two bacterial assay systems, Kada's *Bacillus subtilis* rec⁻ assay and Ames' *Salmonella typhimur-*

ium assay. Shamberger *et al*. (1979) have demonstrated increased mutagenicity with increasing concentrations of malonaldehyde and β-propiolactone. The increased mutagenicity was observed in five *S. typhimurium* strains mutated by a frame-shift mechanism and two *S. typhimurium* strains mutated through a basepair substitution. Coexposure of the bacterial cells to mutagen and increasing concentrations of Se or antioxidants including vitamin C, vitamin E, and BHT markedly reduced mutagenesis in strains mutated by the frame-shift mechanism.

The multiplicity of inhibitory and inducing effects of selenium compounds on mutagenesis and carcinogenesis reflects the properties of different redox states of selenium. In the presence of agents such as ascorbic acid, Se(VI) can easily be reduced to Se(IV). *In vivo*, Se(IV) is readily converted to Se(-II). In the Ames assay, selenate, Se(VI), was mutagenic, giving rise to base pair substitutions, whereas selenite was not mutagenic (Lofroth and Ames, 1977). The above observation illustrates the importance of clearly defining all parameters in each *in vivo* and *in vitro* test system. When adequate documentation is provided, seemingly contradictory reports on the effects of "selenium" on carcinogenesis, mutagenesis, chromosome aberrations, mitosis, unscheduled DNA repair, etc. may in fact all be correct and in concert.

In order to elucidate altered biochemical events through which selenite inhibits tumorigenesis, our laboratories investigated the effects of this form of Se in bacterial and human lymphocyte culture systems. Selenium decreased the mutagenicity of 2-acetylaminofluorine (AAF), N-hydroxyacetylaminofluorene (N-OH-AAF), and N-hydroxyaminofluorine (N-OH-AF) in the *Salmonella typhimurium* TA1538 tester strain (Jacobs *et al*. 1977b). An effective molar ratio of Se/AFF = 10, Se/N-OH-AAF = 10, and Se/N-OH-AF = 300 reduced the mutagenicity to 65, 68, and 61% of their respective controls with mutagen alone. With a molar ratio of Se/N-OH-AAF = 100, selenite reduced the activity to 28% of the mutagenicity of N-OH-AF alone. In control studies, the viable cell count per plate in all assays with Se (Na_2SeO_3) alone and of mutagens in the presence and absence of Se remained contant (2–3 $\times$ 10^8 cells per plate). In addition, an average background of 14 spontaneous revertants per plate was observed with 0.1 to 40 mM Se and no mutagen. The S9 fraction was included in the assay for microsomal activation of AAF. A microsome-free fraction from rat liver homogenate was incubated with N-OH-AAF in the Ames assays. In future studies it would be interesting to determine whether or not there is a reduction in N-hydroxylase activity and formation of 3-OH-AAF in the bacterial assay as was observed in the animal models. Essential factors to be considered in evaluating mutagenicity tests and relating mutagenic events to neoplastic events in mammalian tests have been reviewed by Matter (1976).

D. Other in Vitro Systems

Inorganic selenium can induce DNA fragmentation, DNA-repair synthesis, chromosome aberrations, and mitotic inhibition in cell culture systems. In comparing the cytogenetic effect of Se compounds in cultured human lymphocytes, Nakamuro et al. (1976) noted the decreasing order in chromosome-breaking activity: $H_2SEO_3 > Na_2SeO_3 > SeO_3 > H_2SeO_4 > Na_2SeO_4$. Frequently, the above undesirable events are elicited in cell culture/mutagenic systems by inordinately high concentrations of the test compound. In contrast, in vitro models as well as in vivo animal models require Se as an essential nutrient for optimal growth and survival. Selenium was reported by McKeehan et al. (1976) to be essential for clonal growth of diploid fibroblasts from human fetal lung (WI38) in media containing small amounts of serum proteins. Maximum growth was obtained when 30 nM neutralized selenious acid was added to the synthetic medium. Selenium was also required by a Chinese hamster cell line grown in a protein-free synthetic culture medium. The requirement for Se compounds is better understood when we recognize Se as a normal component of subcellular elements involved in normal biochemical activities, e.g., glutathione peroxidase (Flohe et al., 1973), selenobases in transfer RNA (Saelinger et al., 1972), and selenouridine (Hoffman and McConnell, 1974).

In cultured human fibroblasts and xeroderma pigmentosum, 8×10^{-5} to 3×10^{-3} M sodium selenite induced DNA fragmentation, chromosome aberrations, mitotic inhibition, and DNA-repair synthesis (Lo et al., 1978). Incubation with mouse liver S9 fraction increased the capacity of selenite to induce chromosomal aberrations with DNA-repair synthesis. In order to obtain these observations, concentrations of sodium selenate (Na_2SeO_4) in the dose range of 8×10^{-5} to 3×10^{-3} M were required.

Another in vitro assay in wide use today is the sister chromatid exchange (SCE) frequency of cells in culture. Although the biochemistry of SCE formation is unknown, it has been suggested that SCEs reflect some aspect of DNA repair. Ray et al. (1978) have studied the effects of short- and long-term exposures of human whole blood cultures to increasing concentration of selenite. Although Se did induce an increased level of SCEs at the higher concentrations, we found 1.58×10^{-6} to 1.19×10^{-5} M a suitable concentration range for investigating the effects of Se on methylmethansulfonate (MMS) and N-OH-AAF activities (Ray et al., 1978). Selenium reduced MMS- and N-OH-AAF-induced SCE frequencies in human blood cultures. Exposure of lymphocytes to 1×10^{-4} M MMS for the last 19 hr of culture yielded an average SCE frequency of 30.17 ± 0.75. Exposure of lymphocytes to 2.7×10^{-5} M N-OH-AAF resulted in 13.61 ± 0.43 SCEs/cell. Simultaneous addition of 1.19×10^{-5} Na$_2$SeO$_3$ and MMS or N-OH-AAF to the cultures resulted in SCE frequencies that were 30% and 11%, respectively, below the sum of the SCE frequencies produced by the individual compounds.

In further studies from our laboratories, selenium caused a 50% reduction in the aryl hydrocarbon hydroxylase (AHH) activity from human lymphocytes using benzo(a)pyrene as substrate (Rasco et al., 1977). Human lymphocytes were cultured in the presence and absence of inducers of AHH. The presence of 10^{-5} M Se as Na$_2$SeO$_3$ in the culture medium had no effect on induced and noninduced levels of AHH. When Se was added directly to the AHH assay, the enzyme activity was inhibited by more than 50%. The inhibition was observed with 1, 3, 10, and 100 μM benzo(a)pyrene (BP) and 0.1, 0.3, 1, and 10 mM Se. In addition to inhibiting the AHH activity, subsequent studies indicate that in the presence of Se, BP is metabolized to less carcinogenic forms (M. M. Jacobs, unpublished data). This observation is supportive of the earlier observation that the antitumorigenic effect of Se with respect to AAF in male Sprague–Dawley rats is attributed to a reduction in N-hydroxylase activity, reduced N-OH-AAF, and formation of the 3-OH-AAF metabolite (Marshall et al., 1978). The function and role of selenium in the chemoprevention of cancer have been reviewed recently by Griffin (1979).

III. Zinc

Zinc (Zn)-supplemented and Zn-deficient diets both give rise to a reduced tumor incidence in experimental animal systems. Duncan and Droesti (1975) report a reduction in neoplastic DNA synthesis and tumor growth in both rats and mice fed high- and low-Zn diets. In one experiment (Duncan et al., 1974), female Wistar rats received implants of hepatoma induced by 3'-methyl-4-dimethylaminoazobenzene. Test groups were given semisynthetic diets containing 0.4 to 2500 μg Zn/g ration. Control animals received the same diet with 60 μg Zn/g ration. After 3 weeks, labeled thymidine was injected i.p., and 2 hr later the tumors were excised. DNA synthesis in the tumors was reduced in rats maintained on low-Zn (0.4 μg/g) and high-Zn (500 μg/g) diets compared to control animals. In a second experiment,

Duncan and Droesti (1975) fed Swiss mice the same experimental diets for 10 weeks. During this time the mice were painted with 0.5% methylcholanthrene (MC) twice weekly in the shaved interscapular region. Papilloma development and the incidence of malignancy were significantly reduced in mice consuming either Zn-deficient or -supplemented diets. The authors suggest that the reduced DNA synthesis observed in tumors transplanted in rats supports an earlier proposal that decreased tumor growth arises from a block in the cell division cycle at the level of DNA replication.

Poswillo and Cohen (1971) demonstrated Zn inhibition of dimethylbenzanthracene-induced carcinogenesis in hamsters. Young Syrian golden hamsters were provided 21.9 ppm Zn supplements in either the diet or the drinking water. After 4 days, painting of DMBA on the cheek pouch was initiated. Dimethylbenzanthracene treatments were three times weekly for 4 weeks. The Zn supplement in either the diet or water inhibited tumor formation. After 10 months, there was no increase in tumor formation in hamsters provided supplemental Zn in the drinking water.

Supplemental Zn in the drinking water retarded tumor growth induced by DMBA implants in rats (Ciapparelli *et al.*, 1972). Wistar albino rats, 4–5 months old, were given 50-, 100-, and 250-ppm Zn supplements in their drinking water. Dimethylbenzanthracene pellets were implanted in the submandibular gland. Three months later, the glands were dissected and examined histologically. Control rats receiving deionized water and no added Zn developed well-differentiated squamous carcinomas. Increasing concentrations of Zn progressively decreased the amount of squamous epithelium, while an imflammatory response became more marked. Ciapparelli *et al.* (1972) suggested that the increase in lymphatic tissue in tumors from rats on high Zn could indicate an immune response to the developing carcinoma.

DeWys and Pories (1972) and Pories *et al.* (1977) inhibited a variety of tumors in CDF and C57BL/6 mice and Sprague–Dawley rats by dietary Zn deficiency. In their studies, weanlings were fed either a Zn-deficient (1.3 ppm) or Zn-adequate (50 ppm) diet for 7 to 21 days prior to inoculation with tumor cells. Growth of Lewis lung tumor in C57BL/6 mice was markedly reduced in mice receiving Zn-deficient diets compared to Zn-adequate controls. Pretreatment with a Zn-deficient diet also inhibited tumor growth and prolonged survival in mice inoculated with mouse leukemia L5178gt, L1210, or B388 cells. In other experiments (DeWys and Pories, 1972), the effects of Zn deficiency on ascites and solid tumor forms of Walker 256 carcinoma in male Sprague–Dawley rats were studied. Tumor growth inhibition and prolonged survival were observed to the same extent for the two forms. The investigators concluded that "tumor inhibition is a general effect of Zn deficiency, irrespective of cell type, cell growth rate, or site of growth."

IV. Copper

Supplements of copper salts in the diet or drinking water of rats and mice inhibit a variety of chemical carcinogens. Changes in enzyme activities affecting the metabolism of the carcinogens and observations on increased liver retention of copper and liver pathology accompany the majority of reports on antitumorigenic properties of copper compounds. Fare (1964), Fare and Woodhouse (1963), and Fare and Howell (1964) fed albino rats 0.09% 3-methoxy-4-aminoazobenzene in corn diets. Addition of 0.5% copper as cupric oxyacetate hexahydrate to the diets reduced liver tumors from 5/10 in controls to 0/10 in the groups receiving copper (Fare and Howell, 1964). In a second report with dimethylaminoazobenzene (DAB) and the same form of copper (Fare, 1964), the author observed that the amount of azo dye-bound liver protein peaked at 100 days and progressively decreased thereafter. The amount of copper in the liver increased 40% after 315 days in dye-plus-copper-fed groups. The copper content increased 40-fold after 330 days in rats fed copper only. The stored copper was primarily bound to protein. The mean serum optical rotations in rats fed corn diet only, corn diet plus DAB, and corn diet plus DAB plus copper were 46.2, 43.1, and 39.0, respectively (Fare, 1963). In further studies, these authors noted a decrease in liver succinoxidase activity and an accompanying change in the distribution of protein and RNA in DAB-only-treated rats as compared to controls and copper-treated animals (Fare and Woodhouse, 1963).

Yamane and Sakai (1974) and Yamane *et al.* (1969, 1970) investigated biochemical changes in livers of Wistar rats fed DAB and copper acetate. Dimethylaminoazobenzene alone decreased the total lactate dehydrogenase (LDH) activity with the appearance of the LDH isozyme 3. Neither change was seen in rats fed DAB plus copper (Yamane *et al.*, 1970). In another study these authors reported that azo-reduction activity in liver was enhanced by copper. The enhanced N-dimethylase activity in rats fed DAB was reduced by copper. Although the total DAB-metabolizing activities were increased in rats fed DAB plus copper plus phenobarbital (Yamane and Sakai, 1974), the elevated ring hydroxylation was most significant. Finally, these workers reported that 3-methylcholanthrene added to the diets of DAB-plus-copper-treated rats elevated both the azo-reduction and N-dimethylation activities. The increases in ring hydroxylase and azo reductase levels were seen primarily in microsomal fractions and were accompanied by increased microsomal copper.

Brada et al. (1974) report an increase in S-adenosylethionine in the liver of rats fed ethionine plus copper (copper acetate) as compared to rats fed ethionine only. Liver analyses are compounded by the fact that only about 70% of the ethionine is absorbed during passage through the gastrointestinal tract. Analysis of the soluble part of the lumen showed a rise in ethionine metabolites during passage. Copper supplements prevented formation of the new metabolites. Kamamoto et al. (1973) demonstrated that inhibition of ethionine induction of hepatomas after 24 weeks of diet could be completely prevented by addition of copper for 12, 16, or 20 weeks but not by copper addition for only 4 or 8 weeks. From biochemical examination of the liver, these workers suggested that copper was bound to ethionine and deposited in the nuclei, thus affording the protective effect of copper against ethionine carcinogenesis.

Copper sulfate and 7,12-dimethylbenzanthracene (DMBA) were fed to 3- to 6-month-old C57BL/6J and virgin and pseudopregnant strain A mice. Although there was no reduction in ovarian or breast tumors, Burki and Okita (1973) suggested the copper "appeared to prolong survival and may have delayed the development of granulosa cell tumors."

The effects of copper-supplemented (800 ppm) and copper-deficient (1 ppm) diets on the induction of neoplasms by acetylaminofluorene (AAF) and dimethylnitrosamine (DMN) in rats were reported by Carlton and Price (1973). The incidence of kidney neoplasms was 57% in the DMN–copper-deficient group and 0.0% in the DMN–copper-supplemented group. The incidence of extrahepatic neoplasms in AAF-fed rats was 40% in copper-difficient rats but reduced to 17% in copper-supplemented animals.

V. Other Trace Elements and Metals

A. Metal–Metal Anticarcinogenicity

Metal carcinogenesis and metal toxicity have been much more widely publicized than metal anticarcinogenicity and metal detoxification. Over 20 years ago the phenomenon of subcutaneous carcinogenesis was described by Oppenheimer et al. (1956). They observed that subcutaneous injection of metals, plastics, and various other materials can induce sarcomas at the site of implant. The sarcomas are caused by the physical rather than the chemical characteristics of the injected material. Metals can be carcinogenic when provided by routes of administration other than subcutaneous. Nevertheless, simultaneous exposure to metal combinations can give rise to reduced tumor formation and/or mutual detoxification. The classic example of metal–metal anticarcinogenicity is that of selenium (Se) protection against cadmium (Cd)-induced testicular injury (Griffin, 1979). Presumably Se forms complexes with Cd, thereby reducing the available free Cd and hence the tumor incidence (Gunn *et al.*, 1968).

Gunn *et al.* (1963) reported that single subcutaneous injections of cadmium chloride to rats and mice selectively damaged the vascular supply of the testis and results in necrosis of the seminiferous tubules and interstitial tissue. After 1 year, 70–80% of the animals exhibited interstitial cell tumors. The induction of these tumors by Cd is prevented by simultaneous administration of zinc. In another study by Gunn *et al.* (1964), Wistar rats were given one s.c. injection of Cd in the interscapular region and after 10 months had a 41% (9/22) incidence of pleomorphic sarcomas at that site. Animals receiving one Cd injection plus zinc acetate injections before, simultaneously with Cd, and after Cd at the same site had only a 12% (2/17) incidence of sarcomas at the injection site. It is postulated that Cd may interfere with growth-regulating mechanisms in cells by deleting an essential Zn complex. The authors suggest that the administration of excessive Zn is preventing this effect, thereby conferring an anticarcinogenic action of Zn.

There is evidence that cancer results from decompartmentalization of iron (Fe) in cells before or during cell division, resulting in uncontrolled proliferation (R. Wilson, 1977). Zinc can protect against the Fe-induced decompartmentalization, against Fe-catalyzed free radical production, and therefore against cell damage.

The inhibition of nickel (Ni)-induced muscle tumorigenesis by manganese (Mn) has been demonstrated by Sunderman *et al.* (1974). Fisher rats were given a single i.m. injection of a penicillin suspension of nickel subsulfide dust alone or in combination with Mn dust. After 2 years, the incidence of sarcomas at the injection site was 96% (39/40) in Ni-only-treated rats and 63% (15/24) in Ni-plus-Mn-treated rats.

The role of metal interactions in carcinogenesis is a new and fascinating research area. Metal protection against metal carcinogens has been briefly illustrated with four examples, Se–Cd, Zn–Cd, Zn–Fe, and Mn–Ni. An integral part of these and future studies will be consideration of metal toxicities and the profound effect of the nutritional status on the response of the animal to metal or other carcinogens.

B. Nutritional Factors

Nutritional components, including metals and trace elements, can markedly affect carcinogenesis and should be considered in the design and interpretation of a carcinogenicity-testing system. A few examples of nutritional effects serve to illustrate this point. Caloric restriction can reduce chemically induced and spontaneous tumors (Tannenbaum, 1942). Increased dietary protein can protect against the hepatocarcinogen 4-dimethylaminoazobenzene (Tannenbaum and Silvertone, 1957). High-fat diets have been shown to increase chemically induced and spontaneous tumors in mice (Tannenbaum and Silverstone, 1957). Other dietary components including vitamin C (Mirvish *et al.*, 1975; DeCosse *et al.*, 1975), selenium (Griffin and Jacobs, 1977; Jacobs, 1977; Jacobs and Griffin, 1979; Marshall *et al.*, 1979), and food preservatives (Wattenberg, 1979) are known to inhibit chemical carcinogens. The modifying action of dietary constituents cannot be overlooked when elucidating mechanisms of carcinogenesis.

Because there is disparity between the direct correlation between carcinogenicity tests in animals and *in vitro* tests for mutagenicity, cell transformation, unscheduled DNA repair, cytogenicity, etc., we have emphasized animal studies throughout this chapter. A large volume of literature exists on trace element effects on enzyme activities, chromosomes, mutagens, and other short-term tests. Much of the data has been used to propose possible mechanisms of carcinogenesis and anticarcinogenesis observed in animal models. The remaining examples of trace element effects on initiation and tumor development are presented with this relationship in mind.

C. Other Trace Element Effects

The property of platinum (Pt) compounds to inhibit cell division has been successfully put to use in clinical trials. *Cis* Pt(II) is an effective agent in the treatment of metastatic osteogenic sarcoma. Toxicity from the Pt compound results in depressed white counts and platelets in addition to elevated BUN, creatinine, and transaminase levels (Ochs *et al.*, 1977).

With radiolabeled iodine in the form of 5-iododeoxyuridine (IUDR), an antineoplastic effect was observed against an experimental murine tumor (Bloomer and Adelstein, 1975). Injection of C_3HcB/FeJ mice with ovarian embryonal cell carcinoma followed by subsequent i.p. administration of IUDR at 12, 24, and 36 hr resulted in 50% disease-free survival at 150 days.

Germanium (Ge) supplements to the drinking water of Charles River Swiss mice reduced the spontaneous tumor incidence (Kanisawa and Schroeder, 1967). The incidence was reduced from 32% (15/170) in unsupplemented controls to 19% (7/131) in Ge-treated mice. Kanisawa and Schroeder (1969) also reported a reduction in tumors in Ge-fed Long–Evans rats.

The role of magnesium (Mg) on the induction of neoplasia by various experimental conditions has been reviewed by Durlach et al. (1973). Rats placed on Mg-deficient diets do not develop spontaneous lesions. On the other hand, in clinical studies Mg administration has been effective in the treatment of breast cancer.

The effect of cobalt (Co) salts on established tumors in mice has been reported (O'Hara et al., 1971). Mice were treated twice weekly for 21 weeks with methylcholanthrene (MC). After MC treatments were terminated, the mice were then given i.p. injections of cobalt salts biweekly for 5 weeks. The group of mice receiving cobalt nitrite had twice as many tumor regressions and less than half the number of new tumors than controls receiving no cobalt. This finding was not statistically significant. The fact that Co did regress established tumors and prevent the development of new tumors suggests that had the authors provided the cobalt either before or during MC treatment a significant antitumorigenic response might have been observed.

Kobayashi et al. (1970) have demonstrated that aluminum compounds reduce lung tumor induction in mice. They injected female dd mice subcutaneously once weekly for 5 weeks with 4-nitroquinoline-1-oxide. The mice were allowed to inhale 0.2% solutions of either $AlCl_3$ or Al_2O_3 twice weekly for 7 months. Compared to controls receiving no aluminum, the lung adenoma incidence was reduced to 60% ($AlCl_3$) and 70% (Al_2O_3).

In skin-painting studies, vanadium (V) decreased the papilloma incidence as well as the progression of the papillomas to squamous cell carcinomas in polycyclic hydrocarbon-treated mice (Gorski, 1968). Painting of BALB/c × CBA hybrid mice with methylcholanthrene (MC) resulted in 72.5% (29/40) papillomas, 21 of which progressed to carcinomas. A second group of mice painted with MC and vanadium pentoxide in a molar ratio of 1:1000 (MC:V_2O_5) developed only 48.2% (14/29) papillomas, and only 8/14 progressed to carcinomas. The V_2O_5-catalyzed oxidation of several carcinogens was investigated. Four carcinogens were catalytically oxidized, and two were not.

The influence of a variety of trace metals on the hydroxylation of benzo-(a)pyrene (BP) was studied by Calop et al. (1977). Swiss mice were treated with methylcholanthrene, sacrificed 2 days later, and the livers isolated. The aryl hydrocarbon hydroxylase (AHH) activity was measured in *in vitro* liver cultures containing 0.01 to 100 ppm concentrations of each trace element. The investigators report AHH inhibition by Zn, Cu, Ni, Cr, V, Mn, and Cd.

VI. Closing Remarks

The focus of this chapter has been on the anticarcinogenic and other inhibiting properties of trace elements and metals. For many years the balance has been top-heavy with reports on toxic, carcinogenic, and other less desirable effects of trace elements. Furst (1977) and Sunderman (1977) have provided comprehensive reviews of metal carcinogenesis, illustrating the prolonged interest in adverse metal effects. Clearly from this review, at least 16 elements (and others not discussed) can inhibit some stage of carcinogenesis.

The bias with which our review has been written is intended to encourage a reexamination of the nutritional, chemopreventive, and chemotherapeutic potential of many members of the metallo-compound family. Exciting research on the inhibitory effects of trace elements and metals on tumor induction and development has only just begun.

ACKNOWLEDGMENTS. This work was supported in part by grants from the National Large Bowel Cancer Project, National Cancer Institute grant number R26 CA25699, the Selenium–Tellurium Development Association, and the Robert A. Welch Foundation.

References

Atkins, H. L., and Som, P., 1979, Growth-hormone and somatostatin effects on selenomethionine-^{75}Se uptake by the pancreas, *J. Nucl. Med.* **20**:543.
Bloomer, W. D., and Adelstein, S. J., 1975, Antineoplastic effect of iodine-125-labelled iododeoxyuridine, *Int. J. Radiat. Biol.* **27**:509.
Brada, Z., Altman, N. H., and Bulba, S., 1974, Effect of cupric acetate on ethionine metabolism, *Proc. Am. Assoc. Cancer Res.* **15**:145.
Broghamer, W. L., Jr., McConnell, K. P., and Blotcky, A. L., 1976, Relationship between serum selenium levels and patients with carcinoma, *Cancer* **37**:1384.
Burki, H. R., and Okita, G. T., 1973, Effect of oral copper sulfate on 7,12-dimethylbenz(alpha)anthracene carcinogenesis in mice, *Br. J. Cancer* **23**:591.
Calop, J., Burckhart, M. F., and Fontanges, R., 1977, The influence of trace elements on the hydroxylation of benzo(a)pyrene, *Eur. J. Toxicol.* **9**:271.
Carlton, W. W., and Price, P. S., 1973, Dietary copper and the induction of neoplasms in the rat by acetylaminofluorene and dimethylnitrosamine, *Food Cosmet. Toxicol.* **11**:827.

Ciapparelli, L., Retief, D. H., and Fatti, L. P., 1972, The effect of zinc on 9,10-dimethyl-1,2-benzanthracene (DMBA) induced salivary gland tumors in the albino rat—a preliminary study, *S. Afr. J. Med. Sci.* **37**:85.
Clayton, C. C., and Baumann, C. A., 1949, Diet and azo dye tumors: Effect of diet during a period when the dye is not fed, *Cancer Res.* **9**:575.
DeCosse, J. J., Adams, M. B., Kuzma, J. F., LoGerfo, P., and Condon, R., 1975, Effects of ascorbic acid on rectal polyps of patients with familial polyposis, *Surgery* **78**:608.
DeWys, W., and Pories, W., 1972, Inhibition of a spectrum of animal tumors by dietary zinc deficiency, *J. Natl. Cancer Inst.* **48**:375.
Diplock, A. T., 1976, Metabolic aspects of selenium action and toxicity, *CRC Crit. Rev. Toxicol.* **4**:271.
Duncan, J. R., and Droesti, I. E., 1975, Zinc intake, neoplastic DNA synthesis, and chemical carcinogenesis in rats and mice, *J. Natl. Cancer Inst.* **55**:195.
Duncan, J. R., Droesti, I. E., and Albrecht, C. F., 1974, Zinc intake and growth of a transplanted hepatoma induced by 3'-methyl-4-dimethyl-aminoazobenzene in rats, *J. Natl. Cancer Inst.* **53**:277.
Durlach, J., Larvor, P., Augusti, Y., and Albengres-Moineau, E., 1973, Magnesium and cancer, *Concours Med.* **95**:6295.
Eakins, M. N., 1979, The distribution of ^{75}Se-adenosyl selenomethionine in the rat with observations on its potential as a prostate scanning agent, *Eur. J. Nucl. Med.* **4**:101.
Fare, G., 1963, Serum optical rotation during the development of rat tumours induced by feeding 4-dimethylaminoazobenzene, *Nature* **200**:481.
Fare, G., 1964, The effect of cupric oxyacetate on the binding of azo-dye by protein during the induction of liver tumours in the rat, *Biochem. J.* **91**:473.
Fare, G., and Howell, J. S., 1964, The effect of dietary copper on rat carcinogenesis by 3-methoxy dyes. 1. Tumors induced at various sites by feeding 3-methoxy-4-aminoazobenzene and its N-methyl derivative, *Cancer Res.* **24**:1279.
Fare, G., and Woodhouse, D. L., 1963, The effect of copper acetate on biochemical changes induced in the rat liver by p-dimethylaminoazobenzene, *Br. J. Cancer* **17**:512.
Flohe, L., Gunzler, W. A., and Schock, H. H., 1973, Glutathione peroxidase: A selenoenzyme, *FEBS Lett.* **32**:132.
Furst, A., 1977, Inorganic agents as carcinogens, in: *Advances in Modern Toxicology, Environmental Cancer*, Vol. 3 (H. F. Kraybill and M. A. Mehlman, eds.), pp. 209–229, John Wiley & Sons, New York.
Gorski, T., 1968, The catalytic influence of V_2O_5 on the oxidation and on the disappearance of carcinogenic properties of some polycyclic hydrocarbons, *Neoplasia* **15**:267.
Grant, K. E., Conner, M. W., and Newberne, P. M., 1977, Effect of dietary sodium selenite upon lesions induced by repeated small doses of aflatoxin B_1, *Toxicol. Appl. Pharmacol.* **41**:166.
Griffin, A. C., 1979, Role of selenium in the chemoprevention of cancer, *Adv. Cancer Res.* **29**:419.
Griffin, A. C., and Jacobs, M. M., 1977, Effects of selenium on azo dye hepatocarcinogenesis, *Cancer Lett.* **3**:177.
Gunn, S. A., Gould, T. C., and Anderson, W. A., 1963, Cadmium-induced interstitial cell tumors in rats and mice and their prevention by zinc, *J. Natl. Cancer Inst.* **31**:745.
Gunn, S. A., Gould, T. C., and Anderson, W. A., 1964, Effect of zinc on carcinogenesis by cadmium, *Proc. Soc. Exp. Biol. Med.* **115**:653.
Gunn, S. A., Gould, T. C., and Anderson, W. A. D., 1968, Mechanisms of zinc, cysteine and selenium protection against cadmium-induced vascular injury to mouse testis, *J. Reprod. Fertil.* **15**:65.
Harr, J. R., Exon, J. H., Weswig, P. H., and Whanger, P. D., 1973, Relationship of dietary selenium concentration; chemical cancer induction, and tissue concentration of selenium in rats, *Clin. Toxicol.* **6**:287.

Hoekstra, W. G., 1975, Biochemical function of selenium and its relation to vitamin E, *Fed. Proc.* **34**:2083.
Hoffman, J. L., and McConnell, K. P., 1974, The presence of 4-selenouridine in *Escherichia coli* tRNA, *Biophys. Biochim. Acta* **366**:109.
Jacobs, M. M., 1977, Inhibitory effects of selenium on 1,2-dimethylhydrazine and methylazoxymethanol colon carcinogenesis. Correlative studies on selenium effects on the mutagenicity and sister chromatid exchange rates of selected carcinogens, *Cancer* **40**:2557.
Jacobs, M. M., and Griffin, A. C., 1979, Effects of selenium on chemical carcinogenesis. Comparative effects of antioxidants, *Biol. Trace Element Res.* **1**:1-13.
Jacobs, M. M., Jansson, B., and Griffin, A. C., 1977a, Inhibitory effects of selenium on 1,2-dimethylhydrazine and methylazoxymethanol acetate induction of colon tumors, *Cancer Lett.* **2**:133.
Jacobs, M. M., Matney, T. S., and Griffin, A. C., 1977b, Inhibitory effects of selenium on the mutagenicity of 2-acetylaminofluorene (AAF) and AAF derivatives, *Cancer Lett.* **2**:319.
Jansson, B., and Jacobs, M. M., 1976, Selenium—a possible inhibitor of colon and rectum cancer. I. Epidemiological aspects—B. Jansson. II. Biochemical aspects—M. Jacobs, in: *Proceedings of Symposium on Selenium-Tellurium in the Environment*, pp. 326-340, Industrial Health Foundation Inc., Pittsburgh.
Jansson, B., Seibert, G. B., and Speer, J. F., 1975, Gastrointestinal cancer—Its geographic distribution and correlation to breast cancer, *Cancer* **36**:2373.
Jansson, B., Malahy, M. A., and Seibert, G. B., 1976, Geographical distribution of gastrointestinal cancer and breast cancer and its relation to selenium deficiency, in: *Proceedings of the Third International Symposium on Detection and Prevention of Cancer*, Vol. 1 (H. E. Nieburgs, ed.), pp. 1161-1178, Marcel Dekker, New York.
Kamamoto, Y., Makiura, S., Sugihara, S., Hiasa, Y., Arai, M., and Ito, N., 1973, The inhibitory effect of copper on DL-ethionine carcinogenesis in rats, *Cancer Res.* **33**:1129.
Kanisawa, M., and Schroeder, H. A., 1967, Life term studies on the effects of arsenic, germanium, tin and vanadium on spontaneous tumors in mice, *Cancer Res.* **27**:1192.
Kanisawa, M., and Schroeder, H. A., 1969, Life term studies on the effect of trace elements on spontaneous tumors in mice and rats, *Cancer Res.* **29**:892.
Kobayashi, N., Katsuki, H., and Yamane, Y., 1970, Inhibitory effect of aluminum on the development of experimental lung tumor in mice induced by 4-nitroquinoline-1-oxide, *Gann* **61**:239.
Lo, L. W., Koropatnick, J., and Stich, H. F., 1978, The mutagenicity and cytotoxicity of selenate, "activated" selenite and selenate for normal and DNA repair-deficient human fibroblasts, *Mutat. Res.* **49**:305.
Lofroth, G., and Ames, B. N., 1977, Mutagenicity of inorganic compounds in *Salmonella typhimurium:* Arsenic, chromium and selenium, in: *Eighth Annual Meeting of Environmental Mutagen Society*, Program and Abstracts, p. 30, Aa-1, Colorado Springs.
Marshall, M. V., Jacobs, M. M., and Griffin, A. C., 1978, Reduction in acetylaminofluorene (AAF) hepatocarcinogenesis by selenium, *Proc. Am. Assoc. Cancer Res.* **19**:75.
Marshall, M. V., Arnott, M. S., Jacobs, M. M., and Griffin, A. C., 1979, Selenium effects on the carcinogenicity and metabolism of 2-acetylaminofluorene, *Cancer Lett.* **7**:331.
Matter, B. E., 1976, Problems of testing drugs for potential mutagenicity, *Mutat. Res.* **38**:243.
McConnell, K. P., Broghamer, W. L., Blotcky, A. L., and Hurt, O. J., 1975, Selenium levels in human blood and tissue in health and disease, *J. Nutr.* **105**:1026.
McKeehan, W. L., Hamilton, W. G., and Ham, R. G., 1976, Selenium is an essential trace nutrient for growth of WI-38 diploid human fibroblasts, *Proc. Natl. Acad. Sci. USA* **73**:2023.
Mirvish, S. S., Cardesa, A., Wallcave, L., and Shubik, P., 1975, Induction of mouse lung adenomas by amines or urea plus nitrite and by N-nitroso compound: Effects of ascorbate, gallic acid, thiocyanate, and caffeine, *J. Natl. Cancer Inst.* **55**:633.

Nakamuro, K., Yoshikawa, K., Sayato, Y., Kurata, H., Tonomura, M., and Tonomura, M., 1976, Studies on selenium-related compounds. V. Cytogenic effect and reactivity with DNA, *Mutat. Res.* **40:**177.

Noda, M., Takano, T., and Sakurai, H., 1979, Mutagenic activity of selenium compounds, *Mutat. Res.* **66:**175.

Ochs, J., Freeman, A., and Douglass, H., 1977, Clinical trial of *cis*-diamine dichloroplatinum (*cis* Pt II) in osteogenic sarcoma, *Proc. Am. Assoc. Cancer Res.* **18:**167.

O'Hara, G. P., Mann, D. E., and Gautieri, R. F., 1971, Effect of cobalt chloride and sodium cobalt nitrite on the growth of established epithelial tumors induced by methylcholanthrene, *J. Pharm. Sci.* **60:**473.

Oppenheimer, B. S., Oppenheimer, E. T., Danishefsky, I., and Stout, A. P., 1956, Carcinogenic effect of metals in rodents, *Cancer Res.* **16:**439.

Pories, W. J., DeWys, W. D., Flynn, A., Mansour, E. G., and Strain, W. H., 1977, Implication of the inhibition of animal tumors by dietary zinc deficiency, *Adv. Exp. Med. Biol.* **91:**243.

Poswillo, D. E., and Cohen, B., 1971, Inhibition of carcinogenesis by dietary zinc, *Nature* **231:** 447.

Rasco, M. A., Jacobs, M. M., and Griffin, A. C., 1977, Effects of selenium on aryl hydrocarbon hydroxylase activity in cultured human lumphocytes, *Cancer Lett.* **3:**295.

Ray, J. H., Altenburg, L. C., and Jacobs, M. M., 1978, Effect of sodium selenite and methylmethanesulfonate or *N*-hydroxy-2-acetylaminofluorene co-exposure on sister-chromatid exchange production in human whole blood cultures, *Mutat. Res.* **57:**359.

Robinson, M. F., Godfrey, P. J., Thomson, C. D., Rea, H. M., and Van Rij, A. M., 1979, Blood selenium and glutathione peroxidase activity in normal subjects and in surgical patients with and without cancer in New Zealand, *Am. J. Clin. Nutr.* **32:**1477.

Saelinger, D. A., Hoffman, J. L., and McConnell, K. P., 1972, Biosynthesis of selenobases in transfer RNA by *Escherichia coli, J. Mol. Biol.* **69:**9.

Schrauzer, G. N., 1976, Anticarcinogenic action of an essential element, in: *Proceedings of Symposium on Selenium-Tellurium in the Environment,* pp. 293–299, Industrial Health Foundation Inc., Pittsburgh.

Schrauzer, G. N., and Ishmael, D., 1974, Effects of selenium and of arsenic on the genesis of spontaneous mammary tumors in inbred C_3H mice, *Ann. Clin. Lab. Sci.* **2:**441.

Schrauzer, G. N., White, D. A., and Schneider, C. J., 1978a, Selenium and cancer: Effects of selenium and of the diet of the genesis of spontaneous mammary tumors in virgin inbred female C_3H/St mice, *Bioinorg. Chem.* **8:**387.

Schrauzer, G. N., White, D. A., McGinness, J. E., Schneider, C. J., and Bell, L. J., 1978b, Arsenic and cancer: Effects of joint administration of arsenite and selenite on the genesis of mammary adenocarcinoma in inbred female C_3H/St mice, *Bioorg. Khim.* **9:**245.

Schwartz, K., and Foltz, C. M., 1957, Selenium as an integral part of factor 3 against dietary necrotic liver degenerations, *J. Am. Chem. Soc.* **79:**3292.

Shamberger, R. J., 1970, Relationship of selenium to cancer. 1. Inhibitory effect of selenium on carcinogenesis, *J. Natl. Cancer Inst.* **44:**931.

Shamberger, R. J., and Willis, C. E., 1971, Selenium distribution and human cancer mortality, *Clin. Lab. Sci.* **2:**211.

Shamberger, R. J., Rukovena, E., Longfield, A. K., Tytko, S. A., Deodhar, S., and Willis, C. E., 1973, Antioxidants and cancer. 1. Selenium in the blood of normals and cancer patients, *J. Natl. Cancer Inst.* **50:**863.

Shamberger, R. J., Tytko, S. A., and Willis, C. E., 1976, Antioxidants and cancer. Part IV. Selenium and age-adjusted human cancer mortality, *Arch. Environ. Health* **31:**231.

Shamberger, R. J., Corlett, C. L., Beaman, K. D., and Kasten, B. L., 1979, Antioxidants reduce the mutagenic effect of malonaldehyde and β-propiolactone. Part IX. Antioxidants and cancer, *Mutat. Res.* **66:**349.

Shapiro, J. R., 1973, Selenium compounds in nature and medicine, in: *Organic Selenium Com-*

pounds: Their Chemistry and Biology (D. L. Klayman and W. H. H. Gunther, eds.), pp. 693–726, Wiley, New York.

Sunderman, F. W., 1977, Metal carcinogenesis, in: *Advances in Modern Toxicology, Toxicology of Trace Elements,* Vol. 2 (R. A. Goyer and M. A. Mehlman, eds.), pp. 257–295, Wiley, New York.

Sunderman, F. W., Lau, T. J., and Cralley, L. J., 1974, Inhibitory effect of manganese upon muscle tumorigenesis by nickel subsulfide, *Cancer Res.* **34**:92.

Tannenbaum, A., 1942, The genesis and growth of tumors. II. Effects of caloric restriction per se, *Cancer Res.* **2**:460.

Tannenbaum, A., and Silverstone, H., 1957, Nutrition and the genesis of tumors, in *Cancer,* Vol. 1 (R. W. Ravin, ed.), pp. 306–334, Butterworth, London.

Wattenberg, L. W., 1979, Inhibitors of carcinogenesis, in: *Carcinogens: Identification and Mechanisms of Action* (A. C. Griffin and C. R. Shaw, eds.), pp. 299–316, Raven Press, New York.

Wedderburn, J., 1972, Selenium and cancer, *N. Z. Vet. J.* **20**:56.

Weisberger, A. S., and Suhrland, L. G., 1955, Studies on analogues of L-cysteine and L-cystine. III. The effect of selenium cystine on leukemia, *Blood* **10**:19.

Wilson, C. S., and Petrakis, N. L., 1976, Selenium as a protective against breast cancer in Northwestern diets, *Fed. Proc.* **35**:578.

Wilson, R. L., 1977, Iron, zinc, free radicals and oxygen in tissue disorders and cancer control, *Ciba Found. Symp.* **51**:331.

Yamane, Y., and Sakai, K., 1974, Effect of the basic cupric acetate on biochemical changes in the liver of the rat fed carcinogenic aminoazo dye. III. Effect of copper compound with some other metals, phenobarbital and 3-methylcholanthrene on the metabolism of 4-dimethyl-amino-azobenzene, *Chem. Pharm. Bull. (Tokyo)* **22**:1126.

Yamane, Y., Sakai, K., Uchiyama, I., Tabata, M., Taga, N., and Hanaki, A., 1969, Effect of basic cupric acetate on the biochemical changes in the liver of the rat fed carcinogenic aminoazo dye. I. Changes in the activities of DAB metabolism by liver homogenate, *Chem. Pharm. Bull. (Tokyo)* **17**:2488.

Yamane, Y., Sakai, K., Hayashi, M., Matsuzaki, M., and Hanaki, A., 1970, Effect of the basic cupric acetate on the biochemical changes in the liver of the rat fed carcinogenic aminoazo dye. II. Activity and isozyme pattern of lactate dehydrogenase, *Chem. Pharm. Bull. (Tokyo)* **18**:1050.

Zedeck, M. S., Frank, N., and Wiessler, M., 1979, Metabolism of the colon carcinogen methylazoxymethanol acetate, in: *Frontiers of Gastrointestinal Research,* Vol. 4 (L. van der Reis, ed.), pp. 32–37, S. Karger, Basel.

7
Plant Sterols: Protective Role in Chemical Carcinogenesis

BERTRAM IRA COHEN and ROBERT FRANKLIN RAICHT

I. Background

The pathogenesis of colorectal cancer is currently unknown. Epidemiological studies in man and studies in experimental animals have implicated various classes of compounds as potential tumor promoters or tumor inhibitors. Plant sterols, a group of compounds found in vegetables, will be the focus of this review.

Colorectal cancer ranks as the second most commonly occurring cancer in man today. In the United States, approximately 102,000 cases of colorectal cancer were detected in 1978, and 52,000 deaths were attributed to this disease (American Cancer Society, 1978). Important factors are environmental rather than genetic (Armstrong and Doll, 1975; Burkitt, 1975; Doll, 1969) or social. This is well documented by studies that show that first- and second-generation Japanese immigrants in Hawaii have a higher incidence of colon cancer than Japanese in Japan (Wynder et al., 1969; Haenszel et al., 1973; Stemmerman, 1970).

The role of diet in colon cancer has been the subject of intensive investigation (Wynder and Reddy, 1974, 1975; Reddy, 1975; Reddy et al., 1975b, 1977b; Broitman et al., 1977; Reddy and Wynder, 1973; Drasar and

---

BERTRAM IRA COHEN and ROBERT FRANKLIN RAICHT • Veterans Administration Medical Center, New York, New York, 10010; and Department of Medicine, New York University School of Medicine, New York, New York 10016.

Jenkins, 1976). Tumor-promoting as well as tumor-retarding components may be present in the diet. Populations consuming meat-rich diets, which are high in protein and fat, have an increased risk of developing colon cancer compared to populations whose diets are low in these components but high in plant products (e.g., vegetarian diets) (Enstrom, 1975; Phillips, 1975). Metabolic epidemiological studies have shown that high-risk populations have increased concentrations of bile acids and neutral sterols in the feces (Haenszel *et al.*, 1973; Reddy and Wynder, 1973, 1977; Reddy *et al.*, 1976, 1977b). Others have demonstrated that placing volunteers on meat-rich diets increased the fecal concentrations of bile acids and neutral sterols (Reddy *et al.*, 1977b; Reddy, 1980). This has led investigators to suggest that these compounds play a role in the etiology of large bowel cancer.

Animal models have been used to investigate potential promoters and inhibitors of colon cancer. For example, in animals treated with a carcinogen, it has been shown that manipulations designed to increase colonic concentrations of bile acids will enhance colon cancer incidence (Cohen *et al.*, 1980; Sarwal *et al.*, 1979; Reddy *et al.*, 1976b,c, 1977a,c, 1978a,b; Chomchai *et al.*, 1974; Nigro *et al.*, 1973). Tumor inhibitors have been studied in similar models; compounds such as antioxidants, isothiocyanates, and selenium, which are present in varying amounts in our diet, have been shown to be tumor inhibitors (Wattenberg, 1972, 1977; Jacobs, 1977).

Populations consuming diets rich in vegetable products have relatively low incidences of colon cancer (Phillips, 1975). There are several possible explanations for this. First, diets high in vegetables are low in animal fat, and this may be partially responsible for the decreased colonic cancer incidence. Second, fiber, an important constituent of vegetables, is thought to be one of the protective components in our diet (Burkitt *et al.*, 1972). Recent studies in Finland have shown that fiber may play a role in diluting potentially tumorigenic compounds in feces (Reddy *et al.*, 1978a). Third, tumor-inhibiting substances like the isothiocyanates present in certain vegetables may also play a role (Wattenberg, 1977). Another group of compounds present mainly in vegetables consists of the plant sterols. This review will deal with the plant sterols (β-sitosterol in particular) as potential tumor inhibitors.

II. Plant Sterols: Structure and Function

Plant sterols resemble the animal sterol cholesterol (I) (Fig. 1), having a cyclopentenophenanthrene ring, a $\Delta^{5,6}$ double bond, and a 3β-hydroxyl group in the molecule. In the sterol side chain, the plant sterols contain one or two more carbon atoms than cholesterol (as either methyl or ethyl groups). The major sterols belonging to the plant sterol class have been identified as campesterol (II), β-sitosterol (III), and stigmasterol (IV) (Fig. 1) (Subbiah, 1971).

Plant sterols comprise about 20% of all sterols and 1% of the adult diet. β-Sitosterol has been the plant sterol studied most extensively since the early 1950s. In man, absorption of β-sitosterol from orally administered doses was usually no higher than 5% of the total sterol ingested (Borgstrom, 1969; Grundy *et al.*, 1968). When absorbed, β-sitosterol distribution in the total body sterol pool is similar to that of cholesterol. Absorbed β-sitosterol has been reported to be converted to both neutral products and acidic steroids (Subbiah *et al.*, 1969). However, the majority of the absorbed sterol is excreted unchanged as β-sitosterol (Subbiah *et al.*, 1969).

Orally administered β-sitosterol reduced levels of plasma cholesterol in man by as much as 40% (Best *et al.*, 1958). These preparations of β-sitosterol, particularly Cytellin® (Eli Lilly & Co.), have been used for this therapeutic effect. Several possible explanations for the hypocholesterolemic effect of β-sitosterol have been proposed. Most of the evidence suggests that β-sitosterol interferes with the uptake of cholesterol into membranes (Glover and Green, 1957). β-Sitosterol can be incorporated into membranes but not as readily as cholesterol (Edwards and Green, 1972). The biological effects of the incorporation of plant sterols into membranes have not been determined.

The possible role of plant sterols in tumor development has not been examined. Plant sterols have been found in certain malignant tissues, but their origin was unclear (Mellias *et al.*, 1977; Gordan *et al.*, 1967). We have chosen

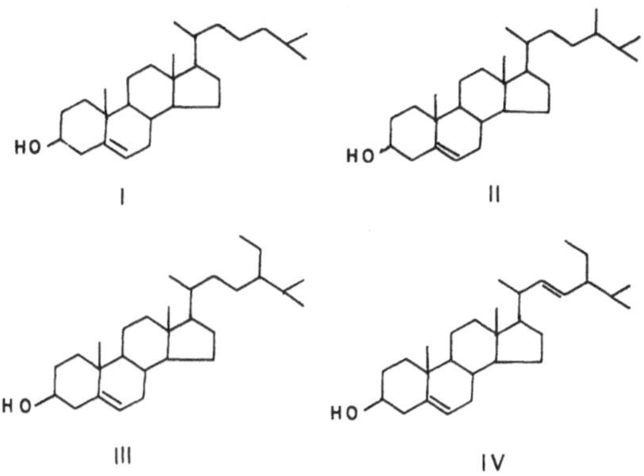

FIGURE 1. Major sterols in animals and plants: I, cholesterol; II, campesterol; III, β-sitosterol; IV, stigmasterol.

to study plant sterols as tumor inhibitors for several reasons. Epidemiological evidence suggests that populations consuming diets high in plant sterols have a lower incidence of colon cancer. Second, plant sterols are absorbed only to a limited extent; ingested plant sterols, therefore, would be present in high concentrations in the colon (Miettinen and Tarpila, 1978). This would increase the amount of plant sterols that could potentially be incorporated into colonic epithelial cell membranes. The biological effect of changing membrane structure is not clear, but changes in cell proliferation may occur.

III. Animal Test Systems

There are several well-described animal models of colon carcinogenesis that employ direct- and indirect-acting chemical carcinogens (Reddy *et al.*, 1975a; LaMont and O'Gorman, 1978). Inhibitors of chemical carcinogenesis can be examined in the same animal model systems. Among the direct-acting carcinogens (no metabolic activation required) are N-methyl-N-nitrosourea (MNU) and N-methyl-N'-nitro-N-nitrosoguanidine (MNNG). Indirect-acting carcinogens (metabolic activation required) include such compounds as 1,2-dimethylhydrazine (DMH) and azoxymethanol (AOM). Our experiments with rats employ the direct-acting carcinogen MNU which is administered intrarectally. Reasons for using this system include: (1) tumors are produced only in the colon and histologically resemble colon cancer in man; and (2) MNU is direct acting, and any changes in tumorigenicity could not be attributed to carcinogen metabolism.

N-Methyl-N-nitrosourea is administered intrarectally in sterile saline (2 mg/0.5 ml per rat) on days 1, 4, 7, and 10 of the experiment. This dose produced a tumor incidence of about 50% in all animals. The total amount of carcinogen administered on any one day (2 mg) as well as the absolute amount of carcinogen given for the entire experiment (8 mg) are critical factors, as one might overwhelm the potential inhibitory capacity of the compound being tested if excessive amounts of carcinogen are given. In our system, in which we obtain a baseline tumor incidence of 50%, we are capable of detecting reductions as well as elevations in tumor incidence.

There are many ways of administering chemical inhibitors to animals. In studies of colon carcinogenesis, it is appropriate to administer the potential inhibitor in the diet, as epidemiological studies have suggested dietary differences between populations may influence colon cancer development. A critical question is the relation of these models to colon tumors in man. It is

TABLE 1. Animal Model for N-Methyl-N-Nitrosourea Sterol Carcinogenesis Study[a]

Diet	Number of rats	Carcinogen treatment
Control chow	30	None; saline given on days 1, 4, 7, 10
Control chow	30	MNU given, 2 mg on days 1, 4, 7, 10
Sterol-supplemented diet	30	None; saline given on days 1, 4, 7, 10
Sterol-supplemented diet	80	MNU given, 2 mg on days 1, 4, 7, 10

[a] Fisher CD 344 rats of similar age were randomly divided into four groups at the start of the study. At 6 weeks of age, each animal was treated with carcinogen or saline, and the experimental diet was begun. The study lasted 28 weeks, at which time animals were sacrificed and their colons examined grossly and microscopically for type and position of tumors.

speculated that human colon cancer is caused by the exposure of colonic epithelial cells to low doses of carcinogens over long periods of time. Although the animal model is unlike the hypothesized situation in man in that a carcinogen is given over a short period of time in a relatively high dose, this technique is essential in designing experiments of reasonable lengths.

The experimental design for our studies employing the Fisher CD 344 male rat is outlined in Table 1. The animals are fed the inhibitor (or other

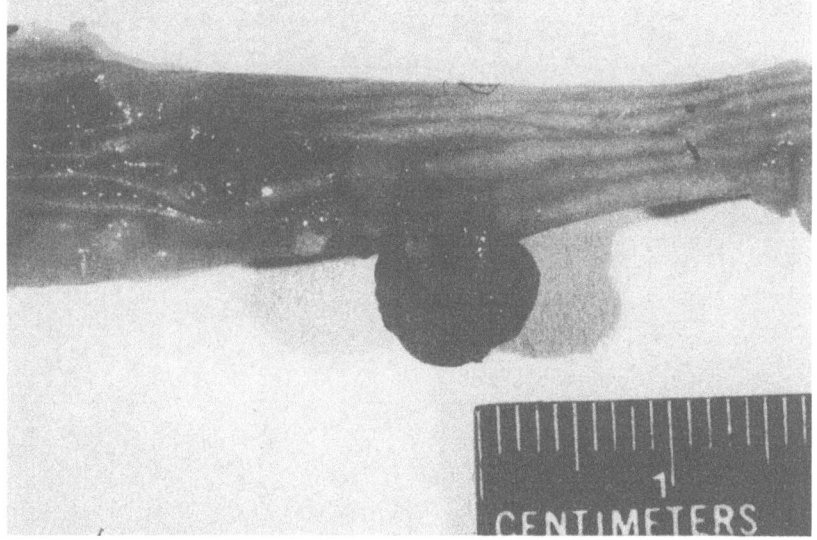

FIGURE 2. At week 28, the colon of each animal was opened and photographed. Tumors were observed in the animals treated with the carcinogen (MNU). Most of the tumors were discrete polypoid excresences.

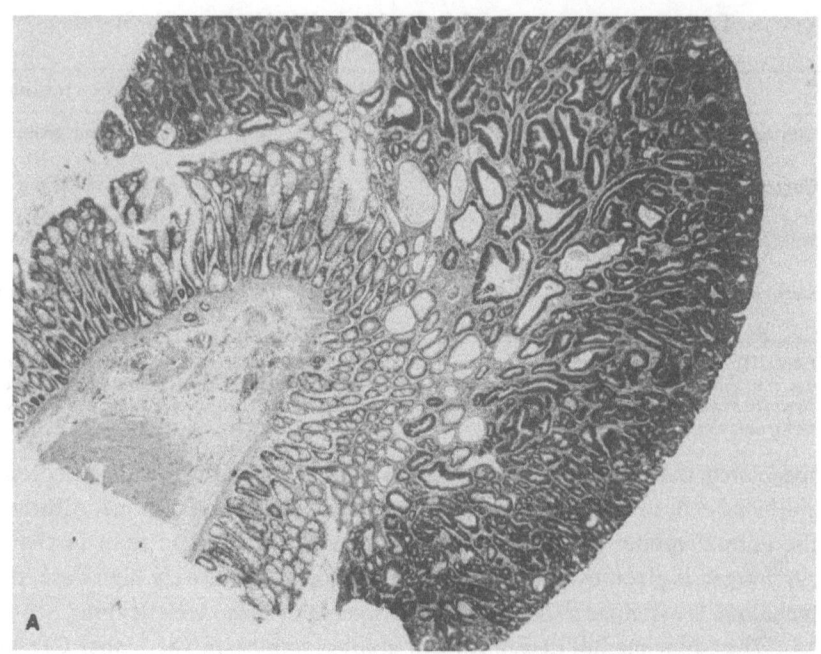

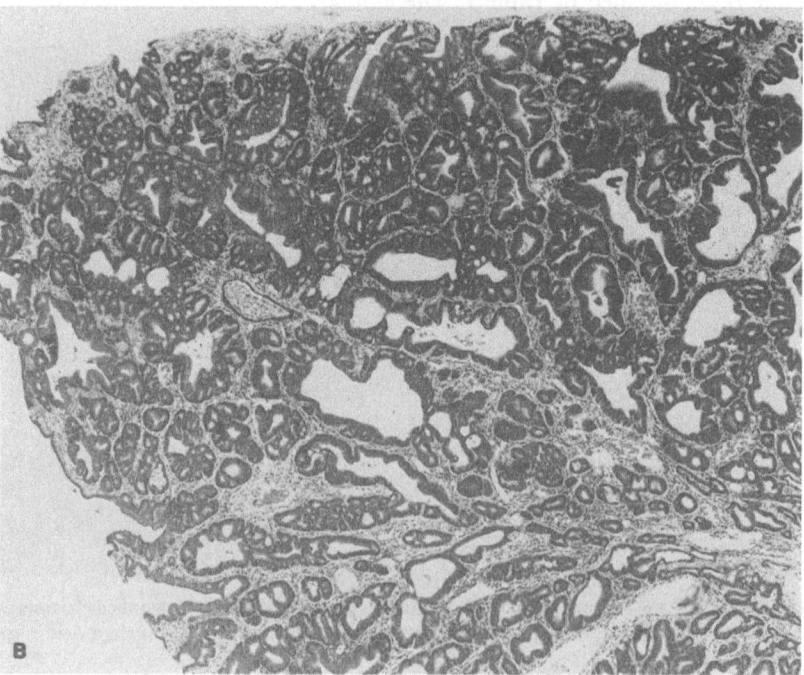

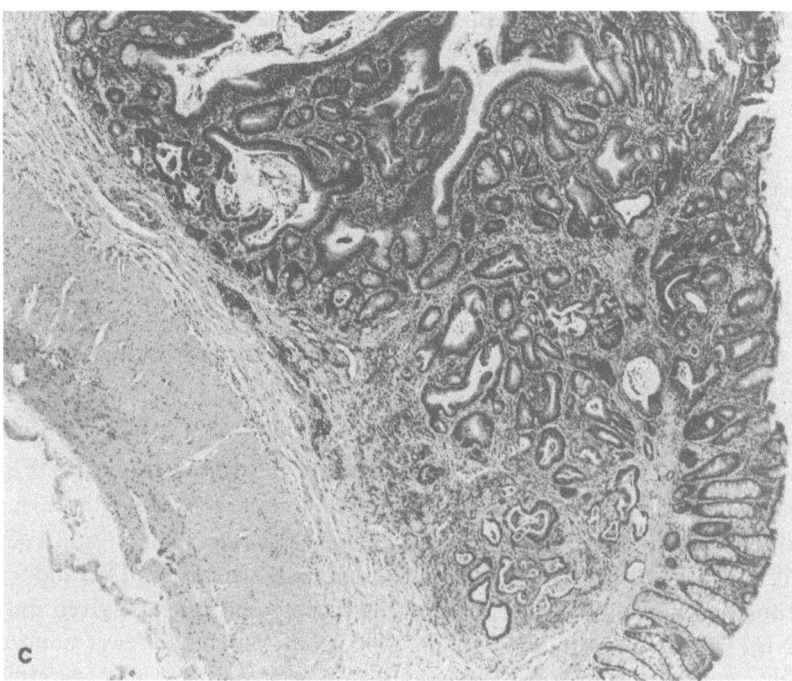

FIGURE 3. Histological and pathological examination was performed on each tumor. The tumors were either adenoma (A), carcinoma in situ (B), or invasive carcinoma (C).

compound) in the diet simultaneously with the first carcinogen treatment. The animals are kept for 28 weeks, after which time they are sacrificed and evaluated for colon cancer formation.

IV. Results

A. Effect of N-Methyl-N-nitrosourea on Tumor Formation in Animals Given Plant Sterol and/or Bile Acid

Utilizing the MNU animal model described above, we examined the potential tumor-inhibitory effect of β-sitosterol. β-Sitosterol was fed at the 0.2% level (see Table 1). No adverse affects and no deaths occurred during the 28-week experiment. Fecal steroid analysis revealed no significant changes in fecal acidic steroid composition or concentration. Fecal cholesterol concentration was also unaffected. However, there was a seven to eightfold increase in fecal concentration of β-sitosterol and its bacterial metabolites.

TABLE 2. Effects of 0.2% β-Sitosterol on Tumor Incidence in Rats Treated with 8 mg N-Methyl-N-Nitrosourea[a]

Group	Diet	Number of animals	Carcinogen	Animals with tumors Number	Animals with tumors %	Tumors/ animal	Tumors/ tumor-bearing animals
1	Control	30	—	0	—	0	—
2	β-Sitosterol	30	—	0	—	0	—
3	Control	71	+	38	54	1.10	1.92
4	β-Sitosterol	48	+	16	33[b]	0.44[b]	1.31[c]

[a] Animals were treated with carcinogen or saline and fed the plant sterol or control diet. Each animal was scored for position and type of tumor.
[b] Differs from group 3, $p < 0.05$ by Chi-square test.
[c] Differs from group 3, $p < 0.01$ by modified Chi-square test.

At 28 weeks, all tumors noted were discrete polypoid excrescences (Fig. 2). Microscopic examination revealed that the tumors progressed through a pattern of adenoma, to carcinoma in situ, to invasive carcinoma (Figs. 3A–C) (Hill et al., 1978). The data in Table 2 show that animals given MNU and fed β-sitosterol had significantly fewer tumors compared to those given only MNU (33% vs. 54%). In addition, the β-sitosterol group had fewer tumors/ animal and tumors/tumor-bearing animal. This experiment demonstrated that β-sitosterol feeding can decrease colon tumors in this animal model. Since it appeared that plant sterols could act to inhibit tumor formation, we decided to determine if plant sterols could exert an inhibitory effect in the presence of a tumor-promoting agent (bile acids).

A typical promoting experiment is outlined in Table 3. In this study, it is evident that supplementing the diet of rats with 0.2% cholic acid resulted in enhancement of colonic tumor formation. Thus, when cholic acid was added to the diet, the number of tumors/animal increased from 1.1 to 1.8, and the number of tumors/tumor-bearing animal increased from 1.92 to 2.92.

In the next experiment designed to challenge the promoting effect of cholic acid, both β-sitosterol and cholic acid were added to the diet (Table 3). In this experiment, the number of tumors/animal was 1.20, and the number of tumors/tumor-bearing animal was 1.86. Thus, the tumor-promotional affects of bile acids previously observed have been eliminated.

V. Discussion

Current data suggest that chemical carcinogens play a very significant role in the etiology of cancer in man. Cancer comes about through a

TABLE 3. Effect of Bile Acid and Plant Sterol on Tumor Incidence in Rats[a]

Group	Diet	Number of animals	Carcinogen	Animals with tumors		Tumors/ animal	Tumors/ tumor-bearing animal
				Number	%		
1	Control	36	−	—	—	—	—
2	Cholic acid (0.2%)	10	−	—	—	—	—
3	β-Sitosterol (0.2%) + cholic acid (0.2%)	36	−	—	—	—	—
4	Control	71	+	38	54	1.10	1.92
5	Cholic acid (0.2%)	42	+	26	62	1.80	2.92[b]
6	β-Sitosterol (0.2%) + cholic acid (0.2%)	75	+	49	65	1.20	1.86[c]

[a] Animals were treated with carcinogen or saline and fed the sterol bile acid or control diet for 28 weeks. Animals were examined at week 28 for position and type of tumor.
[b] Differs from group 4, $p < 0.05$ by t test.
[c] Differs from group 5, $p < 0.05$ by t test.

complicated series of steps that are not easily distinguishable from each other. Current thought delineates the process as consisting of initiation, followed by promotion, and eventually cancer. Initiation in colon carcinogenesis is probably caused by a carcinogen (or carcinogens) present in the intestinal lumen at low concentration for long periods of time. This is supported by the fact that colon cancer tends to be a cancer that is concentrated in the older age group. In addition, recent innovative studies have demonstrated mutagens in the intestinal tract of man (Bruce et al., 1979). Of particular interest is the fact that the level of mutagens is influenced by dietary factors as well as other manipulations. The nature of the mutagens in the intestinal lumen in their origin are as yet unknown and represent an area of extreme interest that demands future intensive study. Promotion follows initiation and is as important as the initiation step. Studies of animal models of colon cancer have clearly shown that bile acids can act as promoters. Both primary and secondary bile acids have this activity, but the secondary bile acids seem to be more potent agents in this regard (Wattenberg, 1977).

Reduction in tumor formation using animal models can occur for a variety of reasons. If one accepts the premise that a lumenal carcinogen and promotional agents may be involved in colon carcinogenesis, then one can postulate ways in which inhibitory agents could exert an influence. Initiation could be interferred with in several ways. Compounds could prevent metabolic activation of a carcinogen or increase inactivation. Binding of a carcinogen to prevent access to the site of action could occur. Dilution of lumenal carcinogens also could impair initiation. At the promotional stage, there are again many possibilities for influencing carcinogenesis. If a promoter is exogenous, decreasing intake would be important. Endogenous promoters could be decreased if their secretion were dependent on exogenous intake of some dietary substance (e.g., bile acids' dependence on fat intake). Other possibilities for inhibiting promotion include binding the promoter or diluting the promoter by increasing fecal bulk.

The above mechanisms are not meant to be exhaustive but to suggest a variety of means by which initiation and promotion could be inhibited. Obviously, other inhibitory mechanisms must exist, and some have been postulated, e.g., stimulation of cellular DNA repair processes, reversal of neoplasms already established (Sporn et al., 1979).

The studies we have presented clearly show that the plant sterol β-sitosterol can inhibit MNU-induced tumor formation in rats and can abolish the promotional effects of bile acids in this animal model. The significance of this finding is evident from the fact that plant sterols are abundant in our diet and thus may be very important as colon cancer-retarding agents. We believe that these agents act at the promotional stage, but it is not yet clear what the mechanism of action might be. Bile acids are membrane-active agents that clearly cause loss of colon epithelial cells leading to proliferative activity (Raicht et al., 1980). We speculated that β-sitosterol's incorporation into membranes lessens this effect, and this is presently being investigated.

ACKNOWLEDGMENTS. The authors wish to thank Miss Rubell Smith for her expert secretarial effort.

References

American Cancer Society, 1978, *Cancer Facts and Figures*, American Cancer Society, Washington.
Armstrong, B., and Doll, R., 1975, Environmental factors and cancer incidence and mortality in different countries with special reference to dietary factors, *Int. J. Cancer* 15:617.
Best, M. M., Duncan, C. H., and VanLoon, E. J., 1958, Lowering of serum cholesterol by the administration of a plant sterol, *Circulation* 10:201.
Borgstrom, B., 1969, Quantification of cholesterol absorption in man by fecal analysis after the feeding of a single isotope labeled meal, *J. Lipid Res.* 10:331.
Broitman, S. A., Vitale, J. J., Vourousek-Jakuba, E., and Gottlieb, L. S., 1977, Polyunsaturated fat, cholesterol and large bowel tumorigenesis, *Cancer* 40:2455.
Bruce, W. R., Dion, P. D., Kakizoe, T., and Land, P. C., 1979, A strategy using short term assays to identify carcinogens that act in man, *Nutr. Cancer* 1:4.
Burkitt, D. P., 1975, Large bowel carcinogenesis—an epidemiological jigsaw puzzle, *J. Natl. Cancer Inst.* 54:3.
Burkitt, D. P., Walker, A. R. P., and Pointer, N. S., 1972, Effect of dietary fibre on stools and transit times, and its role in the causation of diseases, *Lancet* 2:1408.
Chomchai, C., Bhadrochari, N., and Nigro, N. D., 1979, The effect of bile on the induction of experimental intestinal tumors in rats, *Dis. Colon Rectum* 17:310.
Cohen, B. I., Raicht, R. F., Deschner, E. E., Takahashi, M., Sarwal, A. N., and Fazzini, E., 1980, Effect of cholic acid feeding on N-methyl-N-nitrosourea-induced colon tumors and cell kinetics in rats, *J. Natl. Cancer Inst.* 64:573.
Doll, R., 1969, The geographic distribution of cancer, *Br. J. Cancer* 23:1.
Drasar, B. S., and Jenkins, D. J. A., 1976, Bacteria, diet and large bowel cancer, *Am. J. Clin. Nutr.* 29:1410.
Edwards, P. A., and Green, C., 1972, Incorporation of plant sterols into membranes and its relationship to sterol absorption, *FEBS Lett.* 20:97.
Enstrom, J. E., 1975, Colorectal cancer and consumption of beef and fat, *Br. J. Cancer* 32:432.
Glover, J., and Green, C., 1957, Sterol metabolism 3. The distribution and transport of sterols across the intestinal mucosa of the guinea pig, *Biochem. J.* 67:308.
Gordan, G. S., Fitzpatrick, M. E., and Lubich, W. P., 1967, Identification of osteolytic sterols in human breast cancer, *Trans. Assoc. Am. Physicians* 50:183.
Grundy, S. M., Ahrens, E. H., Jr., and Salen, G., 1968, Dietary β-sitosterol as an internal standard to correct for cholesterol losses in sterol balance studies, *J. Lipid Res.* 9:374.
Haenszel, W., Berg, J. W., Segi, M., Kurihara, M., and Locke, F. B., 1973, Large bowel cancer in Hawaiian Japanese, *J. Natl. Cancer Inst.* 51:1765.

Hill, M. J., Morson, B. C., and Bussey, H. J. R., 1978, Aetiology of the adenoma-carcinoma sequence in large bowel, *Lancet* **1**:245.
Jacobs, M. M., 1977, Inhibitory effects of selenium on 1,2-dimethylhydrazine and methylazoxymethanol colon carcinogenesis, *Cancer* **40**:2557.
LaMont, J. T., and O'Gorman, T. A., 1978, Experimental colon cancer, *Gastroenterology* **75**:1157.
Mellias, M. J., Ishikawa, T. T., Glueck, C. J., and Crissman, J. P., 1977, Phytosterols and cholesterol in malignant and benign breast tumors, *Cancer Res.* **37**:3034.
Miettinen, T. A., and Tarpila, S., 1978, Fecal β-sitosterol in patients with diverticular disease of the colon and in vegetarians, *Scand. J. Gastroenterol.* **13**:573.
Nigro, N. D., Bhadrochari, N., and Chomchai, C., 1973, A rat model for studying colonic cancer: Effect of cholestyramine on induced tumors, *Dis. Colon Rectum* **16**:438.
Phillips, R. L., 1975, Role of life style and dietary habits in risk of cancer among Seventh-Day Adventists, *Cancer Res.* **35**:3513.
Raicht, R. F., Cohen, B. I., Fazzini, E. P., Sarwal, A. N., and Takahashi, M., 1980, Protective effect of plant sterols against chemically induced colon tumors in rats, *Cancer Res.* **40**:403.
Reddy, B. S., 1975, Role of bile metabolites in colon carcinogenesis, *Cancer* **36**:2401.
Reddy, B. S., 1980, Effect of diet on excretion of bile acids in the feces, in: *1980 Workshop on Bile Acids and Large Bowel Carcinogenesis*, M. D. Anderson Hospital and Tumor Institute, Houston.
Reddy, B. S., and Wynder, E. L., 1973, Large bowel carcinogenesis: Fecal constituents of populations with diverse incidence rates of colon cancer, *J. Natl. Cancer Inst.* **50**:1437.
Reddy, B. S., and Wynder, E. L., 1977, Metabolic epidemiology of colon cancer: Fecal bile acids with neutral sterols in colon cancer patients and patients with adenomatous polyps, *Cancer* **39**:2533.
Reddy, B. S., Narisawa, T., Maronpot, R., Weisburger, J. H., and Wynder, E. L., 1975a, Animal models for the study of dietary factors and cancer of the large bowel, *Cancer Res.* **35**:3421.
Reddy, B. S., Weisburger, J. H., and Wynder, E. L., 1975b, Effects of high risk and low risk diets for colon carcinogenesis on fecal microflora and steroids in man, *J. Nutr.* **105**:878.
Reddy, B. S., Mastromarino, A., Gustafson, C., Lipkin, M., and Wynder, E. L., 1976a, Fecal bile acids and neutral sterols in patients with familial polyposis, *Cancer* **38**:1694.
Reddy, B. S., Narisawa, T., Weisburger, J. H., and Wynder, E. L., 1976b, Promoting effect of sodium deoxycholate on colon adenocarcinomas in germ free rats, *J. Natl. Cancer Inst.* **56**:441.
Reddy, B. S., Narisawa, T., and Weisburger, J. H., 1976c, Effect of a diet with high levels of protein and fat on colon carcinogenesis in F344 rats treated with 1,2-dimethylhydrazine, *J. Natl. Cancer Inst.* **57**:567.
Reddy, B. S., Mangot, S., Sheinfel, A., Weisburger, J. H., and Wynder, E. L., 1977a, Effect of type and amount of dietary fat and 1,2-dimethylhydrazine and biliary bile acids, fecal bile acid and neutral sterols in rats, *Cancer Res.* **37**:2132.
Reddy, B. S., Martin, C. W., and Wynder, E. L., 1977b, Fecal bile acids and cholesterol metabolites of patients with ulcerative colitis, a high risk group for development of colon cancer, *Cancer Res.* **37**:1697.
Reddy, B. S., Watanabe, K., Weisburger, J. H., and Wynder, E. L., 1977c, Promoting effect of bile acids in colon carcinogenesis in germ free and conventional F344 rats, *Cancer Res.* **37**:3238.
Reddy, B. S., Hedge, A. R., Laakso, K., and Wynder, E. L., 1978a, Metabolic epidemiology of large bowel cancer, *Cancer* **41**:2832.
Reddy, B. S., Weisburger, J. H., and Wynder, E. L., 1978b, Colon Cancer: Bile salts as tumor promoters, *Mechanism of Tumor Promotion and Cocarcinogenesis* (T. J. Slage, A. Swok, and R. K. Botwell, eds.), pp. 453-464, Raven Press, New York.

Sarwal, A. N., Cohen, B. I., Raicht, R. F., Takahashi, M., and Fazzini, E., 1979, Effects of dietary administration of chenodeoxycholic acid on N-methyl-N-nitrosourea-induced colon cancer in rats, *Biochim. Biophys. Acta* **574**:423.

Sporn, M. B., Newton, D. L., Smith, J. M., Acton, N., Jacobson, A. E., and Brossi, A. 1979, Retinoids in cancer prevention, in: *Carcinogens: Identification and Mechanisms of Action, The University of Texas System Cancer Center, 31st Annual Symposium on Fundamental Cancer Research*, (A. Clark Griffin and Charles R. Shaw, eds.), pp. 441-453, Raven Press, New York.

Stemmerman, G. N., 1970, Patterns of disease among Japanese living in Hawaii, *Arch. Environ. Health* **20**:266.

Subbiah, M. T. R., 1971, Significance of dietary plant sterols in man and experimental animals, *Mayo Clin. Proc.* **46**:549.

Subbiah, M. T. R., Kuksis, A., and Moorkeryea, S., 1969, Secretion of bile salts by intact and isolated rat livers, *Can. J. Biochem.* **47**:847.

Wattenberg, L. W., 1972, Inhibition of carcinogenic and toxic effects of polycyclic hydrocarbons by phenolic antioxidants and ethoxyquin, *J. Natl. Cancer Inst.* **48**:1425.

Wattenberg, L. W., 1977, Inhibition of carcinogenic effects of polycyclic hydrocarbons by benzyl isothiocyanates and related compounds, *J. Natl. Cancer Inst.* **58**:395.

Wynder, E. L., and Reddy, B. S., 1974, Metabolic epidemiology of colorectal cancer, *Cancer* **34**:801.

Wynder, E. L., and Reddy, B. S., 1975, Dietary fat and colon cancer, *J. Natl. Cancer Inst.* **53**:7.

Wynder, E. L., Kajitani, T., Ishikawa, S., Dodo, H., and Takano, A., 1969, Environmental factors of cancer of the colon and rectum II, Japanese epidemiological data, *Cancer* **23**:1210.

8

Immunoprevention

HANS OLOV SJÖGREN

I. Introduction

Prevention of large bowel cancer by immunological mechanisms has not yet been attempted in humans. Various approaches to achieve a basis for judgment of the feasability of immunoprophylaxis are best worked out in animal models such as the DMH-induced bowel cancer of the rat. Preventive interventions are ideally directed against the inducing agents. At present it does not appear possible to use immunological methods for that purpose. Instead, various approaches involving stimulation of immunity to tumor cell antigens have been investigated. A fundamental requirement is the presence of tumor-associated antigens (TAA) on large bowel cancer cells. The *in vitro* and *in vivo* evidence for the existence of tumor-associated antigens in rat bowel cancer will be reviewed in Section II. It has been reported that in this model stimulation of immunity before a tumor has developed and also after tumor appearance may lead to prevention of tumor growth. Preventive effects have been achieved both by stimulation of immunity to transplantable colon carcinoma cells and to embryonic cells at certain stages of differentiation. This evidence will be reviewed and some implications discussed.

II. Detection of Tumor-Associated Antigens in Experimental Rat Bowel Carcinomas

Bowel carcinomas may be induced in rats with various chemical carcinogens, among which 1,2-dimethylhydrazine (DMH) has been most widely used

---

HANS OLOV SJÖGREN • The Wallenberg Laboratory, University of Lund, Lund, Sweden.

(Druckrey, 1970). Histologically, the induced carcinomas are closely similar to the human counterparts (Lindström, 1978). However, at the dose levels used, multiple rather than single neoplasms usually appear. A striking difference is also that liver metastasis is only very rarely seen in this model.

Bowel carcinomas induced in rats with 1,2-dimethylhydrazine or N-methyl-N'-nitrosoguanidine (MNNG) possess tumor-associated antigens demonstrable by *in vitro* techniques (Steele and Sjögren, 1974a; Sjögren and Steele, 1975). Cellular immunity and humoral antibodies against antigens with tissue type specificity are induced in rats developing primary bowel carcinomas, in recipients of isografts of such tumors, and in animals immunized with several doses of irradiated colorectal cancer cells (Sjögren, 1978). This immunity has been demonstrated by lymphocyte cytotoxicity assays with lymph node cells and blood lymphocytes (Steele and Sjögren, 1974a), complement dependent cytotoxicity tests with sera (Steele *et al.*, 1974b; Sjögren, 1979), antibody-binding assays (T. Brodin and H. O. Sjögren, unpublished), and antibody-dependent cellular cytotoxicity (ADCC) tests (Sjögren, 1979; Table 1). Sera of tumor-bearing rats were found to block specifically the lymphocyte cytotoxicity against the tumor cells (Steele and Sjögren, 1974a). Evidence for immunity to unique antigens and tissue type-specific antigens has also been obtained in neutralization tests with lymphocytes (so called Winn tests) (H. O. Sjögren and P. Flodgren, unpublished) and in isograft-rejection tests *in vivo* (Steele, 1975; Sjögren, 1978). The isograft resistance induced on the basis of common tissue type-specific antigens was found to be rather weak compared to that induced on the basis of unique antigens.

III. Evidence that Embryonic Antigens Are Associated with Bowel Carcinomas

Several lines of evidence indicate that some tumor-associated antigens that are shared by various bowel carcinomas are also expressed on embryonic cells at certain stages of development (Table 2). Lymph node cells of rats bearing bowel carcinoma are cytotoxic to gut cells of 13- to 15- day-old fetuses (Steele and Sjogren, 1974b). Similarly, the sera contain antibodies to embryonic cells (Martin *et al.*, 1975).

Immunity to embryonic cell antigens is also manifested as reactivity to colorectal carcinoma cells. Lymphocytes and sera of multiparous rats are reactive to embryonic cells and to bowel cancer cells as well but not to adult normal cells (Steele and Sjögren, 1974b). Cocultivation of normal spleen cells

TABLE 1. Detection of Immunity to Tumor-Associated Antigens
of Large Bowel Carcinomas in Rats Immunized to or Bearing
the Target Tumor or Other Bowel Carcinomas

In vitro
  Complement-dependent serum cytotoxicity to cultured colon carcinoma target cells
  Ig-binding assays
  Antibody-dependent cellular cytotoxicity (ADCC)
  Lymphocyte cytotoxicity

In vivo
  Neutralization of isograft growth by lymphocytes (Winn assay)
  Isograft rejection

---

of virgin females with embryonic cells leads to reactivity to embryonic cells and to bowel carcinoma cells as well (Nelson and Sjögren, 1978). When solubilized colon carcinoma membranes were admixed to lymphocytes of multiparous rats *in vitro*, the cytotoxicity of the lymphocytes to embryonic cells and tumor cells was blocked specifically (Steele *et al.*, 1975). This indicates that embryonic antigens are present in the membrane extracts of the bowel cancer cells. Subcutaneous inoculation of suspended embryonic cells was also shown to induce isograft immunity to a transplantable colon carcinoma (Steele, 1975). A similar isograft rejection was demonstrated as a result of implantation of fetal colon beneath the kidney capsule (Hedlund and Sjögren, 1980). Rats bearing primary large bowel carcinomas have also been reported to reject implants of syngeneic embryonic gut cells (B. R. Bansal *et al.*, 1978a).

TABLE 2. Immunological Similarities between
Bowel Cancer Cells and Fetal Cells

Immunization to bowel cancer cells results in immunity also to cultured fetal cells
  Lymphocytes of rats bearing colon cancers are cytotoxic to cultured fetal cells.
  Sera of rats bearing colon cancers contain antibodies reacting with fetal cells.
  Rabbit antisera to rat colon cancers are reactive to fetal bowel cells after appropriate absorption with adult normal bowel tissue.

Immunization to fetal cells results in immunity also to cultured colon carcinoma cells
  Lymphocytes of multiparous females are cytotoxic to cultured colon carcinoma cells.
  Normal lymphocytes cocultivated with syngeneic fetal cells become cytotoxic to cultured colon cancer cells.
  Sera of multiparous females contain antibodies reacting with cultured colon cancer cells.
  Immunization with embryonic cells induces isograft immunity to colon carcinomas.

Extracts of colon cancer tissue contain embryonic antigens
  Partially purified fractions of tumor extracts can block the cytotoxicity of multiparous lymphocytes to fetal cells.

IV. Enhanced 1,2-Dimethylhydrazine-Induced Tumorigenesis in Immunosuppressed Rats

Although most models using tumor viruses successfully demonstrated an increased tumor incidence in immunosuppressed animals (Allison *et al.*, 1974; Stutman, 1975), evidence has been inconclusive in models using chemical carcinogens (Baldwin, 1975; Kroes *et al.*, 1975; Andrews, 1974). It has not been established whether this discrepancy is caused by differences in strength of immune surveillance in the systems or results from an immunosuppressive action of chemical carcinogens obliterating any further effect by additional immunosuppression (Klein, 1975; Stutman, 1969). 1,2-Dimethylhydrazine in the doses given in tumorigenesis experiments does not seem to have an immunosuppressive effect (S. C. Bansal *et al.*, 1978). Provided the tumor-associated antigens detectable in the previously mentioned *in vitro* tests and in isograft-rejection tests *in vivo* are indeed of importance in DMH carcinogenesis, immunosuppression would be expected to cause a facilitated tumor development. On the other hand, prevention or delay of tumor development may be anticipated as a result of bolstering of immunity to the tumor antigens. One efficient way of achieving immunological (T-cell) suppression is to administer antithymocyte immunoglobulin (ATG) (Levey and Medawar, 1966). The effect of such treatment on the induction of bowel cancer by DMH has been studied by S. C. Bansal *et al.* (1978). The proportion of animals developing multiple bowel carcinomas was increased by ATG treatment from 17% to 61% in one series and from 20% to 73% in another series. The frequency of tumors that metastasized within the observation period was also significantly increased. Both the total number of tumors developing and the proportion that grew invasively were augmented in the immunosuppressed rats.

V. Inhibitory Effect on Bowel Carcinogenesis by Immunization with Transplantable Syngeneic Colon Carcinoma

On the basis of the *in vitro* demonstration of common antigens associated with colorectal carcinomas and the fact that these antigens are also detectable in isograft-rejection tests, I investigated whether immunization with a colorectal carcinoma might have a preventive effect on DMH-induced tumorigenesis (Sjögren, 1978). Five groups of rats were given a standardized DMH treatment. One control group received no further treatment. Another group received subcutaneous isografts of a control breast tumor. When the tumor had grown out, it was surgically removed, and carcinogen administration was initiated after 2 weeks. Three further groups were similarly isografted with three different colon carcinomas. After excision and appropriate carcinogen treatment all animals were followed closely for tumor appearance by repeated double-contrast bowel examinations (Rosengren, 1978) and laparotomies. The group of rats pretreated with breast tumor had the same frequency of bowel carcinomas as the control group without pretreatment. The group pretreated with one of the colon carcinomas showed a significantly reduced frequency of rats developing primary bowel carcinomas: 20% developed tumor within 50 weeks as compared to 46% in the control group. The number of tumors per rat was significantly lower in this group than in the control group (0.29 as compared to 0.64 tumors per rat). The groups pretreated with the other two colon carcinomas did not show a significant inhibition of tumorigenesis. It was concluded that immunization against some tumor antigens shared among bowel carcinomas may form a basis for immunopreventive intervention.

These results are compatible with other evidence of immune responses to common tumor-associated antigens early in the latency period, long before detection of primary tumors in carcinogen-treated rats. Figure 1 illustrates the appearance of antibodies detectable in cytotoxicity assays with complement both in rats preimmunized to a transplantable colon carcinoma and in untreated animals as well. Analogous sera of rats that did not develop bowel carcinoma but kidney carcinoma contained no antibody activity. Those preimmunized rats that remained tumor-free developed rather low but significant levels of antibodies. Those preimmunized rats that did develop a primary tumor often had high titers of antibodies by early in the latency period. The cytotoxic activity was associated with the IgM fraction of the sera (Sjögren, 1979). These antibodies were also detectable in binding assays and in ADCC tests (Sjögren, 1979; Brodin and Sjögren, unpublished). Sera of some animals were also tested for antibody activity against cultured embryonic cells as compared to normal adult cells. Antibody activity towards embryonic cells parallelled the activity against bowel carcinoma target cells. A more complete immunological analysis remains to be performed to dissect classes and subclasses of the immunoglobulins that account for the various antibody activities such as complement-dependent cytotoxicity, ADCC, and possibly interference with antibody and lymphocyte cytotoxicity and ADCC. Furthermore, it will also be necessary to distinguish the alterations in the cell-mediated immunity associated with the spontaneously developing immunity from that induced by immunological interventions.

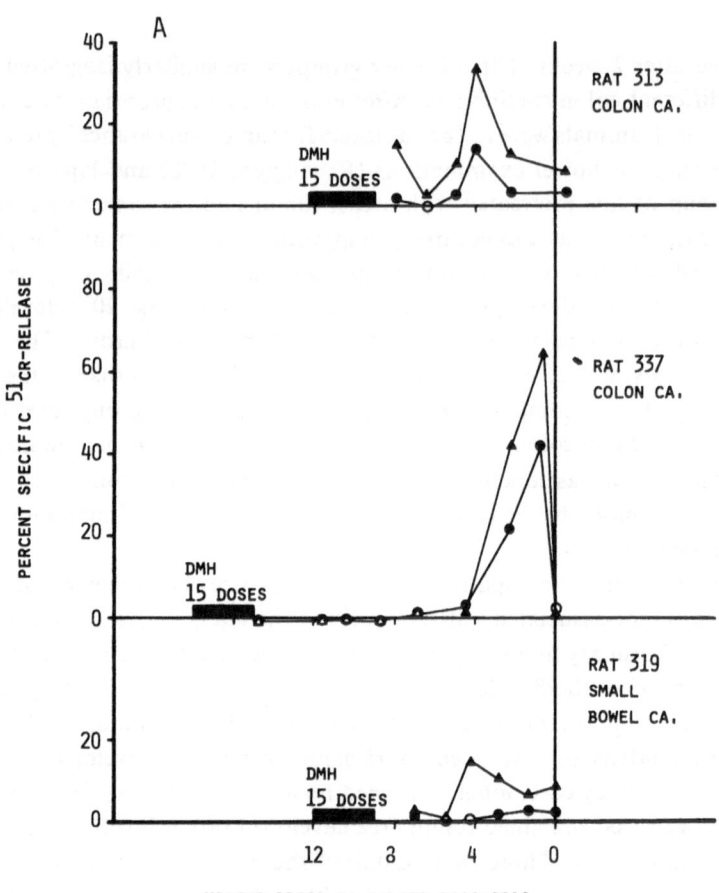

FIGURE 1. Detection of humoral antibodies to bowel cancer cells in rats treated with DMH after preimmunization with colon carcinoma DMH-W49 or without such immunization. Tests for complement-dependent cytotoxicity against syngenic DMH-W163 colon carcinoma cells (measured as percentage of ^{51}Cr release) with sequential sera of rats exposed to DMH with no other treatment (A) or pretreated with colon carcinoma DMH-W49 (B), respectively. All sera were tested at dilutions 1:20 (Δ) and 1:40 (O). Statistically significant values are indicated by filled symbols.

VI. Inhibitory Effect on Bowel Carcinogenesis by Immunization with Fetal Tissue

The effect of repeated immunizations against fetal liver and gut tissue on DMH-induced carcinogenesis has been studied (B. R. Bansal *et al.*, 1978a). After a 9-month period, all of 19 control rats had developed tumors, and the

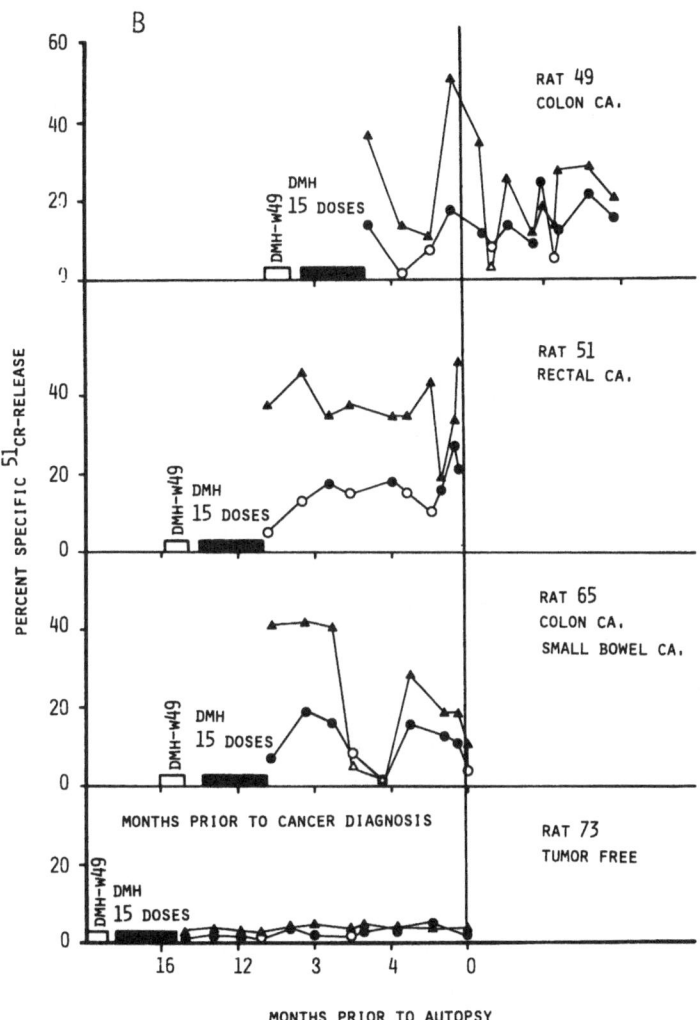

FIGURE 1. (*Continued*)

average number of tumors per rat was 3.1. Only 15 of 31 rats receiving three doses of suspended liver and gut tissue from 12- to 13- day-old embryos had developed tumors within this time period with an average of 0.7 tumors per animal. Twenty-four rats immunized with liver and gut tissue of newborn rats all developed cancer with an average of 2.0 tumors per rat.

It is evident that the tissue of 12- to 13- day-old embryos but not newborn animals induced a significant preventive effect on bowel carcinogenesis. The effect tended to be somewhat stronger in males than in females. This finding agrees with previous reports in other tumor systems, demonstrating the highest concentrations of embryonic antigens of the type appearing in tumor cells in 13- to 15-day-old embryos with a fall to undetectable levels at the end of gestation (Baldwin et al., 1974). These experiments did not explore whether or not the embryonic antigens were organ specific.

VII. Inhibition of 1,2-Dimethylhydrazine-Induced Carcinogenesis in Multiparous Rats

Multiparous females have been shown to develop demonstrable immunity against bowel carcinoma cells *in vitro* (Steele and Sjögren, 1974b). I therefore investigated whether such animals also showed a relative resistance to induction of bowel cancer by DMH (Sjögren, 1977). Two groups of animals were tested. One consisted of breeding females that were mated at the initiation of DMH treatment and had a minimum of three litters in the course of the experiment. The other group contained females that had had a minimum of three litters before the experiment and were not further mated after initiation of DMH treatment. The first group of breeding females showed a reduced tumor frequency (18% tumor-positive rats 50 weeks after DMH treatment versus 46% in controls). In addition, the group of older multiparous females showed a significantly reduced frequency of rats with bowel cancer and fewer tumors per rat compared to age-matched virgin females. One interpretation of these results is that immunization against the embryonic antigens is capable of rejecting early primary tumors. However, alternative interpretations have not yet been ruled out. It has not been studied whether the observed reduction of tumor incidence in these rats was the result of hormonal influences during the pregnancies rather than of immunization against embryonic antigens. However, this explanation would be less likely in those rats that had no pregnancies after carcinogen administration.

VIII. Effect of Tumor Resection on the Development of Additional Primary Tumors

It has been established in rat bowel cancer and in other experimental tumor systems that excision of a primary tumor leads to rather rapid disappearance of the serum-blocking activity against lymphocyte, whereas the lymphocyte cytotoxicity itself is not rapidly decreased in animals subjected to tumor excision (Sjögren and Bansal, 1971). On this basis, it was studied how excision of a first primary tumor in rats treated with DMH affected the appearance of additional tumors (B. R. Bansal *et al.*, 1979). Since removal of a tumor by excision may be regarded as an immunological intervention, decreasing the serum content of factors blocking the lymphocyte cytotoxicity and also leading to the appearance of complement-dependent cytotoxic antibodies, one might expect the early removal of a first tumor to inhibit the appearance of additional tumors.

It was indeed found that the early excision of a first tumor decreased the frequency of rats developing further tumors and also reduced the total number of additional tumors developing. This was evident also when comparison was made to controls undergoing bowel surgery but with the first primary tumor left intact in an isolated segment of colon. That the reduced frequency of additional tumors had an immunological basis was indicated by the fact that when rats subjected to tumor removal were treated with immunosuppressive doses of ATG, the appearance of additional tumors and the frequency of metastasis were significantly increased, approaching the frequency seen in controls.

IX. Regression of Early Primary Bowel Carcinomas by Multimodal Immunological Treatment

Working with the rat colorectal carcinoma model, B. R. Bansal *et al.* (1978b) established a certain DMH dose and administration scheme by which all rats, by 140–150 days after the initiation of DMH, would develop either clinically visible bowel cancer or alterations in bowel mucosa such as carcinoma *in situ* and/or mucosal tumors capable of developing into infiltrating cancer. Various groups of animals were subjected to different immunological treatments initiated 150 days after the first dose of DMH was given (B. R. Bansal *et al.*, 1978b). The aim of the immunological manipulations was threefold: (1) to increase the general immunocompetence of the rats nonspecifically by administering levamisole and *Corynebacterium parvum*; (2) to increase specific cell-mediated immunity by passive transfer of presensitized lymphoid cells; and (3) to counteract the serum-blocking activity of tumor-bearing rats by splenectomy and passive transfer of antitumor antiboides with demonstrated "unblocking activity" (Hellström and Hellström, 1970; S. C. Bansal and Sjögren, 1971). Optimal results were reported by use of a combination of all of these immunological manipulations over a 4-month period. The effect of the

TABLE 3. Immunoprevention of 1,2-Dimethylhydrazine-Induced Carcinogenesis in Rats

Immunological treatment		Prevention effect			
		Reduced frequency of			
Treatment	Scheme in relation to initiation of DMH administration	Rats developing bowel cancer	Tumors per rat	Metastic spread	References
Colon carcinoma isografting	Temporary growth and excision 2 weeks before carcinogen	+	+	−	Sjögren, 1978
Bowel and liver from 12–13 day old fetuses	3 doses after carcinogen	+	+	+	B. R. Bansal et al., 1978a
Multiple pregnancies	Before carcinogen After carcinogen	+ +	+ +	− −	Sjögren, 1977 Sjögren, 1977
Resection of a first bowel carcinoma	After completion of carcinogen treatment	+	+		B. R. Bansal et al., 1979
Combined treatment with *C. parvum* and lavamisole, transfer of sensitized lymphocytes and "unblocking" serum, and splenectomy	After completion of carcinogen treatment when early tumors had already developed	+	+	−	B. R. Bansal et al., 1978b

treatment on development of primary bowel carcinomas was studied by repeated laparotomies once a month until 12 months after initiation of DMH treatment, when all animals were killed and autopsied except for those animals that had already succumbed to progressive tumor growth. In the untreated control group, all ten animals had developed tumors within 10 months. All of these animals were found to have metastatic spread intraperitoneally at the time of autopsy.

The rats subjected to multimodal immunotherapy developed tumors in a significantly lower frequency (six out of ten rats at the time of autopsy). None of these tumors had metastasized. The total number of tumors at autopsy was seven in ten animals, whereas 21 tumors were detected in the ten animals of the control group. Two tumors were temporarily detectable for a 3-month period in the treated group but were macroscopically undetectable at autopsy. Histological investigation detected fibrotic remnants of the recorded tumors. Four of the seven tumors in the treated group had evidence of severe tumor rejection in the form of extensive necrosis, fibrosis, and lymphocyte infiltration. Out of 18 control tumors, only one had evidence of a moderate rejection response.

This investigation indicates that it is possible to entirely protect some animals from tumor development by immunological intervention, to cause complete regression of established tumors in some animals, to markedly inhibit tumor growth, and to totally inhibit metastatic spread. Because of the multimodal form of immunotherapy it is impossible to single out any particular part of the combined therapy as the most efficient component. Rather, the study clearly indicated that the multimodal form of therapy was superior to any of the less extensive modes tested. These results are particularly important since the immunological intervention came rather late, initiated at a stage when most animals would be expected to have already developed an early tumor.

X. Conclusions

The following conclusions may be drawn from the studies in the rat model of DMH-induced bowel cancer.

1. Immunosuppressive treatment facilitates carcinogenesis.
2. Immunization to antigens known to be shared among a majority of bowel cancers has an inhibitory effect on tumorigenesis.
3. Multimodal immunological intervention instituted at a stage when

early primary tumors have already developed may cause a significant decrease in growth rate and may result in tumor regression.
4. The achieved immunoprevention is not complete but rather is only partially effective. There is still no immunological treatment that leads to a complete prophylaxis in all animals even when immunization is allowed to precede carcinogen exposure.

It is not yet known what distinguishes those animals that are protected by the immunological treatment from those that are not. Therefore, it is not yet possible to predict which individuals will remain tumor-free and which will not benefit from the treatment on the basis of immunological tests. The preventive effects so far reported are limited to essentially one animal model, the DMH-induced bowel cancers in rats. It remains to be established which of these procedures have a general applicability.

The obvious possibility of combining the immunoprevention with other preventive treatments in order to achieve higher efficiency has not yet been explored. Such combined ventures are likely to have the greatest potential.

Although animals have tolerated the various immunological manipulations well, there has been no critical evaluation of the possible side effects of the procedures. Some of the procedures used are likely to cause various more or less serious problems, particularly when executed over long periods of time. This aspect will require special consideration if a preventive treatment is to be extended to patients at lower cancer risk.

The most important question of whether human large bowel cancer can be prevented by immunological means cannot be answered on the basis of the presently available data. However, there are a number of similarities between the immunological features of human bowel cancer and the rat colorectal carcinoma model. There is *in vitro* evidence of shared tissue type-specific antigens associated with human colorectal carcinomas which are capable of inducing immunity in the original tumor host (Hellström *et al.,* 1971). The technical difficulties are considerable in demonstrating the specificity of these reactions in individual patients because of the existence of spontaneously cytotoxic lymphocytes (Herberman and Holden, 1978). Comparisons among various groups of patients allow safer conclusions concerning the existence of these antigens. Studies of patients' immunity to their own bowel cancers support the conclusion that immunity to colon cancer antigens does indeed exist. However, the efficiency *in vivo* of such immune reactions is entirely unknown, primarily because of the technical difficulties in performing *in vivo* experiments in human patients. To prove the *in vivo* importance of the immunity demonstrated *in vitro*, it will probably be necessary to achieve successful immunotherapy or immunoprevention.

In view of these technical difficulties in the human application, the work with animal models chosen to be analogous to the human bowel cancer is most important. If efficient immunoprevention of bowel cancer could be achieved in model systems, very precise experiments could be defined to explore the applicability of the same principles in human patients. Several recent developments in tumor immunology remains to be explored in terms of immunotherapy and prevention of large bowel cancer. Among these are various manipulations to increase the efficiency of the cellular effectors by, e.g., elimination of suppressor subpopulations, *in vitro* sensitization and boostering, and prolonged *in vitro* cultivation and multiplication of cytotoxic effector cells followed by reinfusion. Studies of the possible therapeutic use of monoclonal antitumor antibodies and *in vitro* removal of certain interfering factors, including certain immunoglobulins, immune complexes, and circulating tumor antigens, have only recently been initiated.

As long as the etiological condition or agent is not eliminated, it is likely that even a temporarily very efficient immunological treatment would have to be maintained over a very long period of time in order to prevent new tumors from developing. Therefore, immunological prevention is not likely to be developed as a general procedure except when directed against etiological agents. Immunological prevention would rather be feasible for selected, high-risk groups of patients already exposed to the inducing agents.

ACKNOWLEDGMENTS. This work was supported by Public Health Service Grant CA-14924 from the National Cancer Institute through the National Large Bowel Cancer Project and by grants from the Swedish Cancer Society, the John and Augusta Persson's Foundation, and the Medical Faculty, University of Lund.

References

Allison, A. C., Monga, J. N., and Hammond, V., 1974, Increased susceptability to virus oncogenesis of congenitally thymus deprived nude mice, *Nature* 252:746.

Andrews, E. J., 1974, Failure of immunosurveillance against chemically induced in situ tumors in mice, *J. Natl. Cancer Inst.* 52:729.

Baldwin, R. W., 1976, Role of immunosurveillance against chemically induced rat tumors, *Transplant. Rev.* 28:62.

Baldwin, R. W., Embleton, M. J., Price, M. R., and Vose, B. M., 1974, Embryonic antigen expression on experimental rat tumors, *Transplant. Rev.* 20:77.

Bansal, B. R., Mark, R., Rhoads, J. E., and Bansal, S. C., 1978a, Effect of embryonic tissue immunization on chemically induced gastrointestinal tumors in rats. I. Embryonic antigens can act as rejection antigens? *J. Natl. Cancer Inst.* 61:189.

Bansal, B. R., Mobini, J., and Bansal, S. C., 1978b, Multimodal immunotherapy of primary gastrointestinal tumors in rats. I. Histologic correlation, *Cancer* 42:2079.

Bansal, B. R., Mark, R., Mobini, J., Rhoads, J. E., and Bansal, S. C., 1979, Demonstration of antitumor immunity in an autochthonous host bearing 1,2-dimethylhydrazine-induced primary colon tumors, *J. Natl. Cancer Inst.* **63**:127.

Bansal, S. C., and Sjögren, H. O., 1971, "Unblocking" serum activity in in vitro in the polyoma system may correlate with antitumour effects of antiserum in vivo, *Nature* **233**:76.

Bansal, S. C., Mark, R., Bansal, B. R., and Rhoads, J. E., 1978, Immunologic surveillance against chemically induced primary colon carcinoma in rats, *J. Natl. Cancer Inst.* **60**:667.

Druckrey, H., 1970, Production of colonic carcinomas by 1,2-dialkylhydrazines and azoxyalkanes, in: *Carcinoma of the Colon and Antecedent Epithelium* (N. J. Burdette, ed.), pp. 267–279, Thomas, Springfield, Ill.

Hedlund, G., and Sjögren, H. O., 1980, Induction of transplantation immunity to rat colon carcinoma isografts by implantation of intact fetal colon tissue, *Int. J. Cancer* **26**:71–73.

Hellström, I., and Hellström, K. E., 1970, Colony inhibition studies on blocking and non-blocking serum effects on cellular immunity to Moloney sarcomas, *Int. J. Cancer* **5**:195.

Hellström, I., Hellström, K. E., Sjögren, H. O., and Warner, G. A., 1971, Demonstration of cell-mediated immunity to human neoplasms of various histological types, *Int. J. Cancer* **7**:1.

Herberman, R. B., and Holden, H. T., 1978, Natural cell-mediated immunity, *Adv. Cancer Res.* **27**:305–377.

Klein, G., 1975, Immunological surveillance against neoplasia, *Harvey Lect.* **69**:71.

Kroes, R., Berkvens, J. M., and Weisburger, J. H., 1975, Immunosuppression in primary liver and colon tumor induction with N-hydroxy-N-2-fluorenylacetamide and azoxymethane, *Cancer Res.* **35**:2651.

Levey, R. H., and Medawar, P. B., 1966, Some experiments on the action of antilymphocyte sera, *Ann. N. Y. Acad. Sci.* **129**:164.

Lindstrom, C. G., 1978, Experimental colo-rectal tumours in the rat, *Acta Pathol. Microbiol. Scand.* [*Suppl.*] **268**:1–75.

Martin, F., Knobel, S., Martin, M., and Bordes, M., 1975, A carcinofetal antigen located on the membrane of cells from rat intestinal carcinoma in culture, *Cancer Res.* **35**:333.

Nelson, K. A., and Sjögren, H. O., 1978, Effects of presensitization in vivo on cell-mediated responses to embryonic antigens in vitro, *Int. J. Cancer* **21**:108.

Nelson, K. A., Sjögren, H. O., and Rosengren, J. E., 1977, Detection of antibodies to embryonic antigens in sera of multiparous or colon tumor-bearing rats by a new indirect immunofluorescence assay, *Int. J. Cancer* **20**:227.

Rosengren, J. E., 1978, Experimental colonic tumors in the rat. I. Preparation and technique of examination, *Acta Radiol.* [*Diagn.*] **19**:353.

Sjögren, H. O., 1977, Overview: The application of immunology of the development of immunotherapeutic programs for patients with large bowel cancer, *Cancer* **40**:2710.

Sjögren, H. O., 1978, Immunology of experimentally induced large bowel bowel cancer, in: *Carcinoma of the Colon and Rectum* (W. E. Enker, ed.), pp. 247–258, Year Book Medical Publishers, Chicago.

Sjögren, H. O., 1979, Immunologic studies on rat bowel carcinomas, *Immunodiagnosis and Immunotherapy of Malignant Tumors* (H.-D. Flad, Ch. Herfarth, and M. Betzler, eds.), pp. 20–28, Springer-Verlag, New York.

Sjögren, H. O., and Bansal, S. C., 1971, Antigens in virally induced tumors, in: *Progress in Immunology* (B. Amos, ed.), pp. 921–938, Academic Press, New York.

Sjögren, H. O., and Steele, G., Jr., 1975, Colon carcinoma antigens in the rat, *Ann. N. Y. Acad. Sci.* **259**:404.

Steele, G., Jr., 1975, *Immunologic Studies of Chemically Induced Rat Bowel Tumors*, Thesis, University of Lund.

Steele, G., Jr., and Sjögren, H. O., 1974a, Cross-reacting tumor-associated antigen(s) among chemically induced rat colon carcinomas, *Cancer Res.* **34**:1801.

Steele, G., Jr., and Sjögren, H. O., 1974b, Embryonic antigens associated with chemically induced colon carcinomas in rats, *Int. J. Cancer* **14**:435.

Steele, G., Jr., Ankerst, J., and Sjögren, H. O., 1974, Alteration of in vitro anti-tumor activity of tumor-bearer sera by absorption with *Staphylococcus aureus, Cowan I, Int. J. Cancer* **14**:83.

Steele, G. Jr., Sjögren, H. O., and Price, M. R., 1975, Tumor-associated and embryonic antigens in soluble fractions of a chemically-induced rat colon carcinoma, *Int. J. Cancer* **16**:33.

Stutman, O., 1969, Carcinogen-induced immunodepression: Absence in mice resistant to chemical carcinogenesis, *Science* **166**:620.

Stutman, O. 1975, Tumor development after polyoma infection in a thymic nude mice, *J. Immunol.* **114**:1213.

9
Summation and Future Challenges

RULON W. RAWSON, MARTIN
LIPKIN, and MORRIS S. ZEDECK

I. Introduction

The foregoing chapters have described a variety of studies on the prevention of tumor induction in experimental animals using a wide spectrum of naturally occurring and synthetic compounds. These substances act in different ways to inhibit the actions of carcinogenic agents in many organ systems. Studies of immunoprevention have also been described.

Of considerable interest is the finding that these inhibitors of tumor development differ in their mechanism of action. The mechanisms of tumor inhibition include inhibition of the formation of carcinogens, inhibition of the activation of procarcinogens to proximate and ultimate carcinogens, enhancement of the detoxification of carcinogens, prevention of the interaction of ultimate carcinogens with macromolecules such as DNA and RNA, and prevention of the progression of chemically altered cells to the state of neoplasia.

It may be anticipated that other mechanisms of tumor inhibition are also possible and that many different types of compounds will be needed to inhibit tumor development. This is especially important in considering the future

---

RULON W. RAWSON • Bonneville Center for Research on Cancer Cause and Prevention, University of Utah Research Institute, Salt Lake City, Utah 84108. MARTIN LIPKIN and MORRIS S. ZEDECK • Memorial Sloan-Kettering Cancer Center, New York, New York 10021.

extension of these studies to human populations where agents presumed to be responsible for at least part of the total incidence of human cancer are very diverse in structure and activity.

II. Challenges to Chemists and Molecular and Cell Biologists

A large and important group of chemical carcinogens whose formation and/or actions will have to be inhibited are those that occur naturally in the environment. These may originate as products of combustion, such as polycyclic aromatic hydrocarbons, as products of modern processes such as food preservation, or as natural products of the plant kingdom. The physical decomposition of organic cellular components also leads to carcinogen formation; this was recently demonstrated in the pyrolysis of free and protein-bound amino acids at high temperatures during charring of food substances. Synthetic chemicals, pharmacologic agents, and many compounds needed for, or products of, modern technology play an important role in the induction of human cancer.

The potential carcinogens that man may be exposed to belong to numerous chemical classes that seem to have no common characteristics. Although this does not readily suggest the possibility of a common mechanism of carcinogenesis, many of the chemical carcinogens require cellular metabolic conversions in order to progress to their final carcinogenic forms. An important characteristic of these metabolic products is that, unlike their wide-ranging procarcinogen counterparts, they have similar electrical characteristics; specifically, they are strongly electrophilic and can interact with cellular macromolecules. Other alkylating and acylating chemical carcinogens tend to be highly reactive as such and nonenzymatically form covalent adducts rather indiscriminately with many nucleophilic, electron-rich cellular molecules. Nucleic acids and proteins have been the most actively studied targets of this reaction because of their informational properties and because chemical carcinogens are often mutagenic. Since the covalent binding of ultimate carcinogens can occur not only with DNA but also with cellular proteins and RNA, chemical tumor inductions may incorporate genetic and epigenetic events. Thus, a primary approach toward inhibition of carcinogenesis must include alterations of the carcinogen-metabolizing system.

Mammalian cells are able to activate and inactivate carcinogens through oxidases in the endoplasmic reticulum and, in some cases, even in the nuclear membranes. Chemical carcinogenesis *in vivo* can be markedly inhibited by inducers of such microsomal enzymes. The amount of ultimate reactive carcinogenic electrophiles formed in a tissue is determined by the relative balance between the activated and inactivated forms. Also, the levels of ultimate chemical carcinogens in test systems and in man are influenced by the pharmacodynamic systems of conjugation and excretion. Substances that either inhibit activation of carcinogens or enhance their detoxification will be very useful for prevention of tumor development, and identification and complete understanding of the carcinogen-metabolizing enzymes should be major efforts.

Other challenges to biologists and chemists in the area of tumor prevention include the following topics: detection of man-made and natural chemical carcinogens that appear in the environment; continued synthetic development and localization of naturally occurring tumor-prevention substances and the further development of rapid *in vitro* and *in vivo* test systems for assay of these compounds; expanded studies designed to clarify interactions of genotoxic ultimate carcinogens with DNA and RNA; expanded studies designed to clarify mechanisms of normal repair of nucleic acids following genotoxic interactions with carcinogens; and investigations of the metabolism of carcinogens in susceptible experimental animals compared to animals that are resistant to actions of carcinogens.

In this discussion, we have emphasized the initial events in the process of carcinogenesis: carcinogen activation and interaction with cellular components. It is known from experimental studies, however, that cancer can also develop following exposure of animals to promotor agents. These substances, while not being carcinogenic by themselves, are able to affect carcinogen-exposed cells that might otherwise not proceed to become cancer cells so that they express properties of autonomy and eventually develop into a tumor. This promotion of cells previously altered by carcinogens is now being studied in great detail, and substances will be needed to inhibit the chemical and biochemical steps induced by promotors that are part of the transformation process. This might be of special importance in populations at increased risk for cancer where the cause for susceptibility of individuals to neoplasia is associated with inheritance.

Attempts to inhibit the development of cancer will also have to be directed to physical carcinogens. The various forms of radiation that have been reported to be carcinogens include ultraviolet, gamma, neutron, alpha, and beta. Other naturally occurring physical agents, such as asbestos and fiberglass, also contribute to the development of human cancer, and all of these problems will need to be addressed.

Another area worthy of study is the effect of using combinations of tumor-preventive agents. In this regard, it will be necessary not only to monitor enhanced protection but to determine whether any toxicity develops as a result of using two or more agents.

Cancer prevention via manipulation of the host's immunological systems is an exciting approach. Success in this area will depend largely on furthering our understanding of normal immunological mechanisms. Although limited in scope, the examples of immunoprevention described above suggest that this form of cancer prevention may be feasible. A considerable increase in effort in this area is needed and worthwhile.

III. Challenges to Epidemiologists and Oncologists

Studies in the field of epidemiology have provided us with important leads to the possible inhibition of cancer from natural causes. These leads have given unique opportunities to develop more rational guidelines for the future. Much of the important information acquired by modern cancer epidemiologists has come through demographic studies on incidence and mortality rates of certain cancers correlated with regional exposure, air or water pollutants, proximity to certain industrial plants, and occupational exposures or cultural practices. There is a need to expand on these efforts to consider the total environment. Such studies require structured interviews with afflicted subjects and possibly with their families. In the future, epidemiologists will need to examine the total environment of an individual afflicted with cancer, including life styles and dietary practices, complete histories of residence, of occupation and of avocation, family histories and cultural practices. Innovative and comprehensive studies on the epidemiology of health may lead to new information not only on causal factors but to the identification of previously unrecognized protective practices or of environments providing inhibitors of carcinogenesis.

A major question is whether variations in the incidence of certain cancers among population groups reflect variations in exposure to tumor-prevention agents as well as to carcinogens. The question can be rephrased in the following way: do variations in the balance of carcinogens and inhibitors of carcinogenesis determine whether or not someone will have cancer?

A particularly noteworthy study is the natural trend of a decrease in primary stomach cancer in the United States in the past four decades. The same trend has been observed in several other countries including Japan which for centuries has been a center of unusually high stomach cancer incidence. The tumor-inhibitory compounds noted above are widely distributed in the environment. Other inhibitors undoubtedly exist, and it is likely that their wide diversity and distribution will have an important role in the incidence of cancer.

Exogenous environmental factors almost totally determine activities of the metabolizing systems of carcinogens in tissues such as intestinal tract and lungs. Thus, diet and environmental exposures can determine the enzyme activities in tissues that make contact with chemical carcinogens. The inverse relationship between colon cancer and cabbage consumption is such an example. Individuals with high cabbage consumption had one-third the risk of cancer of those with little or no cabbage consumption. Other studies have shown an inverse relationship between consumption of lettuce, celery, and tomatoes and precursor lesion or cancer of the stomach. There is a reduced incidence of cancer in Seventh Day Adventists, a vegetarian group. However, exact interpretation of these findings is hampered by a lack of extensive evidence that high consumption of vegetables alone has actually enhanced the effectiveness of these protective systems against chemical carcinogens, and quantitative data are needed to firmly establish relationships between risk and diet.

Prior to the use of tumor-inhibiting substances in the human population at large, toxicological studies will need to be done to determine whether any adverse effects result from acute or chronic treatments. Following this, it will be necessary to design controlled studies to determine whether nontoxic levels of these substances are capable of preventing the development of cancer in humans. These studies should include subjects in higher than normal risk groups such as those with genetic or familial predisposition of cancer.

There seems to be little doubt at this time that prevention of tumor induction and development is a viable area for future research. The accomplishments to date using experimental systems are very encouraging, and the data obtained from individual efforts of biologists and epidemiologists support each other's findings. The knowledge that there are some substances in the natural environment capable of preventing cancer serves as an enticement to seek other such agents. All in all, there is enough evidence to give hope that within the near future we will need only to direct our efforts toward finding better ways of preventing cancer rather than attempting to treat it.

Index

AAF, *see* 2-Acetylaminofluorine
Acetaldehyde, disulfiram and, 52
2-Acetylaminofluorene, 16
   carcinogenicity of, 52–54
   disulfiram and, 53–54
   mutagenicity of, 175
   selenium and, 174
N-Acetyl-L-methionine, in DMBA-induced mammary tumors, 34
Acidic dissociation constant, of nitrous acid, 102
ADCC tests, *see* Antibody-dependent cellular cytotoxicity tests
S-Adenosylmethionine, 28
[^{75}Se]Adenosyl selenomethionine, 171
AF, *see* 2-Aminofluorene
AHH activity, *see* Aryl hydrocarbon hydroxylase activity
Alcoholism, disulfiram and, 24–25
Alkylating agents
   carcinogenesis and, 128–129
   tumor inhibition and, 128
Alkylated nucleic acid bases, 135
5,6-All-*trans*-epoxyretinoids, structure and activity of, 89
All-*trans*-retinal, structure and activity of, 83
All-*trans*-retinamides, as carcinogenesis inhibitors, 87–88
All-*trans*-retinoic acid
   isomerization of, 87
   ketoretinoic acids and, 89
   mouse skin carcinogenesis and, 79
   oral use of in man, 80
   retinamides and, 87
   ring-modified analogues and, 78–79
All-*trans*-retinoic acid (*cont.*)
   side-chain-modified analogues of, 80
   structure and activity of, 77
   toxic effects of, 95
All-*trans*-retinoic acid amides, structure and activity of, 84–85
All-*trans*-retinol, structure and activity of, 81
All-*trans*-retinyl amine derivatives, structure and activity of, 82–83
Allyl isothiocyanate, 11
Aluminum compounds, in lung tumor inhibition, 183
American Cancer Society, 189
2-Aminofluorene, 132
3-Amino-1,2,4-triazole, 49
Aminopyrine
   ASC and, 105
   DMN formation and, 111
   nitrosation of, 107
α-Angelicalactone, inhibition of DMBA-induced neoplasms by, 10
Animals, administration of chemical inhibitors to, 192
Animal tumors, selenium and, 172–174
Antabuse®, *see* Disulfiram
Antibody-dependent cellular cytotoxicity
   humoral antibodies and, 207–208
   tests for, 204
Anticarcinogens, trace elements and metals as, 169–184
Antioxidant compounds, nitrile consumption by, 142–143
Antitumor antibodies, unblocking activity of, 211
Aqueous systems, nitrosation in, 138–139

Arene oxide, 131
Aromatic isothiocyanates, as carcinogen inhibitors, 10–12
Arylamines, 52–55
Aryl hydrocarbon hydroxylase activity
 flavone effect on, 12
 increase in, 6–8
 indoles and, 14
 methylcholanthrene and, 184
 selenium and, 177
ASC, see Ascorbic acid
Ascorbate, in meat industry, 108–110
D-Ascorbate, 109
Ascorbate anion, oxidation of, 103–104
Ascorbic acid
 and carcinogenesis in man, 119–120
 carcinogenicity and mutagenicity tests for, 116–117
 conversion to dehydroascorbic acid, 104
 inhibition of N-nitroso compound formation by, 101–122
 in vivo nitrosation and, 115
 lung tumorigenesis and, 118
 mutagenicity of, 116–117, 121
 in nitrite ion competition, 141
 in nitrosated drugs, 105
 nitrous acid and, 103
 in NMOR formation, 105–106
 and NNO compound carcinogenicity or mutagenicity, 117–119
 oxidation of by nitrite, 106
 preformed nitrosamines and, 158–159
 as reducing agent, 150
L-Ascorbic acid, 9
Ascorbic acid/morpholine ratio, 105
Azo dyes, carcinogenicity of, 55–57
Azomethane, 36, 41
Azoxymethane, ^{14}C-labeled, 42–44
Azoxymethane hydroxylation, inhibition of, 43
Azoxymethane metabolism, disulfiram inhibition of, 42
Azoxy carcinogens, 35–47
Azoxymethanol, 192

Bacillus subtilis, 174
Bacon
 nitrosamine formation in, 153
 NPYR production in, 109
 sodium nitrite in, 152–153

Bacterial systems, selenium as inhibitor in, 174–176
5,6-Benzoflavone, 12
Benzo[*a*]pyrene
 metabolism in, 6, 32–33
 mutagenesis of, 4
 toxicity of, 32–33
Benzyl isothiocyanate, 10–11
BBN, see *N-n*-Butyl-*N*-(4-hydroxybutyl)nitrosamine
Beer, nitrosamines in, 154
BHA, see Butylated hydroxyanisole
BHT, see Butylated hydroxytoluene
Bisethylxanthogen, azomethane and, 41
Bladder cancer
 nitrosamines and, 156–157
 synthetic retinoids in prevention of, 90–91
Blocking agents, in N-nitroso formation, 145–150
Blocking systems, integration of, 150–152
Blood, N-nitroso compounds in, 157
Bowel cancer
 embryonic antigens and, 204–205
 regression of by multimodal immunological treatment, 211–213
Bowel cancer cells, immunological similarities with fetal cells, 205
Bowel carcinogenesis
 inhibitory effect of immunization with fetal tissue in, 208–210
 and transplantable syngeneic colon carcinoma, 206–207
BP, see Benzo[*a*]pyrene
Breast cancer
 selenium and, 171
 synthetic retinoids in prevention of, 90–91
Broccoli, indoles in, 13
2-Bromoergocryptine, 92
Bronopol™, 140
Brussels sprouts, indoles in, 13, 17
Butylated hydroxyanisole
 as antioxidant, 143
 group reactions with, 8
 inhibitory effects of, 4
 mechanism of, 5–8
 UV light and, 129
Butylated hydroxytoluene, 4
 as antioxidant, 143
 microsomal monooxygenase activity and, 16

Index

Butylated hydroxytoluene (*cont.*)
  selenium and, 173
N-n-Butyl-*N*-(4-hydroxybutyl)nitrosamine, 51-52
Di-*n*-Butylnitrosamine, selective carcinogenicity of, 51

Cabbage, indoles in, 13, 17
Caffeic acid, nitrile and, 150
Calcium carbimide, 25
Cancer (*see also* Carcinogenesis; Carcinogens; Breast cancer; Gastric cancer; Lung cancer; Skin cancer)
  ascorbic acid inhibition of, 119-120
  bowel, *see* Bowel cancer
  colorectal, *see* Colorectal cancer
  and decompartmentalization of iron, 181
  nasopharyngeal, 121
  retinoid mechanism in chemoprevention of, 90-94
Carbon disulfide
  azomethane and, 41
  industrial use of, 30-31
  metabolism of, 28
Carbon tetrachloride, diethyldithiocarbamate and, 59
Carbonyl sulfide, 28
Carcinogenesis
  alkylating agent in, 128-129
  ascorbic acid and, 119-120
  chemical, *see* Chemical carcinogenesis
  common mechanism in, 220
  metal interactions in, 181
  natural retinoids in prevention of, 77-80
  pickling and, 154
  retinoid deficiency and, 76
  UV light in, 129-130
Carcinogenesis Testing Program, 57
Carcinogenic electrophiles, 2
Carcinogen metabolism, inhibition of, 23-60
Carcinogens
  chemical, *see* Chemical carcinogens
  DNA and, 219
Cauliflower, indoles in, 13, 17
Chemical carcinogenesis
  aromatic isothiocyanates in inhibition of, 10-12
  flavones in inhibition of, 12-13
  in human cancer etiology, 196-199

Chemical carcinogenesis (*cont.*)
  inhibition of by phenols and related substances, 1-19
  plant sterols as protection from, 189-199
  stages in, 23
  thiono sulfur compounds and, 33-35
Chemical carcinogens (*see also* Chemical carcinogenesis)
  indoles as inhibitors of, 13-14
  origin of, 220
  precursor-product relationship of, 36
Chemist, challenge to, 220-221
Chemoprophylaxis, alkylating agent and, 128
Cholesterol, plant sterols and, 190
Cigarette smoke, lung cancer and, 155
Clostridium botulinum, 108
Coal tar, toxic action of, 130
Cobalt, as antitumor agent, 183
Colon cancer
  colonic epithelial cells and, 193
  selenium in, 171
Colon carcinogenesis
  animal models of, 192
  initiation of, 198
  nitrate production and, 154-155
Colorectal cancer
  autoimmunity in, 214
  diet in, 189
  incidence of, 189
  nitrosamides and, 120
  pathogenesis of, 189
Combination chemoprevention, with retinoids, 95-96
Copper, as anticarcinogen, 179-180
Copper sulfate, antitumor effect of, 180
Corynebacterium parvum, 211
Coumarins, as carcinogenesis inhibitors, 9-10
Cystine, 34

DAB, *see* 3-Methyl-4-dimethylaminoazobenzene
DBN, *see* di-*n*-Butylnitrosamine
Dehydroascorbic acid, ascorbic acid conversion to, 104, 141, 150-152
1,2-Dialkylhydrazines, 47
Diet
  in colon cancer, 189-190
  fiber in, 190

Diethyldithiocarbamate, 26, 28
  carcinogen inhibition by, 43
  DNA and, 49
  vinylidene chloride and, 59
Diethylnitrosamine, 47–49
3,3'-Diindolylmethane, 13
5,7-Dimethoxycoumarin, 9
Dimethylamine, DMN formation and, 111
Dimethylamine hydrochloride, 112
Dimethylaminoazobenzene, copper and, 179
3,2'-Dimethyl-4-aminobiphenyl, carcinogenicity of, 54–55
7,12-Dimethylbenz[a]anthracene
  as carcinogen, 32–34, 78, 91, 131–132
  copper sulfate and, 180
  selenium inhibition in, 173
Dimethyldithiocarbamate, DMBA-induced tumors and, 35
1,2-Dimethylhydrazine
  as carcinogen, 35–45, 192
  disulfiram and, 39–40, 42
  kidney tumors and, 35–36
  metabolism of, 36–39
  oxidizing to azomethane, 36
  in rat bowel carcinomas, 203–204
  selenium and, 172
1,2-Dimethylhydrazine-induced carcinogenesis
  fetal tissue immunization in, 208–210
  inhibition of in multiparous rats, 210
1,2-Dimethylhydrazine-induced tumorigenesis, in immunosuppressed rats, 206, 212–214
1,2-Diethylhydrazine metabolism, inhibition of, 41
Dimethylnitrosamine
  ASC and, 118
  copper and, 180
  disulfiram and, 47–50
  formation of, 102, 136
  human blood levels of, 135
  inhibitors of, 110
  intragastric formation of, 111
  in lung tumorigenesis, 118
  microsome-mediated mutagenicity of, 118
Dimethylsulfoxide, retinoid solutions in, 85–86
Dinitrogen tetroxide, 139
Diol-epoxides, 131
Diphenylmethyl thiocyanate, 11
Disodium ethylene bis-(dithiocarbamate), 29

Disulfiram
  AAF and, 53
  acetaldehyde and, 52
  alcohol and, 25
  BBN and, 51
  carcinogen metabolism inhibition by, 24–28
  commercial and medical use of, 24–25
  dimethylnitrosamine metabolism and, 49
  DMAB and, 54
  DMBA-induced tumors and, 34–35
  enzyme systems and, 25–27
  excretory route for, 28
  inhibition of azoxymethane carcinogenicity by, 42
  inhibition of carcinogenicity of 1,2-dimethylhydrazine by, 39
  metabolism of, 27–28
  nitrosamines and, 47–48
  procarbazine and, 47
  pyrazole and, 44
  in spontaneous tumors, 57–58
  toxicity of, 25
  weight loss and, 51
Dithiocarbamate pesticides, toxicity of, 29
DMAB-induced colon tumors, disulfiram and (see also 3,2'-Dimethyl-4-aminobiphenyl), 54–55
DMBA, see 7,12-Dimethylbenz[a]anthracene
DMBA-induced carcinogenesis, coumarin and, 10
DMBA-induced mammary gland tumor formation
  aromatic isothiocyanate inhibition of, 11–12
  coumarin inhibition of, 9
  indole inhibition of, 13–14
  N-acetyl-L-methionine and, 34
DMN, see Dimethylnitrosamine
DNA
  carcinogen interactions with, 219
  diethyldithiocarbamate and, 49
  tumorigenesis and, 128

EMQ, see Ethoxyquin
Endoplasmic reticulum, carcinogens in, 220
Enzyme systems
  carbon disulfide and, 30–31
  disulfiram and, 25–26
  sodium diethyldithiocarbamate and, 30

Index

Epidemiologist, challenge to, 222-223
Epithelial cell differentiation, retinoids and, 72-73
Epoxide hydratase, 6
Eppley Institute, 102
Erythorbate, 109
Esophageal cancer, nitrosamines in, 120
Ethoxyquin, 15, 159
Ethylnitrosourea, tumor induction and, 113

FANFT (N-[4-(5-nitro-2-furyl)-2-thiazolyl]formamide), 76
Ferbam®, 29
Fermented foods, nitrosamines in, 154
Ferric dimethyldithiocarbamate, 29
Ferulic acid, nitrite and, 150
Fetal cells, bowel cancer cells and, 205
Fetal tissue, immunization with, 208-210
Fiber, in diet, 190
Flavones, as carcinogen inhibitors, 12-13
Flexner-Jobling carcinoma, 131
9-α-Fluoroglucocorticoids, 90
Food and Drug Administration, 108
Fried bacon, NPYR formation in, 108-109

Gastric cancer
  ascorbic acid in prevention of, 119
  decrease in, 222
  nitrosoureas and, 121, 157-158
Glucose-6-phosphate dehydrogenase, 6
Glucuronic acid, 26, 38
Glutathione, UV light and, 57
Glutathione peroxidase activity, 171
Glutathione-S-transferase, 5-6
Griess reaction, in NMOR formation, 106

Hepatocarcinogenesis, 3'-Me-DAB in, 55-57
Hepatomas, α-tocopherol and, 131
5,6,7,8,3',4'-Hexamethoxyflavone, 12
High-pressure liquid chromatography, 5
Hodgkin's disease, procarbazine and, 45
HPLC, see High-pressure liquid chromatography
Hydrazine, 35
Hydrazo carcinogens (see also 1,2-Dimethylhydrazine; Procarbazine), 35-47
3-Hydroxybenzo[a]pyrene, 5

4-Hydroxyketoretinoic acid, 89
7-Hydroxy-6-methoxycoumarin, 9
4-Hydroxyphenyl retinamide, prostaglandin synthesis and, 95
Hypervitaminosis A, 94
Immunological treatment, regression of early carcinomas by, 211-213
Immunoprevention, 203-215, 222
Immunosuppressed rats, enhanced DMH-induced tumorigenesis in, 206
Indole-3-acetonitrile, 13
Indole-3-carbinol, 13
Indoles
  in AHH activity, 14
  as carcinogenesis inhibitors, 13-14
Inhibitors, administration of to animals, 192-193
Intestinal tumors, selection production of, 38
International Agency for Research in Cancer, 24
5-Iododeoxyuridine, antineoplastic effect of, 182
Iron, decompartmentalization of, 181
Isocitric lactone, 9
Isothiocyanates
  aromatic, 10-12
  in vegetables, 190

Jensen sarcoma, 131

Kale, lung cancer and, 17
4-Ketoretinoic acid, 89

Lactate dehydrogenase activity, copper and, 179
Lactones, as carcinogen inhibitors, 9-10
Limettin, 9
Lung adenomas
  induction of in mice, 113
  methylnitrosobenzylamine and, 117
  NNO compounds in, 113
Lung cancer
  cigarette smoke and, 155
  kale and, 17
  mustard greens and, 17
  nitrogen oxides and, 155
  vegetables and, 17-18
Lung neoplasms, DMBA-induced, 11

Malignancy (*see also* Cancer; Carcinogenesis)
Malignant transformation, suppression of by retinoids, 73–77
MAM, *see* Methylazoxymethanol
Mammary gland, retinoid levels in, 79
Mammary gland tumors, DMBA-induced, *see* DMBA-induced mammary gland tumor formation
Maneb®, 29
Manganese, in nickel-induced muscle tumorigenesis, 181
Manganese ethylene bis(dithiocarbamate), 329
Meat industry, ascorbic acid in, 108
3'Me-DAB, *see* 3'-Methyl-4-dimethylaminoazobenzene
Metal–metal anticarcinogenicity, 180–184
Methionine, ^{75}Se-labeled, 171
L-Methionine, DMBA-induced tumors and, 34
Methylazoxymethanol, 36–37
 glucuronic acid and, 38
 selenium and, 172
 urinary level of, 41
Methylazoxymethyl acetate, pyrazole and, 44
N-Methylbenzylamine, in induced rat tumors, 114
3-Methylcholanthrene, 74, 183
 copper and, 179–180
 inhibition of TCDD binding by, 7
 vitamin E and, 130
3'-Methyl-4-dimethylaminoazobenzene, 55, 131
Methylnitrosobenzylamine, lung adenoma and, 117
N-Methyl-*N*'-nitro-*N*-nitrosoguanidine, 192
 tumor-associated antigens and, 204
N-Methyl-*N*-nitrosourea
 as carcinogen, 91, 192
 in tumor formation following plant sterol intake, 195–196
N-Methyl-*N*-nitrosourea sterol carcinogenesis, animal model of, 193
4-Methylpyrazole, 31, 52
Microsomal azoxymethane hydroxylase, inhibition of, 50
Microsomal mixed-function oxidase activity, 15–16
Microsomal monooxygenase system, 15–16
 alteration of, 8
MNNG, *see* *N*-Methyl-*N*'-nitro-*N*-nitrosoguanidine

Molecular cell biologist, challenge to, 220–221
Monolayer cell culture, malignant transformations in, 74
Monomethylhydrazine, 35
Morpholine
 nitrite and, 114
 in rodent tumor induction, 113
Morpholine nitrosation
 ASC-morpholine ratio in, 105
 inhibition of, 103
 tumorigenesis by, 113–114
Mouse forestomach, BP-induced neoplasia in, 9
Mustard greens, lung cancer and, 17
Mutagenicity, thiono sulfur compounds and, 39
Mutagens, as carcinogens, 18

Nabam®, 29
NADPH-cytochrome C, 27
β-Naphthoflavone, 12
Nasopharyngeal cancer, nitrosamines and, 121
National Cancer Institute, 57, 82
Nickel-induced muscle tumorigenesis, 181
Nitric oxide, nitrite reduction to, 103
Nitrite
 morpholine and, 114
 nitric oxide oxidation to, 103
 α-tocopherol and, 144
Nitrite consumption, by antioxidant compounds, 142–143
Nitrite feeding, and tumor formation in rodents, 112–115
Nitrite reduction, to nitric oxide, 103
Nitrogen oxides, lung cancer and, 155
Nitrogen tetroxide and nitrogen trioxide, tautomers of, 138–139
N-Nitrosamines, 47–52
 in aprotic solvents, 140
 in bacon, 153
 in beer, 154
 bladder cancer and, 156–157
 disulfiram and, 47–48
 in esophageal cancer, 120
 in fish, 153–154
 in foods, 153–154
 formation of, 136–141
 in gastric cancer, 157–158

Index

N-Nitrosamines (cont.)
  in human cancer, 119–121
  as reaction products of secondary amines, 137
  in rodent tumor induction, 113
Nitrosation
  in aqueous solution, 138
  in lipids and by nitrogen oxides, 110–111
  in nonaqueous systems, 139–140
  N-Nitroso compound formation, 136–141
  ascorbic acid inhibition of, 101–122
  blocking agents in, 145–150
N-Nitroso compounds (see also N-Nitrosamines), 132–136
  alkylation of, 135
  ASC formation in, 115
  blocking formation of, 141–144
  in blood, 157
  carcinogenicity of, 133
  in gastric cancer, 157
  lung adenomas and, 113
  mutagenicity of, 134
  as nitrosation sources in vivo, 140
  as procarcinogens, 135
  zero time experiment and, 111
Nitrosomethylurea, 92
Nitrosomorpholine
  in vivo production of, 114–115
  liver tumors and, 115–117
Nitrosomorpholine formation, blocking of, 105–106
5-Nitrosopropylimidazole, 141
N-Nitrosopyrrolidine, 50–51
  carcinogenicity of, 49, 108
Nitrous acid
  acidic dissociation constant for, 102
  ascorbic acid and, 103, 141
NMOR, see Nitrosomorpholine
NNO, see N-Nitroso compounds
Nobiletin, 12
Nonaqueous systems, nitrosation in, 139–140
Nonneoplastic normal rat kidney cells, TGFs and, 75–76
NPYR, see N-Nitrosopyrrolidine
NRK cells, see Nonneoplastic normal rat kidney cells

Oncologist, challenge to, 222–223
Organic decomposition, carcinogen formation in, 220

Ornithine decarboxylase, 89

3,3',4',5,7-Pentahydroxyflavone-3-rutinoside, 12
5,6,7,8,4'-Pentamethoxyflavone, 12
Phenethyl isothiocyanate, 10
Phenols
  as blocking agents, 145–146
  inhibition of chemical carcinogenesis by, 4–8
  in transnitrosation, 141
Phenyl isothiocyanate, 11
Pickling, carcinogens and, 154
Piperazine
  ASC and, 105
  nitrosation and, 107
  in rodent tumor induction, 113
Plant sterols, 189–199
  in MNU animal model tumor formation, 195–196
  structure and function of, 190–192
Platinum compounds, cell division and, 182
Polycyclic aromatic hydrocarbons
  carcinogenicity of, 32–35
  as combustion products, 220
  metabolism of, 32–33
  vitamin E and, 130–132
Polypeptides, transforming, 93
Preformed nitrosamines, ascorbic acid and tocopherol effect on, 158–159
Procarbazine
  disulfiram and, 44, 47
  inhibition of carcinogenicity of, 45–47
  metabolism of, 45
Pulmonary neoplasia, isothiocyanate inhibition of (see also Lung adenomas; Lung cancer), 11
Pyrazole
  azoxymethane and, 44–45
  dimethylnitrosamine metabolism and, 49
  toxicity and enzyme inhibition in, 31–32
Pyrrolidine nitrosation, inhibitors of, 109

Quercetin pentamethyl ether, 12

Radiocarbon, 1,2-dimethylhydrazine and, 41
Rats
  bowel cancer in, 203–204

Rats (cont.)
  fibroblast cell density in, 93
  immunosuppressed, 206, 212–213
  nonneoplastic kidney cells of, 75–76
  tumor induction in, 113–114
Rectal cancer, selenium in, 171
Rectal carcinogenesis, nitrite production and, 154–155
Retinamides
  enzymes in hydrolysis of, 90
  toxicity of, 87
Retinoic acid, structure and activity of (see also All-*trans*-retinoic acid), 77–78
13-*cis*-Retinoic acid
  in bladder carcinogenesis, 90–91
  structure and activity of, 87
Retinoid(s)
  as "antipromoting" agents, 90
  combination chemoprevention with, 95–96
  defined, 71
  DMSO solutions of, 85–86
  epithelial cell differentiation and, 72–73
  irritating toxic effects of, 79
  mechanism of action in cancer prevention, 92–94
  natural, 77–81
  polypeptide hormones and, 93
  in skin cancer, 91–92, 95
  suppression of malignancies and tumor promotion by, 73–76
  synthetic, 81–90
  toxicity mechanism in, 94–95
  in tracheal system, 83–89
Retinoid deficiency
  carcinogenesis and, 76
  neoplasia and, 71–72
Retinoid molecule, modifications to polar terminus of, 86
Retinol, epithelial cell differentiation and (see also Vitamin A), 71
Retinoyl chloride, 86
Retinoyl imidazole, 86
Retinyl acetate
  mammary tissue retinoid levels and, 79
  rat fibroblast cell density and, 93
Retinyl methyl ether, 91
Retinyl palmitate, 79
Rutin, 12

Saccharomyces cerevesiae, 173

Safrole, 15–16
Salmonella typhimurium, 4, 51, 55, 116, 118, 170, 174–175
Sarcoma growth factor
  colony-forming ability and, 94
  defined, 74
  rat fibroblast cell density and, 93
Scopoletin, 9
Selenium
  bacterial systems and, 174–176
  in breast cancer, 171
  in colon cancer, 171
  tumor inhibition by, 170
Selenium compounds, mutagenicity and antimutagenicity of, 174
[^{75}Se]Selenomethionine, 171
SGF, see Sarcoma growth factor
Sister chromatid exchange formation, selenium and, 176–177
β-Sitosterol
  cholesterol and, 191
  tumor-inhibiting effect of, 195–196
Skin cancer
  fluorinated glucocorticoids and, 95
  protease inhibitors and, 95
  retinoids and, 91–92
Skin carcinogenesis, all-*trans*-retinoic acid and, 79
Sodium ascorbate, in bacon, 152–153
Sodium diethyldithiocarbamate, 28–30
  enzyme systems and, 30
  spontaneous tumors and, 57–58
Sodium nitrite
  in bacon, 152–153
  in meat industry, 108
Sorbic acid, nitrosamine formation and, 109
Spontaneous tumors, disulfiram and, 57–58
Stomach cancer, see Gastric cancer
Sulfur compounds, as blocking agents, 145
Syngeneic colon carcinoma, transplantable, 206–207
Synthetic retinoids
  cancer prevention with, 90–92
  structure-activity relationships in, 81–90

TAA, see Tumor-associated antigens
Tangeretin, 12
TCDD (2,3,7,8-tetrachlorodibenzo-*p*-dioxin), 6–7
Tetraethylthiuram disulfide, see Disulfiram

Index

Tetrahydro-12-dimethylbenz[a]anthracene, 32–34
Tetramethylthiuram disulfide (Thiram®), 24, 29
TGFs, see Transformation growth factors
Thiocyanate, catalysis of nitrosation by, 108
Thiol-disulfide exchange mechanism, 26
Thiono sulfur compounds (see also Disulfiram)
 carcinogenicity and, 33, 39–43
 other effects of, 59–60
Thiram®, 24, 29
α-Tocopherol
 applications of, 152–158
 in aprotic solvent, 145
 as blocking agent in N-nitroso formation, 146–149
 conversion to α-tocoquinone, 147
 fish carcinogens and, 153–154
 food carcinogens and, 153
 nitrite and, 144
 in nitrite ion competition, 141
 preformed nitrosamines and, 158–159
 structure of, 147
 tumor development and, 127–159
β-Tocopherol, 147
δ-Tocopherol, 147
d-Tocopherol, 148–149
dl-α-Tocopherol, 148–149
γ-Tocopherol, 147
α-Tocoquinone, 147
Trace elements
 as anticarcinogens, 168–184
 cell division and, 182
 in hydroxylation of benzo[a]pyrene, 183
 mutational factors and, 182
Tracheal epithelium culture, retinoids in reverse keratinization of, 83–84
Tracheal organ culture assay, 82–88
Transformation growth factors
 effects of, 75
 retinoids and, 93
Transforming polypeptides, retinoids and, 93
Transnitrosation, 140–141
Tranylcypromine, 51
Tumor-associated antigens
 detection of in rat bowel carcinomas, 203–204
 on large bowel cancer cells, 203
Tumor induction (see also Carcinogenesis)
 α-tocopherol in, 127–159

Tumor induction (cont.)
 mechanism of, 128
 in rodents, 112–115
Tumor inhibition
 alkylating agents and, 128
 future research in, 223
Tumor promotion, retinoids in suppression of, 73–76
Tumor resection, additional tumor development and, 210–211
Tumors, spontaneous, 57–58

UDP glucose dehydrogenase, 26
UDP glucuronate pyrophosphatase, 26
UDP glucuronyl transferase, 5–6, 26
Ultraviolet light, carcinogenicity and, 57, 129–130
Umbelliferone, DMBA-induced neoplasia and, 9
γ-Valerolactone, 9
Vanadium pentoxide, 183
Vegetables
 isothiocyanates in, 190
 lung cancer and, 17–18
 plant sterols and, 190–192
Vegetarian diet, colon cancer and, 190
Vinyl chloride monomer, hepatotoxicity of, 59
Vitamin A, in cancer prevention (see also Retinol), 71, 81
Vitamin-A-deficient diet, 82
Vitamin E (see also α-Tocopherol)
 as antitumor agent, 129–132
 as blocking agent, 146–149
 commercial forms of, 148
 ester form of, 148
 X-ray irradiation of, 130

Walker carcinoma
 tocopherol absorption in, 131
 zinc deficiency and, 178

Zinc
 dimethylbenzanthracene-induced carcinogenesis and, 178
 DNA synthesis and, 177–178
Zinc dimethyldithiocarbamate, 29
Zinc ethylene bis-(dithiocarbamate), 29
Zineb®, 29
Ziram®, 29